Learning Imaging

Series Editors:

R. Ribes • A. Luna • P.R. Ros

John C. Pedrozo Pupo

(Editor)

Learning Chest Imaging

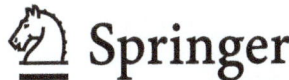 Springer

JOHN C. PEDROZO PUPO
Pulmonologist and Internal Medicine Chief
Respire - Institute for Respiratory Care
Professor at the University of Magdalena
Santa Marta, Colombia

ISBN 978-3-642-34146-5   ISBN 978-3-642-34147-2   (eBook)
DOI 10.1007/978-3-642-34147-2
Springer Heidelberg New York Dordrecht London

Library of Congress Control Number: 2012954871

Printed on acid-free paper

Springer is part of Springer Science+Business Media (www.springer.com)

To all
My wife Deyanira and my children Maria
José and Santiago for being the pillar of my
life and love I have for them
My teachers, for their teachings and
training
My patients, for their trust and respect
My students, for their commitment and
dedication
God for letting me be here and now
My parents (for my father, in memoriam)
My brothers

John C. Pedrozo Pupo

Acknowledgments

The author thanks the department of radiology at the Clinica Mar Caribe, University of Magdalena, and Respire Institute for Respiratory Care in Santa Marta, Colombia.

John C. Pedrozo Pupo

Contents

4 Air Space and Bronchi – I

John C. Pedrozo Pupo, Diego M. Celis Mejía,
Claudia Patricia García Calderón, Victoria Eugenia Murillo,
Bernardo J. Muñoz Palacio, and Carlos de la Rosa Pérez

5 Air Space and Bronchi – II

John C. Pedrozo Pupo, Robin Rada Escobar, Eidelman Gonzalez Mejia,
and Carlos de la Rosa Pérez

6 Trachea and Airway

John C. Pedrozo Pupo, Diego Pardo Pinzón, Manuel Pacheco,
Paulina Ojeda León, Pedro Chaparro Mutis, and Manuel Garay Fernandez

7 Heart and Great Vessels
JOHN C. PEDROZO PUPO AND ALVARO CORAL MARTINEZ

8 Chest Wall and Soft Tissues
JOHN C. PEDROZO PUPO AND ALVARO CORAL MARTINEZ

9 Pulmonary Interstitium
JORGE CARRILLO BAYONA, LILIANA ARIAS ÁLVAREZ, AND PAULINA OJEDA LEÓN

10 Medical Device and Monitoring of the Chest
JOHN C. PEDROZO PUPO, ANA MARÍA PIZARRO,
ALVARO CORAL MARTINEZ, AND JOEL ZABALETA ARROYO

Contributors

Liliana Arias Álvarez, M.D.
Radiology, Santa Clara Hospital,
Bogotá, Colombia

Joel Zabaleta Arroyo, M.D.
Pulmonologist and Critical Care
Medicine,
Medellin, Colombia

Jorge Carrillo Bayona, M.D.
Radiology,
National University of Colombia,
Bogotá, Colombia

Claudia Patricia
García Calderón, M.D.
Internal Medicine, Pulmonologist,
Pablo Tobón Uribe Hospital – Clínical,
Medellín, Colombia

Alfonso Uriza Carrasco, M.D.
Radiology,
Hospital Universitario San Vicente Paul,
Medellín, Colombia

Robin Rada Escobar, M.D.
Internal Medicine, Pulmonologist,
Militar Central Hospital,
Bogotá, Colombia

Manuel Garay Fernandez, M.D.
Internal Medicine, Pulmonologist,
Santa Clara Hospital,
Bogotá, Colombia

Beatriz Aldana Jaramillo, M.D.
Radiology,
Radioimage Radiologists Associated,
Santa Marta, Colombia

Eliana Amaya Lacouture, M.D.
Radiology,
Radioimage Radiologists Associated,
Santa Marta, Colombia

Paulina Ojeda León, M.D.
Pathology, Santa Clara Hospital,
Bogotá, Colombia

Alvaro Coral Martinez, M.D.
Radiology,
Cardiovascular Foundation of
Colombia, Santa Marta, Colombia

Felipe Navas Martinez, M.D.
Intensive Care Medicine,
Sabana University,
Bogotá, Colombia

Diego M. Celis Mejía, FACP, FACCP
Internal Medicine, Pulmonologist,
Pablo Tobón Uribe Hospital,
Medellín, Colombia

Eidelman Gonzalez Mejia, M.D.
Internal Medicine, Pulmonologist,
Metropolitan University Hospital,
Barranquila, Colombia

Elida Laurens Meza, M.D.
Radiology,
Radioimage Radiologists Associated,
Santa Marta, Colombia

Victoria Eugenia Murillo, M.D.
Pathology,
Pablo Tobón Uribe Dinámica
IPS Hospital, Medellín, Colombia

Pedro Chaparro Mutis, M.D.
Internal Medicine and Pulmonologist,
Santa Clara Hospital,
Bogotá, Colombia

Manuel Pacheco, M.D.
Fellow Pulmonologist,
Santa Clara Hospital,
Bogotá, Colombia

BERNARDO J. MUÑOZ PALACIO, M.D.
Internal Medicine, Pulmonologist,
Pablo Tobón Uribe Hospital – Medellín
Clinic, Medellín, Colombia

CARLOS DE LA ROSA PÉREZ, M.D.
Radiology,
North General Clinic,
Santa Marta, Colombia

DIEGO PARDO PINZÓN, M.D.
Thoracic Surgery,
Colombian Cardiothoracic Foundation,
Barranquilla, Colombia

ANA MARÍA PIZARRO, M.D.
Internal Medicine, Marcaribe Clinic,
Santa Marta, Colombia

JOHN C. PEDROZO PUPO, M.D., FCCP
Pulmonologist and Internal Medicine,
Chief Respire - Institute for Respiratory
Care, Professor at the University of
Magdalena, Santa Marta, Colombia

KATIA MEYER, M.D.
Radiology, Clinical El Prado,
Santa Marta, Colombia

Abbreviations

AP	Anterior to posterior
ARDS	Acute respiratory distress syndrome
COPD	Chronic obstructive pulmonary disease
CRX	Chest X-ray
CT	Computed tomography
HRCT	High-resolution CT
LLL	Left lower lobe
LRTI	Lower respiratory tract infection
LUL	Left upper lobe
LV	Left ventricle
LVF	Left ventricular failure
PA	Posterior to anterior
PE	Pulmonary embolus
RA	Right atrium
RLL	Right lower lobe
RML	Right middle lobe
RUL	Right upper lobe
RV	Right ventricle
SOL	Space-occupying lesion
SVC	Superior vena cava
TB	Tuberculosis
TNM	Tumor, nodes, metastases
US	Ultrasound
V/Q	Ventilation-perfusion
XR	X-ray

Pleural and Pleural Space

Joel Zabaleta Arroyo, John C. Pedrozo Pupo, Diego Pardo Pinzón,
and Katia Meyer

Contents

J.C. Pedrozo Pupo (ed.), *Learning Chest Imaging*, Learning Imaging,
DOI 10.1007/978-3-642-34147-2_1, © Springer-Verlag Berlin Heidelberg 2013

Case 1: Pleural Tuberculosis

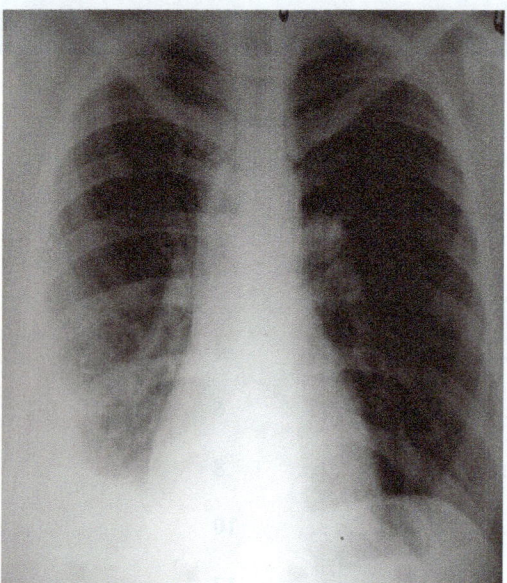

Fig. 1.1.1

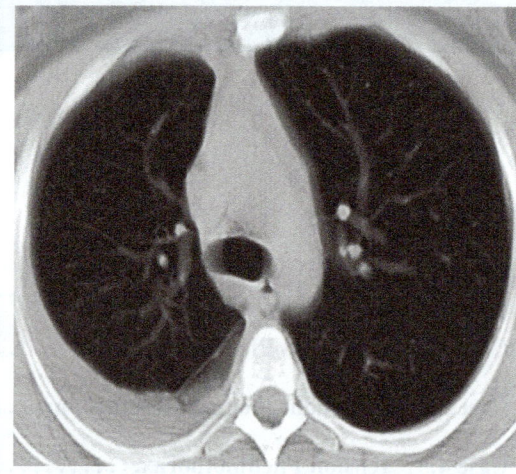

Fig. 1.1.2

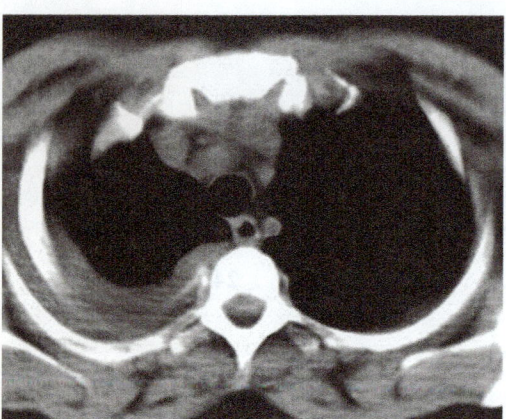

Fig. 1.1.3

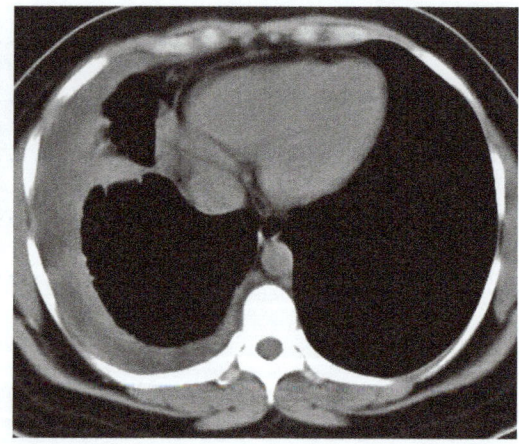

Fig. 1.1.4

A 26-year-old woman with 3-week history of right pleuritic pain, fever, dyspnea, and weight loss. Cytochemical pleural fluid: 90 % mononuclear exudate and adenosine deaminase: 90 U/ml. Pleural biopsy compatible with caseous granulomatous inflammation.

Comments

Pleural tuberculosis (TB) is the most common extrapulmonary manifestation of tuberculosis.

Pleural tuberculosis (TB) should be considered in any patient with an exudative effusion, particularly a lymphocyte-predominant exudative pleural effusion.

The current hypothesis for the pathogenesis of primary tuberculous pleural effusion is that a subpleural caseous focus in the lung ruptures into the pleural space 6–12 weeks after a primary infection. Mycobacterial antigens enter the pleural space and interact with T-cells previously sensitized to mycobacteria, resulting in a delayed hypersensitivity reaction and the accumulation of fluid. It seems that this reaction of the pleura augments the entry of fluid into the pleural space by increasing the permeability of pleural capillaries to serum proteins and thereby increasing the oncotic pressure in the pleural fluid. Involvement of the lymphatic system probably also contributes to the accumulation of pleural fluid. An impaired clearance of proteins from the pleural space has been reported in human tuberculous effusions. It is known that the clearance of proteins and fluid from the pleural space is carried out by lymphatics in the parietal pleura. Fluid gains access to the lymphatics through openings in the parietal pleura called stomata. Since the parietal pleural is diffusely affected with pleural tuberculosis, damage to or obstruction of the stomata could be an important mechanism leading to accumulation of pleural fluid.

Chest radiography typically reveals a small-to-moderate, unilateral pleural effusion in the active pleural TB. The frequency of pleural effusion in these tuberculous patients is currently approximately 31 %; about 20 % of patients have associated pulmonary lesions.

Computed tomography (CT) of the chest may show lymphadenopathy, pulmonary infiltrates, or cavitation not obvious on chest radiography. Pleural thickening of more than 1 cm is seen in most instances. As many as 50 % of patients with tuberculous pleurisy develop pleural thickening 6–12 months after the beginning of the treatment.

True empyema, bronchopleural fistulae, rib or bone erosions, pleurocutaneous fistulae, residual pleural thickening, and calcification are other forms and complications of pleural infection.

Imaging Findings

CRX shows obliteration of the angle cost and cardiophrenic right, occupied by pleural fluid and associated with increased vascular markings in the right lung base (Fig. 1.1.1). CT scan (lung window) shows pleural effusion bordering the lung on the back (Fig. 1.1.2). CT scan (mediastinal window) shows pleural effusion bordering the lung (Figs. 1.1.3 and 1.1.4).

Case 2: Malignant Pleural Effusion

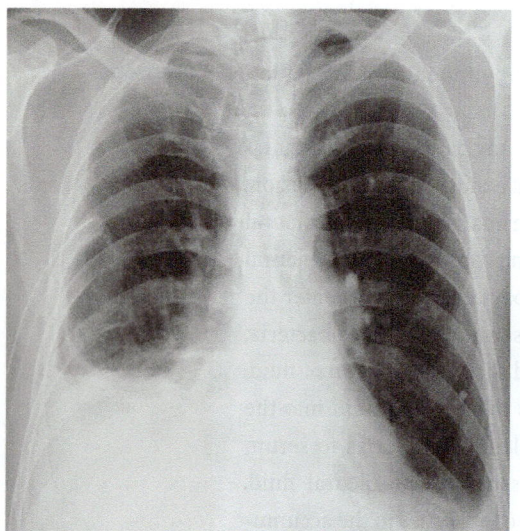

Fig. 1.2.1

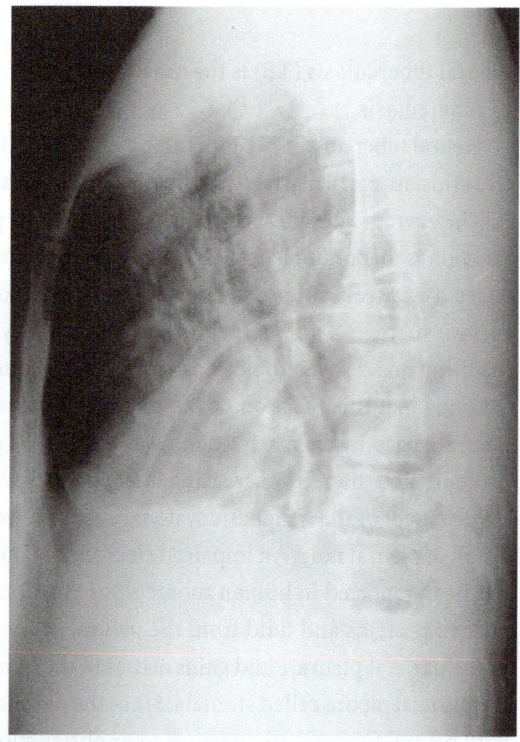

Fig. 1.2.2

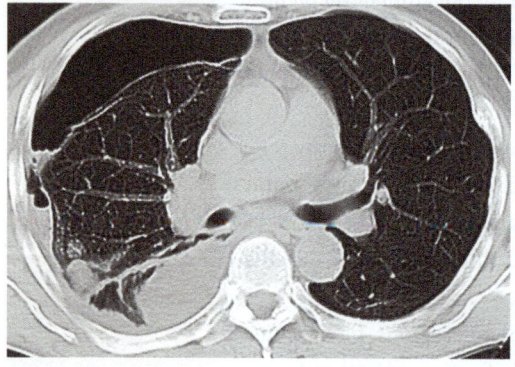

Fig. 1.2.3

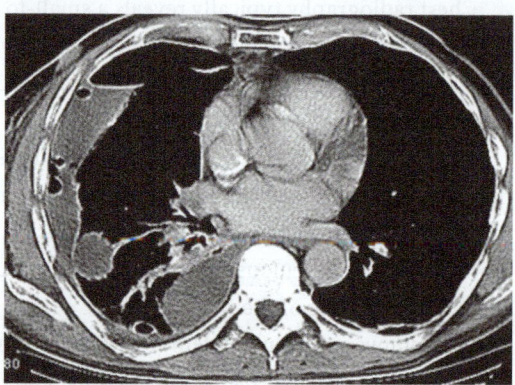

Fig. 1.2.4

A 62-year-old man with history of 2-month grade 2 dyspnea, dry cough, chest pain, and loss of weight. Pleural biopsy and cytology consistent with adenocarcinoma.

Malignant pleural effusions are caused most commonly by carcinomas of the breast, lung, gastrointestinal tract or ovary, and by lymphomas. In male patients, about half of malignant effusions are caused by lung cancer, 20 % by lymphomas or leukemia, 7 % from gastrointestinal primaries, 6 % from genitourinary primaries, and 11 % from tumors of unknown primary site. In female patients, about 40 % of malignant effusions are caused by breast cancer, 20 % from tumors arising in the female genital tract, 15 % from lung primaries, 8 % from lymphomas or leukemia, 4 % from gastrointestinal tract primaries, 3 % from melanoma, and 9 % from tumors of unknown primary site. Effusions may be secondary to impaired pleural lymphatic drainage from mediastinal tumor (especially in lymphomas) and not due to direct pleural invasion.

Effusions may be the presenting sign of cancer, or they may develop after the cancer is diagnosed. Only 50 % of the effusions that develop in cancer patients during the course of their illness are malignant. Correct diagnosis of the cause of pleural effusions is the necessary first step in their management.

A malignant pleural effusion usually signifies advanced metastatic disease and is associated with a poor prognosis with median survival between 3 and 12 months, depending on the primary site.

On CT, metastases may manifest as marked thickening and nodularity of the pleura, usually with an associated pleural effusion. In some cases, the effusion may be large and tumor foci may be difficult to identify. Metastases may mimic malignant mesothelioma, and the two entities cannot be reliably distinguished by cross-sectional imaging.

Certain tumors such as malignant thymoma may produce focal seeding of the pleura. This is usually manifested on CT scanning as localized focal pleural nodules that may be bilateral or unilateral. The differentiation of malignant from benign pleural thickening provides a challenge for the radiologist. There is overlap of the radiologic manifestations of benign and malignant pleural processes. Features that were helpful in distinguishing malignant from benign pleural disease included (a) circumferential pleural thickening, (b) nodular pleural thickening more than 1 cm in thickness, and (c) mediastinal pleural involvement, all of which occurred more consistently with malignant lesions. These features may be seen in mesothelioma and metastatic pleural disease but are unusual in benign pleural disease. The presence of pleural calcification also is suggestive of a benign process. Although calcified pleural plaques may be seen in cases of mesothelioma, they are uncommon.

PA and lateral CRX shows increased lung density by right pleural effusion and presence of chest tube (Figs. 1.2.1 and 1.2.2). CT scan (lung window) shows loculated pleural effusion and presence of residual pneumothorax (Fig. 1.2.3). CT scan (mediastinal window) shows multiloculated pleural effusion (Fig. 1.2.4).

Comments

Imaging Findings

Case 3: Malignant Pleural Mesothelioma

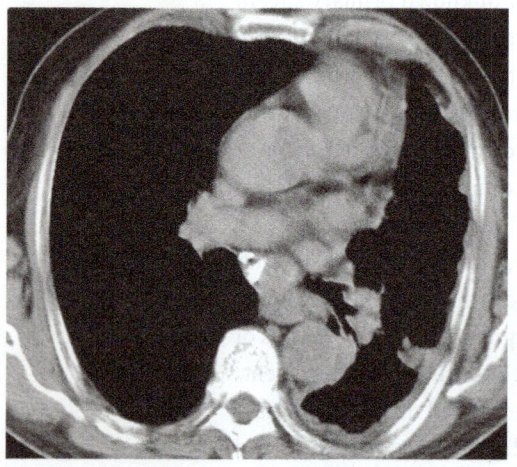

Fig. 1.3.1

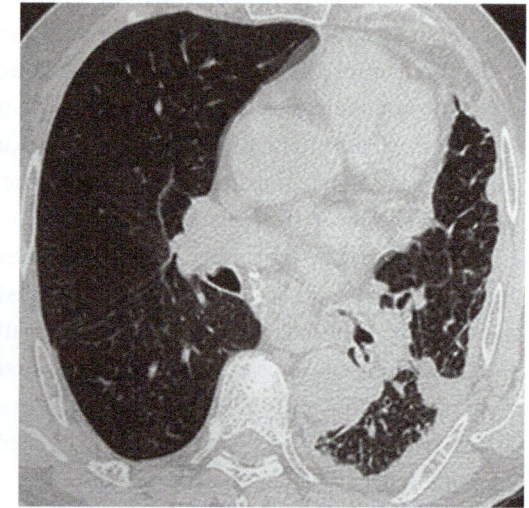

Fig. 1.3.2

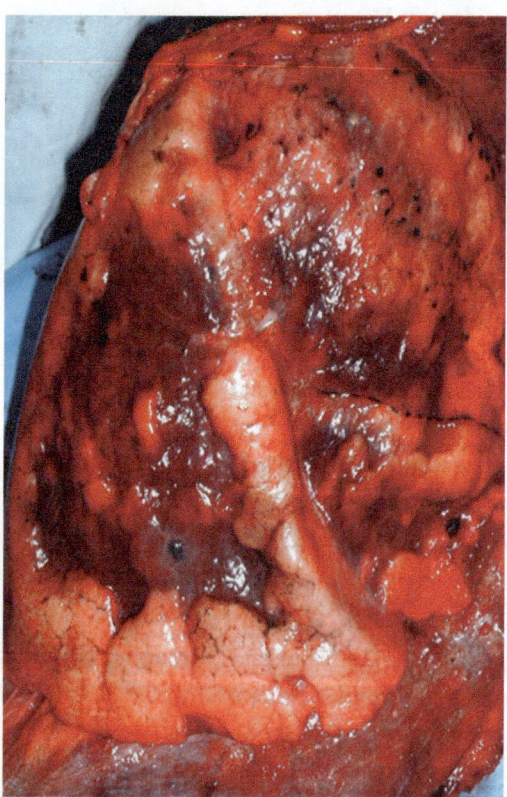

Fig. 1.3.3

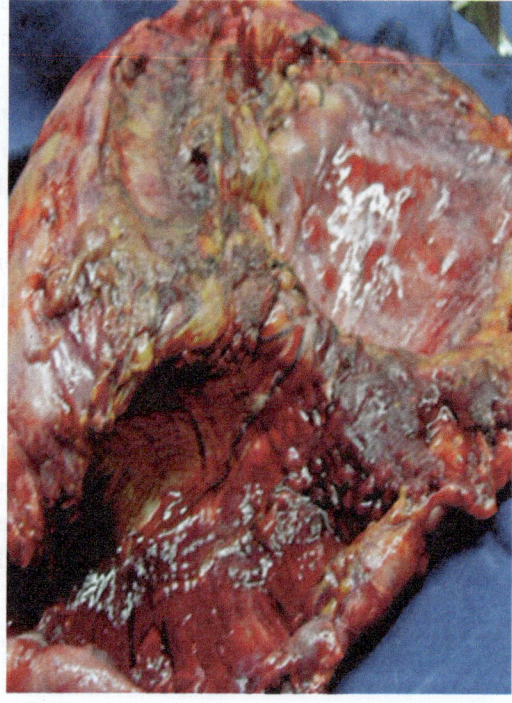

Fig. 1.3.4

A 60-year-old man with epithelial mesothelioma resected with pneumonectomy.

Comments

Malignant pleural mesothelioma (MPM) is a rare tumor. The incidence is 1.25/100,000 in Great Britain and 1.1/100,000 in Germany. Within the next 20 years, the incidence is estimated to double in many countries. Exposure to asbestos is a well-established etiological factor for MPM, with occupational exposure being documented in 70–80 % of those affected.

Cytological examination of the effusion can be diagnostic but often shows equivocal results. Therefore, histology, including immunohistochemistry, is the gold standard. Pleuroscopy, a video-assisted surgical procedure or open pleural biopsy in a fused pleural space may be necessary to provide sufficient material for accurate histological diagnosis. There are three main histological types (epithelial, sarcomatous, and mixed) with ~60 % being epithelial.

CT is accurate for most tumor staging, and MRI is valuable improving detection of tumor extension to chest wall and diaphragm, while PET is used for evaluation of lymph-node involvement and distant metastasis. The characteristic radiographic feature of mesothelioma is unilateral diffuse, irregular, and nodular pleural thickening with or without an associated pleural effusion. Associated asbestos-related pleural disease (e.g., pleural plaques) occurs in 20-25 % of cases. Mediastinal shift towards the involved hemithorax as a result of tumor encasement and volume loss may be identified. Alternatively, massive tumor bulk and large pleural effusions may produce contralateral shift of the mediastinum. Pleural effusion may obscure tumor masses and be the sole or predominant radiographic finding.

CT better characterizes tumor extent and morphology and may demonstrate focal or diffuse pleural masses, nodular pleural thickening, and fissural involvement. Involvement is typically circumferential with involvement of the mediastinal pleura and characteristically extends into the fissures. The cross-sectional imaging features of malignant mesothelioma are often indistinguishable from metastatic involvement of the pleura.

Lobulated thickening of the pleural that exceeds 1 cm in thickness raises the suspicion of a mesothelioma. Loss of volume of the affected hemithorax is pronounced. Invasion of the chest wall, mediastinum, and diaphragm may be demonstrated by CT, but early invasion is often not apparent or may be underestimated.

MRI may better characterize the invasive features of mesothelioma. Tumor typically manifests as minimally increased signal on T1-weighted images and moderately increased signal on T2. The multiplanar capabilities of MR may allow better detection and visualization of chest wall, mediastinal, and diaphragmatic extension of tumor and help predict respectability. Diffuse superficial spread of mesothelioma throughout the pleural space may be difficult to detect by any of the above modalities.

Imaging Findings

CT scan (mediastinal and lung window) shows nodular pleural thickening resulting from loss of volume of the entire left lung (Figs. 1.3.1 and 1.3.2). Shows pleural thickening resected lung parenchyma attached to the lung (Figs. 1.3.3 and 1.3.4).

Case 4: Tension Pneumothorax

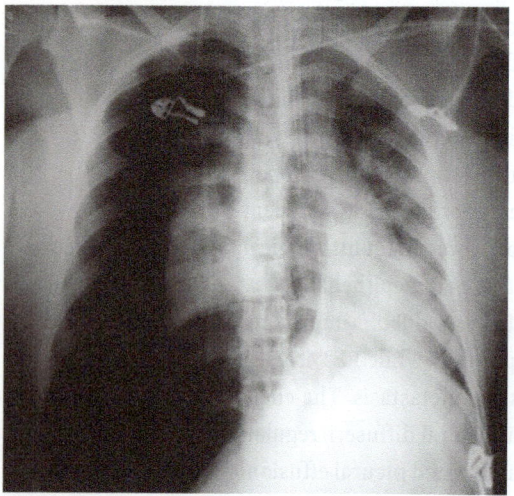

Fig. 1.4.1

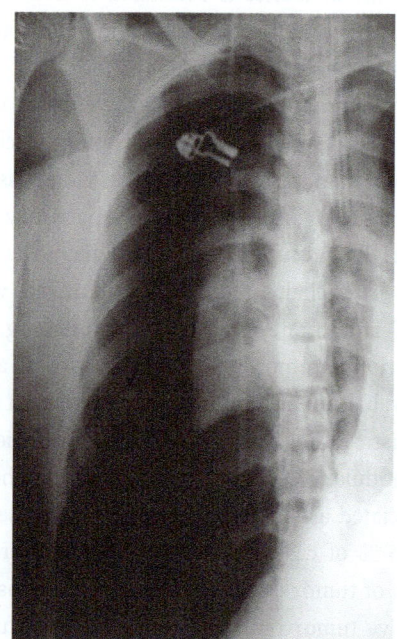

Fig. 1.4.2

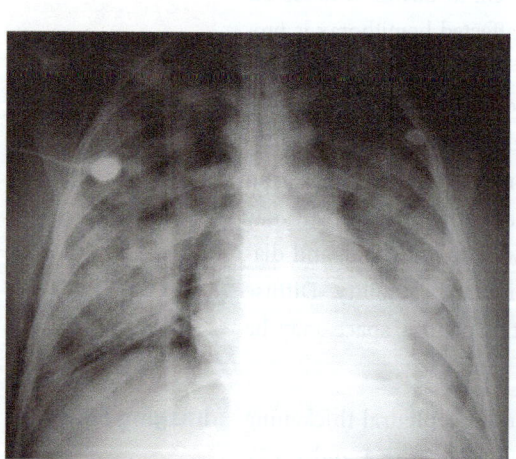

Fig. 1.4.3

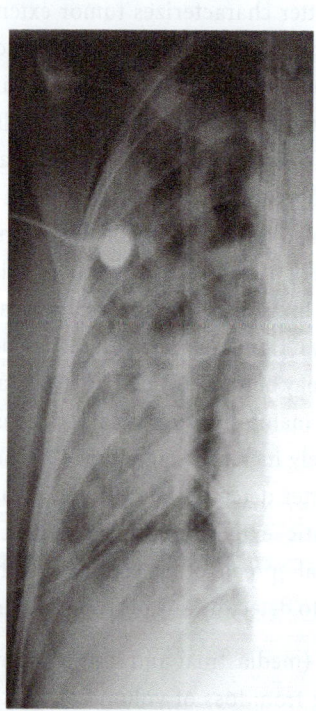

Fig. 1.4.4

A 23-year-old man was admitted to the emergency room with a picture of 5-day history of cough with greenish sputum and grade 3 dyspnea. In impending respiratory failure, blood pressure 70/50, FC 100/min, RR 40/min, O_2 Sat 78 %, and use of intercostal muscles, we performed orotracheal intubation although clinical improvement was not expected. He required tube thoracostomy with right lung re-expansion. There was poor clinical and ventilatory high vasopressor support and he died.

Tension pneumothorax (TPT) is an uncommon disease with a malignant course leading to death if untreated. It is most commonly encountered in prehospital trauma care, emergency departments, and intensive care units (ICUs).

The chest radiological findings of tension pneumothorax. It should be noted that merely looking for mediastinal shift may not give conclusive differentiation of a TPT from a simple pneumothorax as this may occur in both conditions. In rare cases, a loculated anterior TPT may exist that will only be visible on a lateral chest radiography or computed tomography.

Chest radiological findings in tension pneumothorax:

Ipsilateral hyper-expansion:

- Hemidiaphragmatic depression
- Increased rib separation
- Increased thoracic volume

Mediastinal pressure:

- Ipsilateral flattening of heart border
- Contralateral mediastinal deviation

However, the three signs (contralateral mediastinal shift, flattening or inversion of hemidiaphragm, and enlargement of the ipsilateral hemithorax) may be present in most moderate-to-large pneumothoraces due to the release of the effect of negative intrapleural pressure.

The key radiological feature of tension pneumothorax is lung collapse; a partially inflated lung indicates that pneumothorax is not under tension with the exception of stiff lungs in adult respiratory distress syndrome (ARDS), extensive pneumonia, and the rare setting in which bronchial obstruction with a valve mechanism coexists. Therefore, in ARDS, tension pneumothorax should be considered in any patient whose hemodynamic status deteriorates in the presence of high airway pressures.

CRX (AP) shows unilateral hyperlucency associated with the presence of visceral pleural line, increased intercostal spaces, diaphragmatic investment, and deviation contralateral mediastinal structures (Figs. 1.4.1 and 1.4.2). CRX (AP control) shows lung re-expansion by placing a chest tube (Figs. 1.4.3 and 1.4.4).

Case 5: Parapneumonic Pleural Effusions

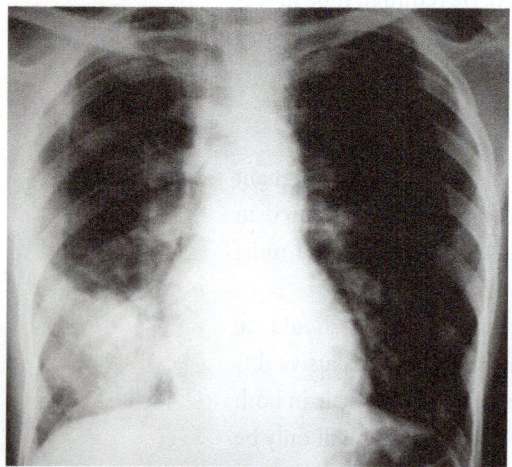

Fig. 1.5.1

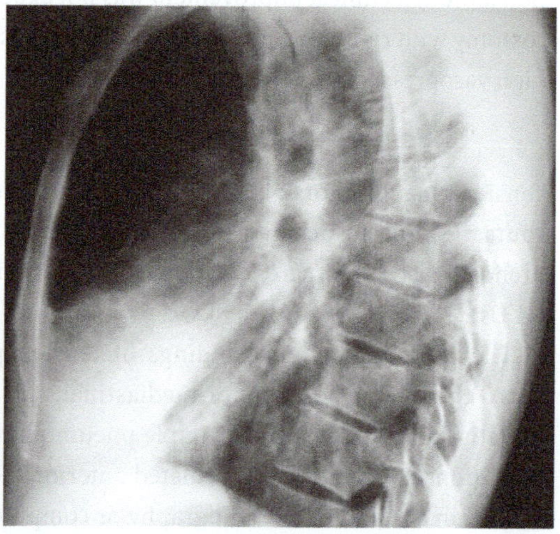

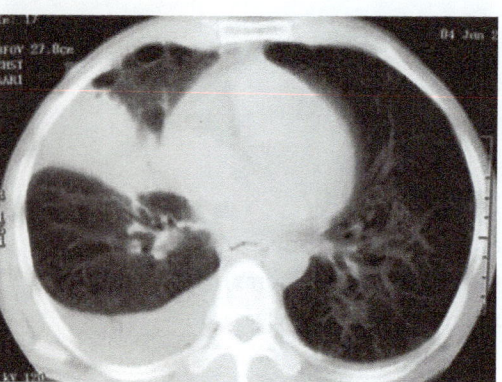

Fig. 1.5.2

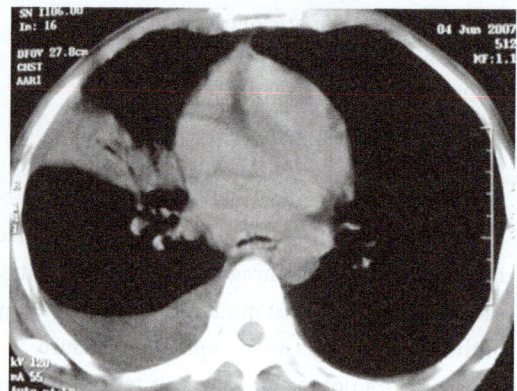

Fig. 1.5.3

Fig. 1.5.4

A 41-year-old man with consultation history of cough with greenish sputum, unquantified fever, and chest pain of 2 weeks duration. 3C AIDS antecedent without good adhesion to handling.

Comments   Parapneumonic effusion is any pleural effusion secondary to pneumonia (bacterial or viral) or lung abscess. Empyema is, by definition, pus in the pleural space. Pus is thick, viscid fluid that appears to be purulent. A complicated parapneumonic effusion is a parapneumonic pleural effusion for which an invasive procedure, such as tube thoracostomy, is necessary for its resolution or a parapneumonic effusion on which the bacterial cultures are positive.

Parapneumonic effusions occur in 20–40 % of patients who are hospitalized with pneumonia. The mortality rate in patients with a parapneumonic effusion is higher than that in patients with pneumonia without a parapneumonic effusion. Some of the excess mortality is due to mismanagement of the parapneumonic effusion. Characteristics of patients that indicate that an invasive procedure will be necessary for its resolution include the following: an effusion occupying more than 50 % of the hemithorax or one that is loculated, a positive Gram stain or culture of the pleural fluid, and a purulent pleural fluid that has a pH below 7.20 or a glucose below 60 or has a lactic acid dehydrogenase level of more than three times the upper normal limit for serum.

The chest radiograph usually shows a small-to-moderate pleural effusion with or without parenchymal infiltrates. There may be evidence of loculations and air-fluid levels. Longstanding empyema may sometimes cause isolated rounded pleural opacities, which may be confused with malignant pathology. It was once considered standard practice to request a lateral decubitus radiograph on all patients with suspected pleural sepsis and to use the lateral thickness of the effusions on these films to guide the decision on the need for a thoracentesis. The pleural effusions less than 1 cm thick on these radiographs resolved with antibiotic therapy alone and did not require pleural aspiration thoracentesis.

Thoracic ultrasound (US), however, is an attractive alternative to a lateral decubitus film, as it can very accurately measure the extent of pleural effusions and yields significantly more information regarding the state of the pleural space. The routine use of thoracic US in patients with suspected pleural sepsis should be encouraged. US is particularly helpful in determining the nature of localized or diffuse pleural opacities and is more sensitive than decubitus expiratory films in identifying small or loculated effusions. Complicated parapneumonic effusions are associated with floating strands of echogenic material which shows mobility with the respiration cycle and denotes advancing stage and chronicity.

Complicated effusions may be subdivided into either septated or non-septated effusions. The presence of septae is clinically relevant: the patients with septated effusions needed longer chest tube drainage, longer hospital care, and were more likely to require fibrinolytic therapy or surgery compared with those with unseptated effusions.

At thoracic computed tomography (CT) scan may be indicated to better delineate pulmonary and pleural anatomy, particularly if there is a suspicion of an alternative diagnosis (e.g., bronchogenic carcinoma) or prior to surgical intervention. It should be appreciated that loculations within a collection are best appreciated on US and often not seen on a chest CT scan. However, collections in interlobar spaces and those adherent to the paramediastinal pleura may escape detection by US and may only be visible on a CT scan.

Imaging Findings

CRX (PA and lateral) shows an increase in density by pneumonic consolidation pulmonary middle lobe level (Figs. 1.5.1 and 1.5.2). CT scan (mediastinal and lung) shows sign of alveolar air bronchograms associated with the presence of free pleural effusion (Figs. 1.5.3 and 1.5.4).

Case 6: Pneumomediastinum

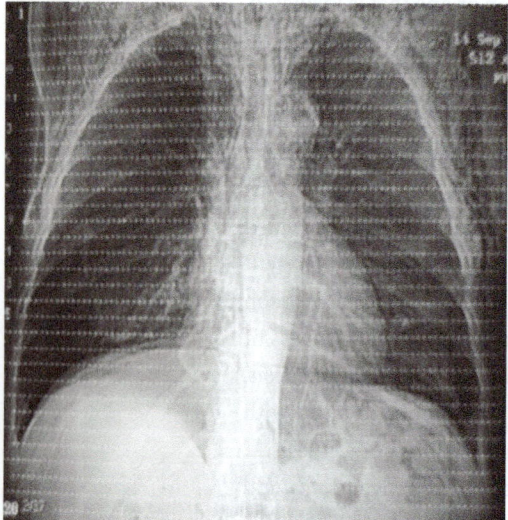

Fig. 1.6.1

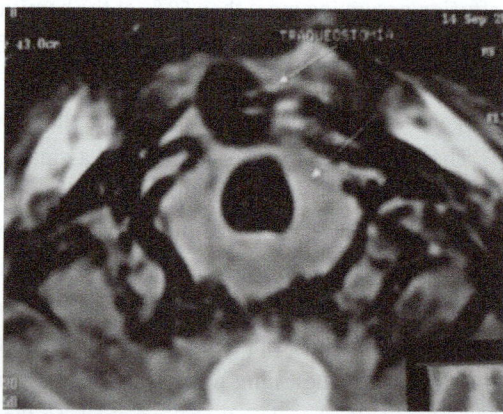

Fig. 1.6.2

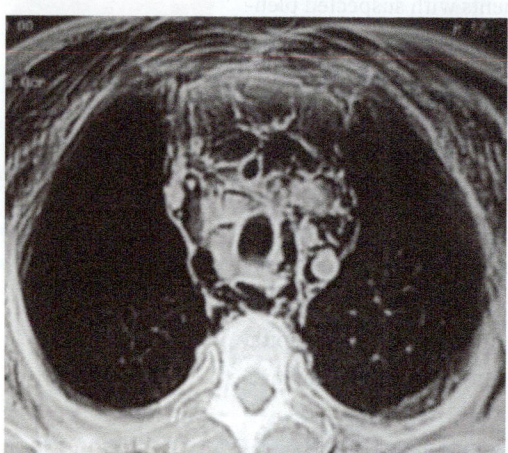

Fig. 1.6.3

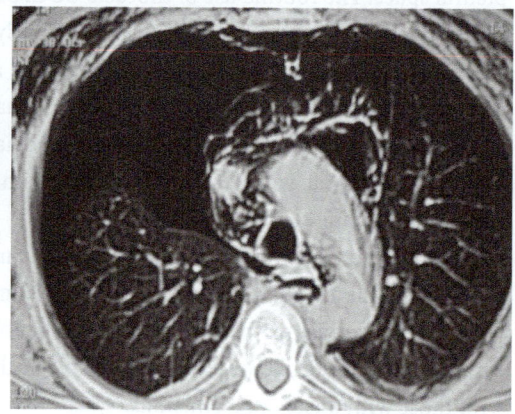

Fig. 1.6.4

A 54-year-old man who 5 days ago had left the institution for sepsis of abdominal origin, hyperosmolar state secondary to mechanical ventilation management controls, and medical surgical abdominal diseases hospitalized in intensive care for 20 days, 15 days of which required mechanical ventilation, and successful extubation. Readmitted with severe dyspnea and stridor at risk of respiratory failure, intubation difficult because it is impossible to pass orotracheal tube is taken to open tracheostomy performed without apparent complication, transferred to ICU. In intensive care it is noted that the patient has subcutaneous emphysema.

Pneumomediastinum, also known as mediastinal emphysema, represents extraluminal gas in the mediastinum. Pneumomediastinum can lead to pneumothorax, pneumopericardium, pneumoperitoneum, or pneumoretroperitoneum.

There are numerous sources of pneumomediastinum. Intrathoracic sources may be encountered in a variety of clinical settings. In asthma, vomiting, parturition, and blunt trauma to the chest.

The radiographic signs of pneumomediastinum depend on the depiction of normal anatomic structures that are outlined by the air as it leaves the mediastinum. If there is sufficient air, the thymus can become elevated to produce the thymic sail sign. Air anterior to the pericardium (pneumopre-cardium) is a frequent manifestation and requires a lateral view of the chest for diagnosis. Air surrounding the pulmonary artery or either of its main branches can result in the ring around the artery sign, particularly when the air surrounds the intramediastinal segment of the right pulmonary artery.

When there is air adjacent to the major branches of the aorta, both sides of the vessel are depicted: Mediastinal air outlines the medial side, and the aer-ated lung marginates the lateral side (tubular artery sign).

Occasionally, air can reside next to a major bronchus, allowing clear depiction of the bronchial wall and producing the double bronchial wall sign. The continuous diaphragm sign is produced by air trapped posterior to the peri-cardium, which gives the appearance of a continuous collection of air at anteroposterior radiography. Air from the mediastinum can extend laterally between the parietal pleura and the diaphragm to produce the extrapleural sign.

In summary the radiographic signs of pneumomediastinum are:
- Subcutaneous emphysema
- Thymic sail sign
- Pneumopericardium
- Ring around the artery sign
- Tubular artery sign
- Double bronchial wall sign
- Continuous diaphragm sign
- Extrapleural sign
- Air in the pulmonary ligament

The differential diagnosis includes pneumothorax, pneumomediastinum, and pneumopericardium.

Comments

CRX PA shows air in the upper mediastinum associated with subcutaneous emphysema (Fig. 1.6.1). CT scan (mediastinal window) shows accumulation of air in the upper mediastinal structures (Fig. 1.6.2). CT scan (lung window) shows hyperlucency by air in bilateral pleural space and mediastinal structures (Figs. 1.6.3 and 1.6.4).

Imaging Findings

Case 7: Empyema

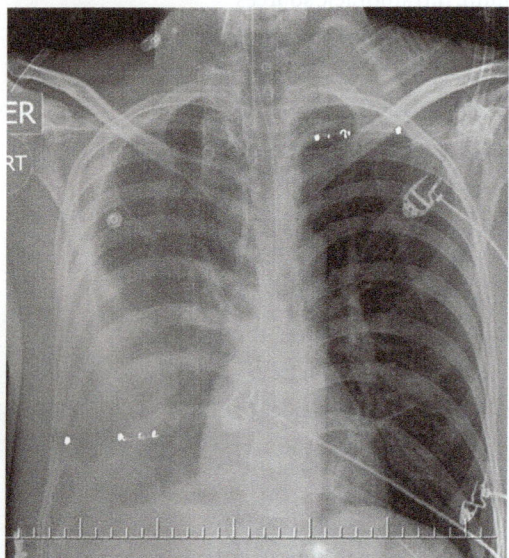

Fig. 1.7.1

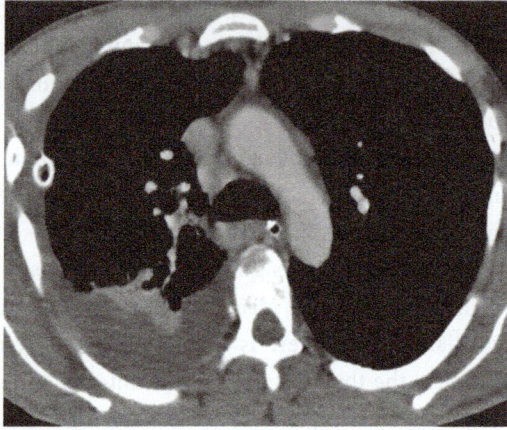

Fig. 1.7.2

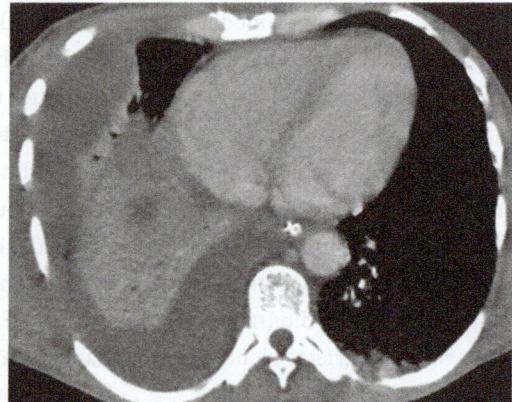

Fig. 1.7.4

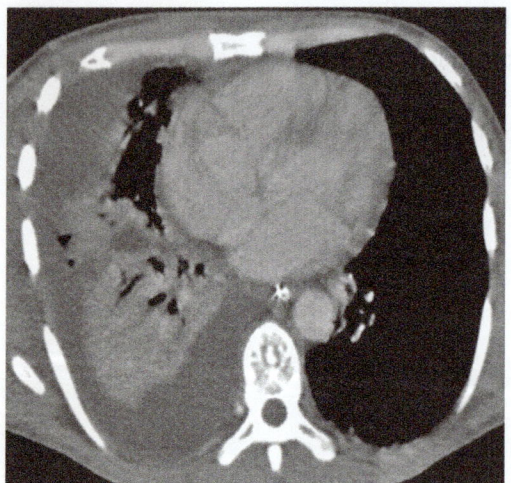

Fig. 1.7.3

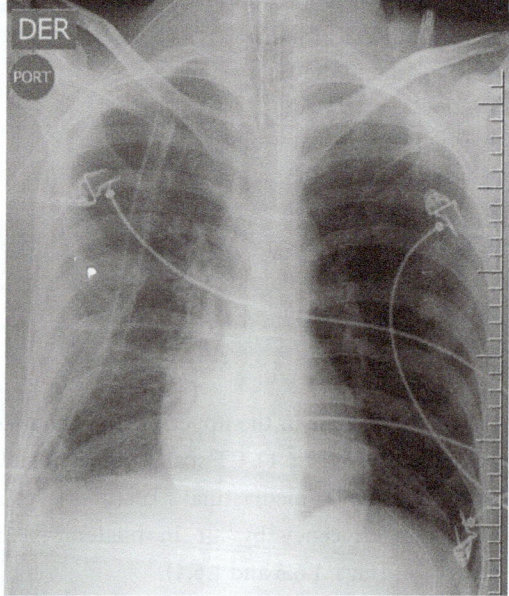

Fig. 1.7.5

A 37-year-old man admitted to ICU for multiple trauma. On the sixth day of hospitalization, showed deterioration in the transfer of oxygen and requires increased ventilator parameters. Right thoracostomy is performed with drainage of purulent fetid. It is carried right thoracotomy for decortication and drainage cavity.

Comments

A pleural empyema refers to an infected purulent and often loculated pleural effusion and is a cause of a large unilateral pleural collection. It is a potentially life-threatening condition requiring prompt diagnosis and treatment. Empyemas are usually the complication of another underlying abnormality, and thus demographics will follow those of the primary cause, e.g., pneumonia, sub-diaphragmatic abscess, and oesophageal perforation. Patients with HIV/AIDS are more likely to have pneumonia and, in turn, are more likely to develop an empyema, which may occur in over 5 % of cases of pneumonia.

Plain Film: Can resemble a pleural effusion and can mimic a peripheral pulmonary abscess, although a number of features usually enable distinction between the two (see empyema vs. lung abscess). Pleural fluid is typically unilateral or markedly asymmetric. Generally empyemas form an obtuse angle with the chest wall and, due to their lenticular shape, are much larger in one projection (e.g., frontal) compared to the orthogonal projection (e.g., lateral)[3]. The lenticular shape (biconvex) is also suggestive of the diagnosis, as transudative/sterile pleural effusions tend to be crescentic in shape (i.e., concave toward the lung; see empyema vs. pleural effusion).

Ultrasound: The appearances of an empyema depend on the composition of the collection. Typically they are not uniformly anechoic and are often septated. Ultrasound has a major role in enabling targeted thoracocentesis.

CT Chest: Typically appears as a fluid density collection in the pleural space, sometimes with locules of gas. They form obtuse angles with the adjacent lung, which is displaced and compressed. The pleura is thickened due to fibrin deposition and ingrowth of vessels with enhancement. At the margins of the empyema, the pleura can be seen dividing into parietal and visceral layers, the so-called split pleura sign, which is the most sensitive and specific sign on CT and is helpful in distinguishing an empyema from a peripheral lung abscess (see empyema vs. lung abscess). The inner walls of the empyema are smooth.

Imaging Findings

CRX PA shows increased radiopacity associated with the presence of right pleural effusion (Fig. 1.7.1). CT scan (mediastinal window) shows moderate pleural effusion and passive atelectasis associated with dilation of the airway (Figs. 1.7.2, 1.7.3, and 1.7.4). CRX PA shows radiopacity right clearance and presence of chest tube (Fig. 1.7.5).

Case 8: Hemothorax

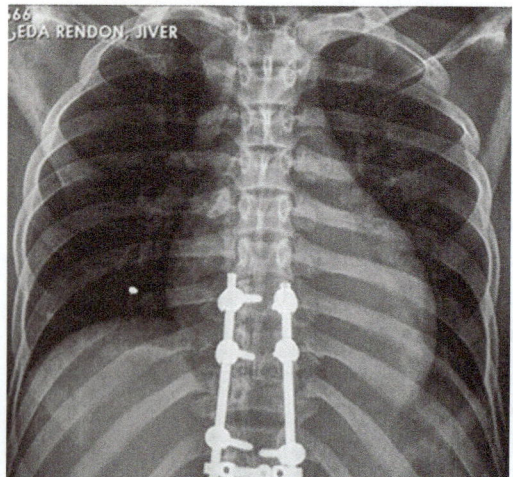

Fig. 1.8.1

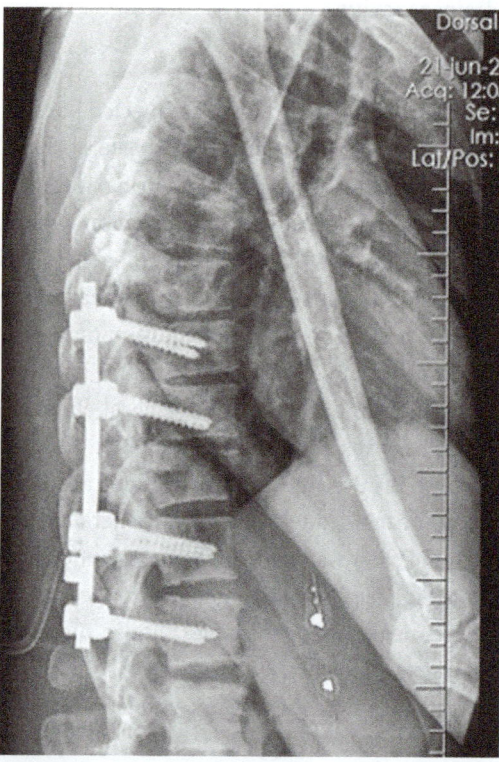

Fig. 1.8.2

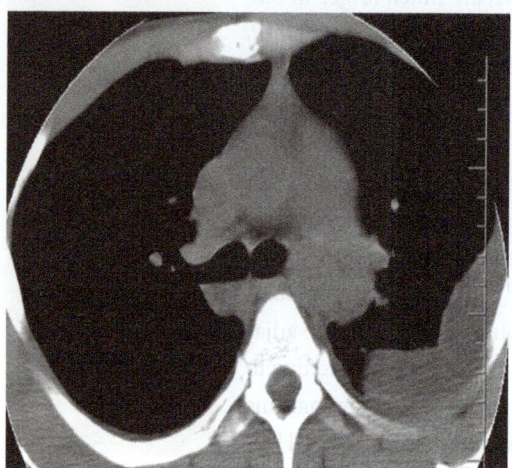

Fig. 1.8.3

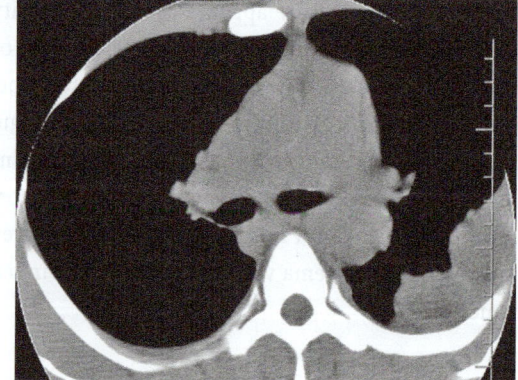

Fig. 1.8.4

A 30-year-old man who suffered multiple injuries after being buried by an avalanche of sand. Is brought to the institution where he is valued by neurosurgery evidence paraplegia with sensory involvement T10, with a fractured spine. It led to fusion of T8 to T12 and decompression by posterior approach.

On day 14, post surgery presents general malaise, fever, and dyspnea. Shown left pleural effusion.

A hemothorax is a collection of blood in the pleural space. It is classified according to the amount of blood. 350 ml or less is considered minimal, 350–1,500 ml is moderate, and greater than 1,500 ml is considered massive. In many cases, blood in the pleural cavity will be diluted by other pleural fluid. In these cases, the pleural fluid hematocrit can be used to diagnose a hemothorax using a hematocrit of greater than half the serum hematocrit as diagnostic of hemothorax.

The upright chest radiograph remains the primary diagnostic study in the acute evaluation of hemothorax. In the normal unscarred pleural space, a hemothorax is noted as a meniscus of fluid blunting the costophrenic angle or diaphragmatic surface and tracking up the pleural margins of the chest wall when viewed on the upright chest X-ray (CRX) film. As much as 400–500 ml of blood is required to obliterate the costophrenic angle as seen on an upright chest radiograph. In the acute trauma setting, the portable supine chest radiograph may be the first and only view available from which to make definitive decisions regarding therapy.

The presence and size of a hemothorax is much more difficult to evaluate on supine films. As much as 1,000 ml of blood may be missed when viewing a portable supine CRX film. CRX has been found to be a poor predictor of patients requiring a VATS.

One drawback of ultrasonography for the identification of traumatic hemothorax is that associated injuries readily seen on chest radiographs in the trauma patient, such as bony injuries, widened mediastinum, and pneumothorax, are not readily identifiable on chest ultrasonography.

Computed tomographic scan is a highly accurate diagnostic study for pleural fluid or blood. In the initial trauma setting, it does not necessarily have a primary role in the diagnosis of hemothorax and pulmonary contusion but is complementary to chest radiography. CT may actually be too sensitive in identifying clinically nonsignificant injuries.

Computed tomographic scan may also be value later in the course of the chest trauma for localization and quantification of any retained collections of clot and potential empyema within the pleural space.

Associated Findings: Rib fractures are the most common chest wall injuries associated with a hemothorax, pulmonary contusion and laceration, and pneumothorax; laceration of intercostal or internal mammary artery can produce persistent bleeding.

CRX film, AP and lateral, shows obliteration of left costophrenic angles (Figs. 1.8.1 and 1.8.2). CT scan (mediastinal window) shows loculated left pleural effusion (Figs. 1.8.3 and 1.8.4).

Case 9: Fibrothorax

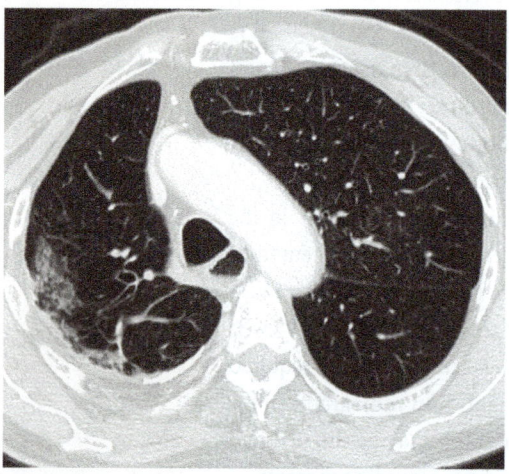

Fig. 1.9.1

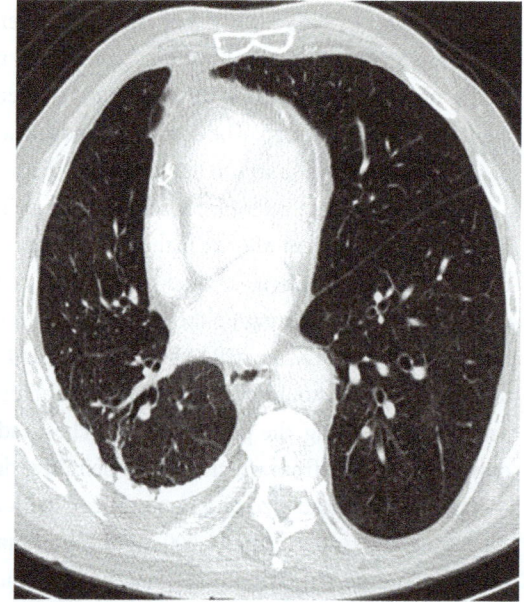

Fig. 1.9.2

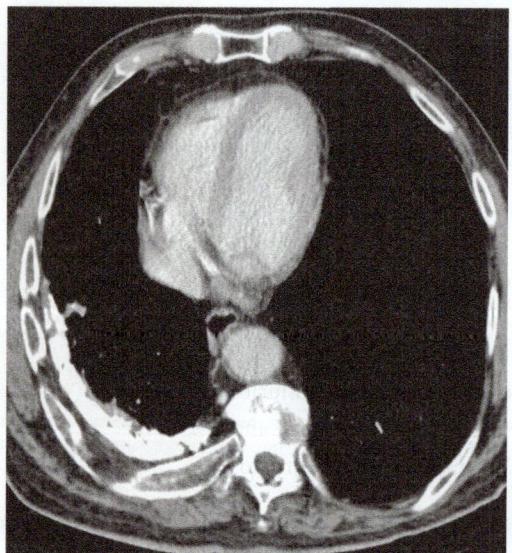

Fig. 1.9.3

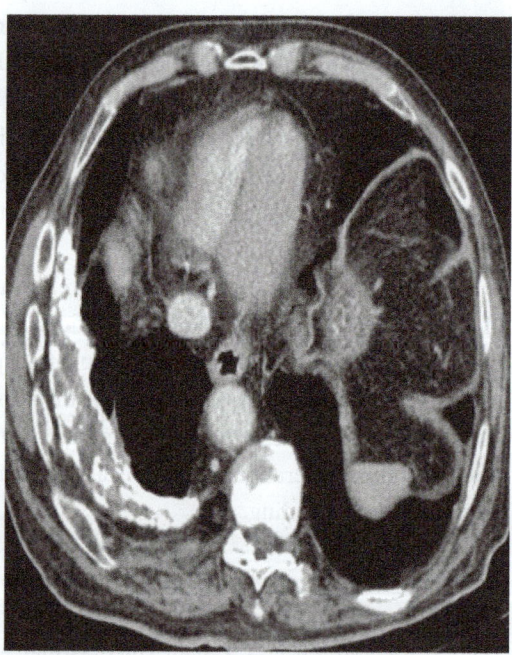

Fig. 1.9.4

A 62-year-old man with a history of pleural tuberculosis for more than 10 years ago.

Fibrothorax or diffuse pleural thickening involving most of the pleural space may develop as the result of previous hemothoraces, tuberculous effusions, and other types of empyema, benign asbestos pleurisy, and occasionally other processes.

The definition of diffuse pleural thickening on chest radiographs as "a smooth, non-interrupted pleural density extending over at least one-fourth of the chest wall" associated or not with costophrenic blunting.

On CT scans, diffuse pleural thickening as "a continuous sheet of pleural thickening more than 5 cm wide, more than 8 cm in craniocaudal extent, and more than 3 mm thick." Diffuse pleural thickening is well studied with CT and MRI.

Diffuse pleural thickening is often associated with a decrease in volume of the ipsilateral lung. Bilateral pleural thickening may be associated with a severe restrictive defect on pulmonary functioning testing.

Tuberculous pleuritis often leaves sequelae ranging from minimal pleural thickening, seen as obliteration of the costophrenic sulcus, to severe thickening, seen as fibrous tissue and calcification encompassing and restricting the lung and referred to as fibrothorax. Fibrothorax may be associated with extensive volume loss of the ipsilateral lung and even with ventilatory impairment.

CT scan (lung window) shows extensive pleural thickening at level of lower right hemithorax, which is decreased in volume (Figs. 1.9.1 and 1.9.2). CT scan (arterial phase) shows extensive pleural thickening at level of lower right hemithorax, which is decreased in volume. Note pleural thickening with heterogeneous attenuation with calcifications (Figs. 1.9.3 and 1.9.4).

Case 10: Benign Tumors of the Pleura

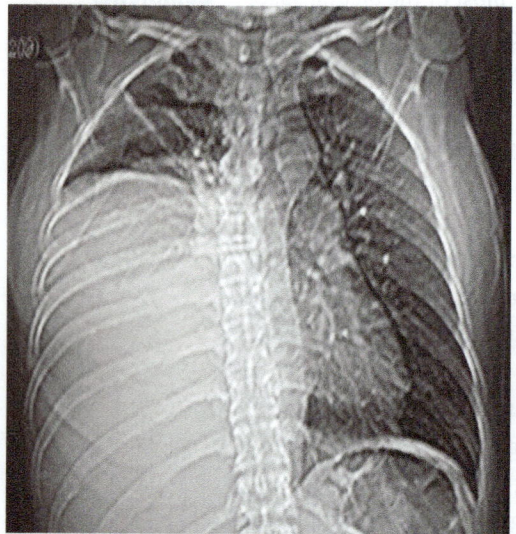

Fig. 1.10.1

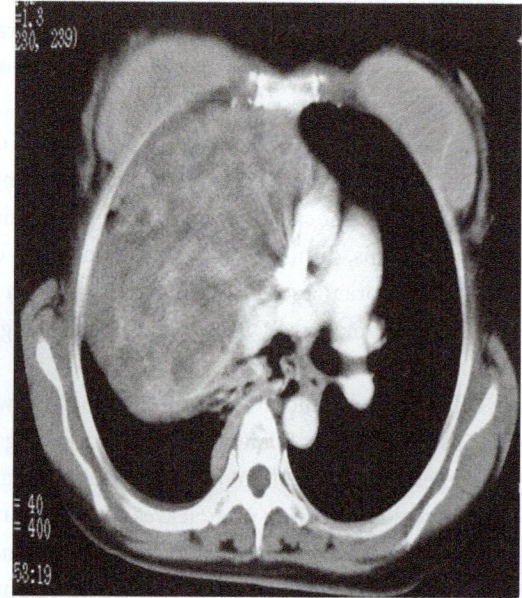

Fig. 1.10.2

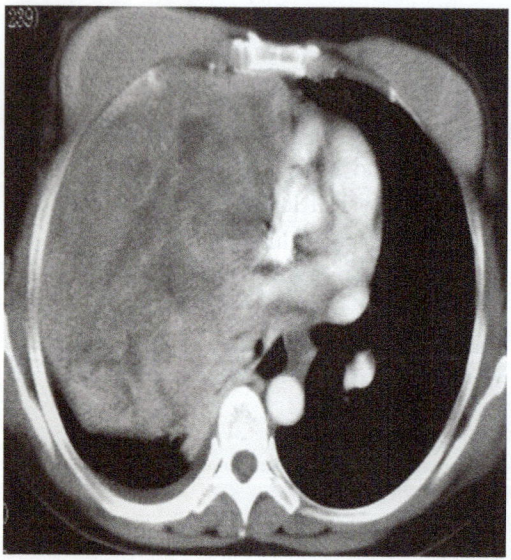

Fig. 1.10.3

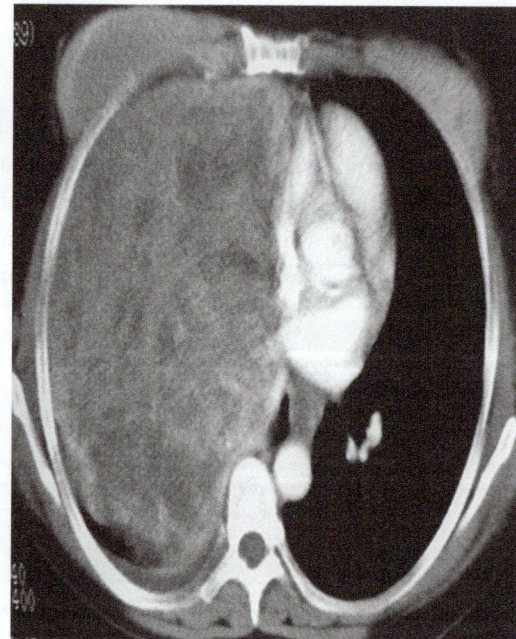

Fig. 1.10.4

A 51-year-old woman referred for cough, dyspnea, and chest pain.

Fibrous tumors of the pleura, also known as benign mesotheliomas, localized fibrous mesotheliomas, and pleural fibromas, are rare tumors, accounting for less than 5 % of all neoplasms involving the pleura. Although these tumors affect men and women of all ages, the mean age is 51 years. These tumors originate from submesoepithelial mesenchymal cells, and approximately 80 % arise from the visceral pleura.

Radiographic findings include a well-delineated mass which may form obtuse angles with the chest wall and mediastinum and which displaces the adjacent lung parenchyma. Frequently the upper edge of the lesion may tend to fade into the lung parenchyma. If the lesion has a pedicle, it may be mobile and change position with different patient posture. These lesions may also occur in the interlobar fissures.

CT findings include a well-delineated often-lobulated soft tissue mass in close relation to the pleural surface. Although an obtuse angle of the mass with respect to the pleural surface may not be identified in every case, a smoothly tapering margin is characteristic and may indicate a pleural location. Calcification is present in 5 % of cases. Homogenous soft tissue lesion (intermediate attenuation similar to muscle and attributable to high collagen density and vascular nature), often abutting chest wall. Heterogeneity may be related to necrosis and hemorrhage. Heterogeneous pattern of enhancement after IV contrast media infusion. Smaller fibromas typically form obtuse angle, larger can form acute angle to pleural surface.

MRI may be helpful in the diagnosis of these lesions. In cases in which there is a fairly high collagen content, fibrous tumors of the pleura may exhibit low single intensity on both T1- and T2-weighted images and enhancement with intravenously administered gadolinium contrast agent. This is in contradistinction to most tumors, which will demonstrate increased signal intensity on T2-weighted images because of high water content.

The differential diagnosis of a calcified mass of the pleura also includes metastatic disease from osteosarcoma, chondrosarcoma, mucinous adenocarcinoma, parosteal osteosarcoma, and calcification-ossification of a mesothelioma. Displacement of adjacent lung parenchyma with compressive atelectasis and bowing of the bronchi and pulmonary vessels around the mass is often noted. Enhancement of the tumor following administration of contrast material is frequent and may be homogenous or heterogenous. In the malignant variety of this tumor, CT may demonstrate local invasion of the chest wall with associated rib destruction. Larger lesions of 10 cm or greater in diameter are more likely to be malignant.

CRX film shows increased radiopacity by mass presence on the right (Fig. 1.10.1). CT scan (arterial phase) shows bulky soft tissue mass with heterogeneous pattern that is closely related to the pleural surface, which occupies the lower 2/3 of the right chest (Figs. 1.10.2, 1.10.3, and 1.10.4).

Case 11: Metastatic Pleural Tumor

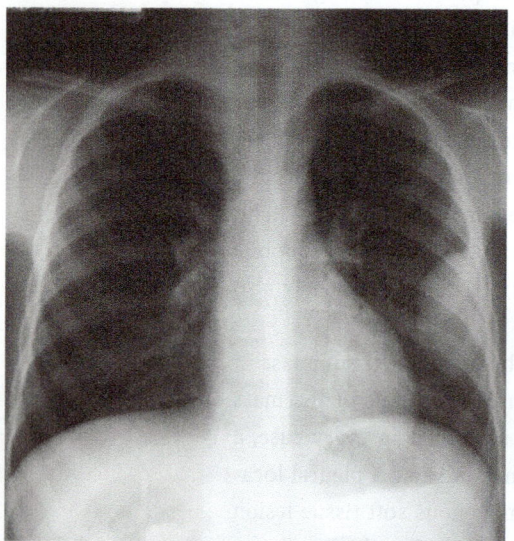

Fig. 1.11.1

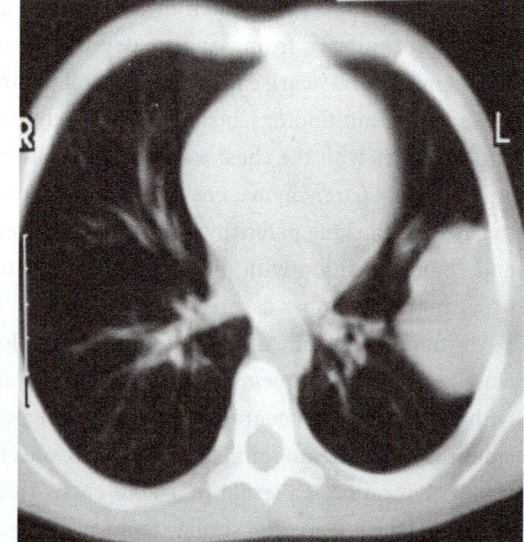

Fig. 1.11.2

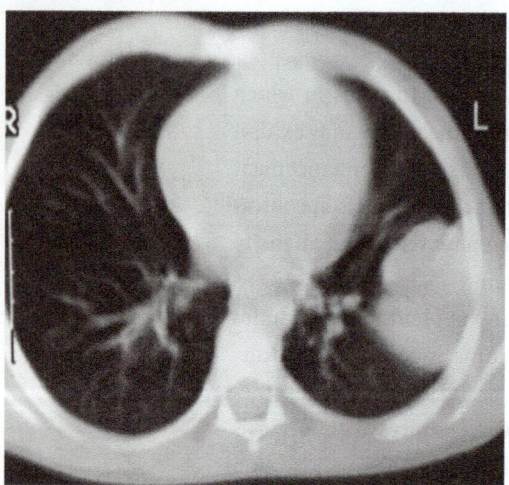

Fig. 1.11.3

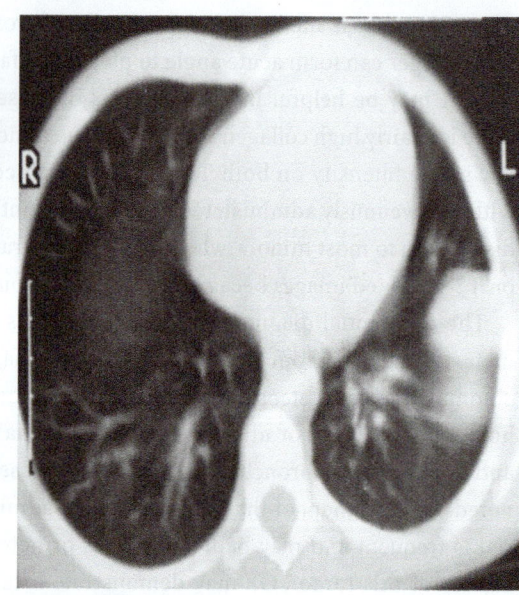

Fig. 1.11.4

A 54-year-old man with 2-month history of left rib pain and weight loss. Percutaneous lung biopsy showed adenocarcinoma.

Metastatic tumor usually involves both the visceral and parietal pleura and often produces malignant pleural effusion. The pleura is a common site of metastases, especially from primary adenocarcinomas. About 40 % are caused by bronchogenic carcinoma, 20 % by breast carcinoma, 10 % by lymphoma, and 10 % by tumors of unknown origin. Although pleural metastases may be asymptomatic in 20 % of patients, they generally cause dyspnea, chest pain, and weight loss. Pleural metastases are the second most common cause of pleural effusion in adults (the first is left heart failure). Other important causes include right heart failure and pulmonary hypertension.

Chest radiography shows pleural metastases as diffuse or focal pleural thickening. This may be nodular thickening, a discrete mass, or circumferential pleural thickening with infiltration into adjacent tissues.

On CT, metastases may manifest as marked thickening and nodularity of the pleura, usually with an associated pleural effusion. In some cases, the effusion may be large and tumor foci may be difficult to identify. Metastases may mimic malignant mesothelioma, and the two entities cannot be reliably distinguished by cross-sectional imaging. Finally, certain tumors such as malignant thymoma may produce focal seeding of the pleura. This is usually manifested on CT scanning as localized focal pleural nodules that may be bilateral or unilateral.

The differentiation of malignant from benign pleural thickening provides a challenge for the radiologist. There is overlap of the radiologic manifestations of benign and malignant pleural processes. Features that were helpful in distinguishing malignant from benign pleural disease included (a) circumferential pleural thickening, (b) nodular pleural thickening more than 1 cm in thickness, and (c) mediastinal pleural involvement, all of which occurred more consistently with malignant lesions.

These features may be seen in mesothelioma and metastatic pleural disease but are unusual in benign pleural disease. The presence of pleural calcification also is suggestive of a benign process. Although calcified pleural plaques may be seen in cases of mesothelioma, they are uncommon.

PET/CT can distinguish benign from malignant pleural thickening and effusion by showing high ^{18}F-FDG uptake in the latter.

CRX film shows soft tissue mass that makes obtuse angles in the right chest (Fig. 1.11.1). CT scan (lung window) shows soft tissue mass of homogeneous density of obtuse angles in the lower left lung (Figs. 1.11.2, 1.11.3, and 1.11.4).

Further Reading

Pleural Tuberculosis

American Thoracic Society (2000) Diagnostic standards and classification of tuberculosis in adult and children. Am J Respir Crit Care Med 161:1376–1395

Barbas CS, Cukier A, de Varvalho CR, Barbas Filho JV, Light RW (1991) The relationship between pleural fluid findings and the development of pleural thickening in patients with pleural tuberculosis. Chest 100:1264–1267

Cordero P, Gil V, Greses J, Soler J, Perpina M, Sanchis F, Sanchis P (1995) The clinical characteristics of pleural tuberculosis in patients with and without human immunodeficiencyvirusinfection.ArchBronconeumol 31(10):512–518

Ferrer J (1997) Pleural tuberculosis. Eur Respir J 10(4):942–947

McAdams HP, Eramus J, Winter JA (1995) Radiologic manifestations of pulmonary tuberculosis. Radiol Clin North Am 33:655–677

Roth J (1999) Searching for tuberculosis in the pleural space. Chest 116:3–5

Trajman A, Kaisermann M, Kritski A et al (2004) Diagnosing pleural tuberculosis. Chest 125:2366–2367

Valdés L, Alvarez D, San José E et al (1998) Tuberculous pleurisy: a study of 254 patients. Arch Intern Med 158:2017–2021

Yilmaz MU, Kumcuoglu Z, Utkaner G, Yalniz O, Erkmen G (1998) Computed tomography findings of tuberculous pleurisy. Int J Tuberc Lung Dis 2:164–167

Malignant Pleural Effusions

Friedman AC, Fiel SB, Redeiki PD et al (1990) Computed tomography of benign pleural and pulmonary parenchymal abnormalities related to asbestos exposure. Semin Ultrasound CT MR 11:393–408

Johnston WW (1985) The malignant pleural effusion: a review of cytopathologic diagnoses of 584 specimens from 472 consecutive patients. Cancer 56(4):905–909

Leung AN, Muller NL, Miller RR (1990) CT in differential diagnosis of diffuse pleural disease. Am J Roentgenol 154:487–492

Roberts ME, Neville E, Berrisford RG, Antunes G, Ali NJ, BTS Pleural Disease Guideline Group (2010) Management of a malignant pleural effusion: British Thoracic Society Pleural Disease Guideline 2010. Thorax 65(suppl 2):ii32–ii40

Malignant Pleural Mesothelioma

Kawashima A, Libshitz HI (1990) Malignant pleural mesothelioma: CT manifestations in 50 cases. Am J Roentgenol 155:965–969

Miller BH, Rosado-de-Christenson ML, Mason AC et al (1996) Malignant pleural mesothelioma: radiologic-pathologic correlation. Radiographics 16:613–644

Stahel RA, Weder W, Lievens Y, Felip E (2010) Malignant pleural mesothelioma: ESMO Clinical Practice Guidelines for diagnosis, treatment and follow-up. Ann Oncol 21(suppl 5):v126–v128

Wechsler RJ, Rao VM, Steiner RM (1983) The radiology of thoracic malignant mesothelioma. Crit Rev Diagn Imaging 20:283–310

Yamamuro M, Gerbaudo VH, Gill RR et al (2007) Morphologic and functional imaging of malignant pleural mesothelioma. Eur J Radiol 64(3):356–366

Zervos MD, Bizekis C, Pass HI (2008) Malignant mesothelioma 2008. Curr Opin Pulm Med 14(4):303–309

Tension Pneumothorax

Barton ED (1999) Tension pneumothorax. Curr Opin Pulm Med 5:269–274

Britten S, Palmer SH (1996) Chest wall thickness may limit adequate drainage of tension pneumothorax by needle thoracocentesis. J Accid Emerg Med 13:426–427

Britten S, Palmer SH, Snow TM (1996) Needle thoracocentesis in tension pneumothorax: insufficient cannula length and potential failure. Injury 27:321–322

Conces DJ Jr, Tarver RD, Gray WC et al (1988) Treatment of pneumothoraces utilizing small caliber chest tubes. Chest 94:55–57

Cullinane DC, Morris JA Jr, Bass JG et al (2001) Needle thoracostomy may not be indicated in the trauma patient. Injury 32:749–752

Dunlop MG, Beattie TF, Preston PG (1989) Clinical assessment and radiography following blunt chest trauma. Arch Emerg Med 6:125–127

Hollins GW, Beattie T, Harper I et al (1994) Tension pneumothorax: report of two cases presenting with acute abdominal symptoms. J Accid Emerg Med 11:43–44

Holloway VJ, Harris JK (2000) Spontaneous pneumothorax: is it under tension? J Accid Emerg Med 17:222–223

Jenkins C, Sudheer PS (2000) Needle thoracocentesis fails to diagnose a large pneumothorax. Anaesthesia 55:925–926

Jones R, Hollingsworth J (2002) Tension pneumothorax not responding to needle thoracocentesis. Emerg Med J 19:176–177

Light RW (1994) Tension pneumothorax. Intensive Care Med 20(7):468–469

Mines D, Abbuhl S (1993) Needle thoracostomy fails to detect a fatal tension pneumothorax [erratum appears in Ann Emerg Med 1993;22:1364]. Ann Emerg Med 22:863–866

Moss HA, Roe PG, Flower CD (2000) Clinical deterioration in ARDS – An unchanged chest radiograph and functioning chest drains do not exclude an acute tension pneumothorax. Clin Radiol 55(8):637–639

Pattison GT (1996) Needle thoracocentesis in tension pneumothorax: insufficient cannula length and potential failure. Injury 27:758

Rojas R, Wasserberger J, Balasubramaniam S (1983) Unsuspected tension pneumothorax as a hidden cause of unsuccessful resuscitation. Ann Emerg Med 12:411–412

Rosen P, Barkin R, Danzl D et al (1999) Emergency medicine – concepts and clinical practice, 4th edn. Mosby, St. Louis

Spiteri MA, Cook DG, Clark SW (1988) Reliability of eliciting physical signs in examination of the chest. Lancet 1:873–875

Steier M, Ching N, Roberts EB et al (1974) Pneumothorax complicating continuous ventilatory support. J Thorac Cardiovasc Surg 67:17–23

Watts BL, Howell MA (2001) Tension pneumothorax: a difficult diagnosis. Emerg Med J 18:319–320

Parapneumonic Pleural Effusions

Aquino SL, Webb WR, Gushiken BJ (1994) Pleural exudates and transudates: diagnosis with contrast-enhanced CT. Radiology 192:803–808

Chapman SJ, Davies RJ (2004) Recent advances in parapneumonic effusions and empyema. Curr Opin Pulm Med 10:299–304

Chen KY, Liaw YS, Wang HC et al (2000) Sonographic septation: a useful prognostic indicator of acute thoracic empyema. J Ultrasound Med 19:837–843

Colice GL, Curtis A, Deslauriers J et al (2000) Medical and surgical treatment of parapneumonic effusions: an evidence-based guideline. Chest 118: 1158–1171

Diacon AH, Brutsche MH, Soler M (2003) Accuracy of pleural puncture sites: a prospective comparison of clinical examination with ultrasound. Chest 123: 436–441

Diacon AH, Theron J, Bolliger CT (2005) Transthoracic ultrasound for the pulmonologist. Curr Opin Pulm Med 11:307–312

Froudarakis ME (2008) Diagnostic work-up of pleural effusions. Respiration 75:4–13, 26

Light RW (2006) Parapneumonic effusions and empyema. Proc Am Thorac Soc 3:75–80

Light RW, Girard WM, Jenkinson SG, George RB (1980) Parapneumonic effusions. Am J Med 69:507–512

Marks WM, Filly RA, Callen PW (1982) Real-time evaluation of pleural lesions: new observations regarding the probability of obtaining free fluid. Radiology 142:163–164

Simmers TA, Jie C, Sie B (1999) Minimally invasive treatment of thoracic empyema. Thorac Cardiovasc Surg 47:77–81

Tsai TH, Yang PC (2003) Ultrasound in the diagnosis and management of pleural disease. Curr Opin Pulm Med 9:282–290

Tu CY, Hsu WH, Hsia TC et al (2004) Pleural effusions in febrile medical ICU patients: chest ultrasound study. Chest 126:1274–1280

Pneumomediastinum

Bejvan SM, David Godwin JD (1996) Pneumomediastinum: old signs and new signs. AJR Am J Roentgenol 166:1041–1048

Zylak CM, Standen JR, Barnes GR, Zylak CJ (2000) Pneumomediastinum revisited. Radiographics 20: 1043–1057

Empyema

Bryant RE, Salmon CJ (1996) Pleural empyema. State-of-the-art clinical article. Clin Infect Dis 22:747–764

Fry W (1998) Surgical management of empyema. In: Kaiser L, Kron IL, Spray TL (eds) Mastery of cardiothoracic surgery. Lippincott-Raven, Philadelphia, pp 247–256

Lee-Chiong TL, Matthay RA (1996) Current diagnostic and medical management of thoracic empyema. In: Faber LP (ed) Empyema, spaces and fistula. Chest Surg Clin North Am 6(3):419–437

Moulton JS (2000) Image-guided management of complicated pleural fluid collections. Radiol Clin North Am 38(2):345–374

Rice TW (2000) Fibrothorax and decortication the lung. In: Shields TW (ed) General thoracic surgery, 5th edn. Lippincott Williams and Wilkins, Philadelphia, pp 729–737

Hemothorax

Blaisdel F (1986) Pneumothorax and hemothorax. In: Blaisdel F, Trunkey D (eds) Trauma management, vol III, Cervicothoracic trauma. Thieme Inc, New York, pp 150–165

Schmidt U (1998) Chest tube decompression of blunt chest injuries by physicians in the field: effectiveness and complications. J Trauma 44(1):98–101

Velmahos G (1999) Predicting the need for thoracoscopic evacuation of residual traumatic hemothorax: chest radiograph is insufficient. J Trauma 46(1):65–70

Weisserg D (1986) Treatment of thoracic injuries. Ann Thorac Surg 42(3):348

Fibrothorax

Choi JA, Hong KT, Oh YW et al (2001) CT manifestations of late sequelae in patients with tuberculous pleuritis. AJR Am J Roentgenol 176(2):441–445

Gevenois PA, de Maertelaer V, Madani A et al (1998) Asbestosis, pleural plaques and diffuse pleural thickening: three distinct benign responses to asbestos exposure. Eur Respir J 11:1021–1027

McLoud TC, Woods BO, Carrington CB et al (1985) Diffuse pleural thickening in an asbestos exposed population: prevalence and causes. Am J Roentgenol 144:9–18

Weber MA, Bock M, Plathow C et al (2004) Asbestos-related pleural disease: value of dedicated magnetic resonance imaging techniques. Invest Radiol 39(9):554–556

Benign Tumors of the Pleura

Abu Arab W (2012) Solitary fibrous tumours of the pleura. Eur J Cardiothorac Surg 41(3):587–597

Dynes MC, White EM, Fry WA, Ghahremani GG (1992) Imaging manifestations of pleural tumors. Radiographics 12:1191–1201

Granville L et al (2005) Review and update of uncommon primary pleural tumors. Arch Pathol Lab Med 129:1428–1443

McLoud T (1998) CT and MR in pleural disease. Clin Chest Med 19(2):261–276

Rosado-de-Christenson ML et al (2003) Localized fibrous tumors of the pleura. Radiographics 23:759–783

Truong M, Munden RF, Kemp BL (2000) Localized fibrous tumor of the pleura. AJR Am J Roentgenol 174:42

Metastatic Pleural Tumor

Bonomo L, Feragalli B, Sacco R, Merlino B, Storto ML (2000) Malignant pleural disease. Eur J Radiol 34:98–118

Hussein-Jelen T, Bankier AA, Eisenberg RL (2012) Solid pleural lesions. AJR Am J Roentgenol 198:W512–W520

Leung AN, Muller NL, Miller RR (1990) CT in differential diagnosis of diffuse pleural disease. AJR Am J Roentgenol 154:487–492

Qureshi NR, Gleeson FV (2006) Imaging of pleural disease. Clin Chest Med 27:193–213

Diaphragm

John C. Pedrozo Pupo and Diego Pardo Pinzón

Contents

J.C. Pedrozo Pupo (ed.), *Learning Chest Imaging*, Learning Imaging,
DOI 10.1007/978-3-642-34147-2_2, © Springer-Verlag Berlin Heidelberg 2013

Case 1: Pneumoperitoneum

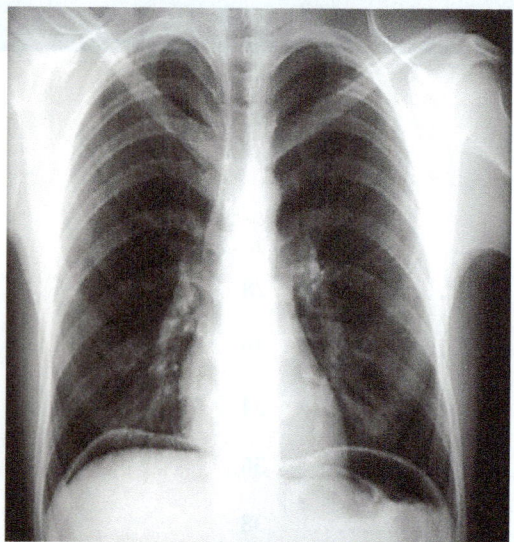

Fig. 2.1.1

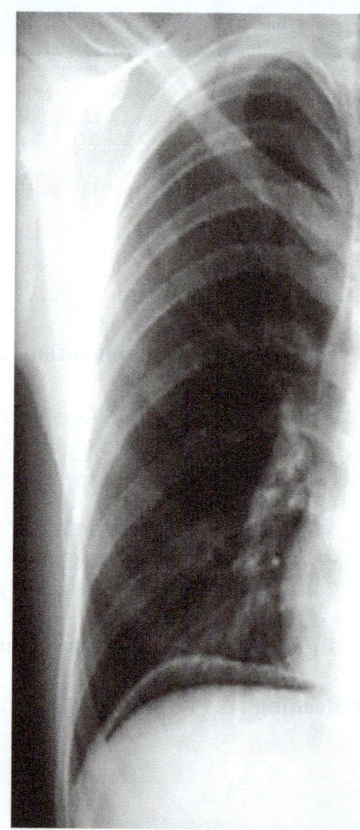

Fig. 2.1.2

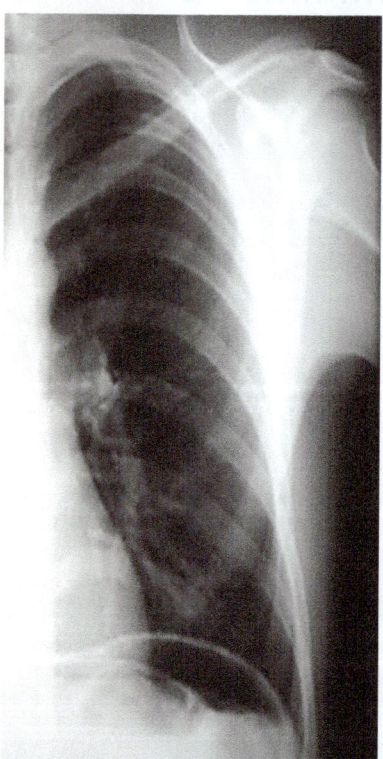

Fig. 2.1.3

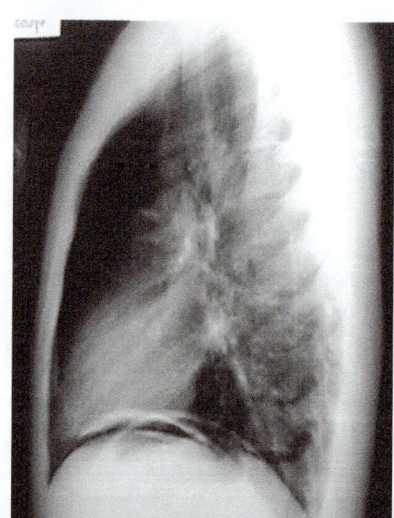

Fig. 2.1.4

A 60-year-old man with abdominal wound opened for exploratory laparotomy, with symptoms of dry cough and dyspnea grade 2 and history of pancreatic carcinoma.

Pneumoperitoneum refers to the presence of air within the peritoneal cavity. **Comments**
The most common cause is a perforation of the abdominal viscus—most commonly, a perforated ulcer, although a pneumoperitoneum may occur as a result of perforation of any part of the bowel; other causes include a benign ulcer, a tumor, or trauma. Likewise, not every bowel perforation results in a pneumoperitoneum; some perforations seal over, allowing little gas to escape. A pneumoperitoneum is common after abdominal surgery; it usually resolves 3–6 days after surgery, although it may persist for as long as 24 days after surgery.

Signs of a large pneumoperitoneum include the following:

The football sign, which usually represents a large collection of air within the greater sac. The air seems to outline the entire abdominal cavity.

The gas-relief sign, the Rigler's sign, and the double-wall sign are all terms applied to the visualization of the outer wall of bowel loops caused by gas outside the bowel loop and normal intraluminal gas. Free intraperitoneal gas and intraperitoneal fluid in excess of 1,000 mL are usually required to elicit this sign.

The urachus is a vestigial peritoneal reflection not normally seen on a plain abdominal radiograph.

The lateral umbilical ligaments, which contain the inferior epigastric vessels, may become visible as an inverted V sign in the pelvis as a result of a large pneumoperitoneum.

A telltale triangle sign represents a triangular pocket of air between 2 loops of bowel and the abdominal wall.

Free air under the diaphragm may depict the diaphragmatic muscle slips as arcuate soft tissue bands, arching parallel to the diaphragmatic dome.

Gas within the lesser sac may be present, particularly with a perforation of the posterior wall of the stomach.

Air may be present around the spleen.

Signs of partial large bowel obstruction with a sigmoid diverticulum perforation may occur in association with signs of a pneumoperitoneum.

On a left lateral decubitus radiograph, free air is apparent around the inferior edge of the liver, which forms the least-dependent part of the abdomen in that position.

CT can readily depict a pneumoperitoneum. It can be an incidental finding on MRI because MRI is not the primary imaging modality.

CRX film (frontal and lateral) shows the air bubble below the left and right **Imaging Findings**
hemidiaphragm (pneumoperitoneum) (Figs. 2.1.1, 2.1.2, 2.1.3, and 2.1.4).

Case 2: Diaphragmatic Eventration

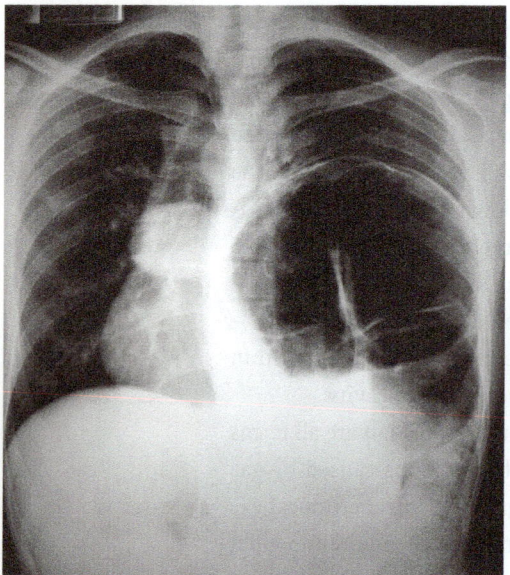

Fig. 2.2.1

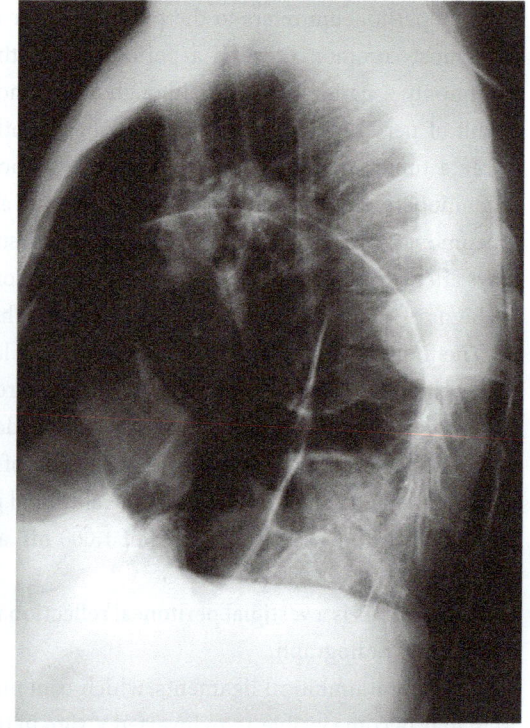

Fig. 2.2.2

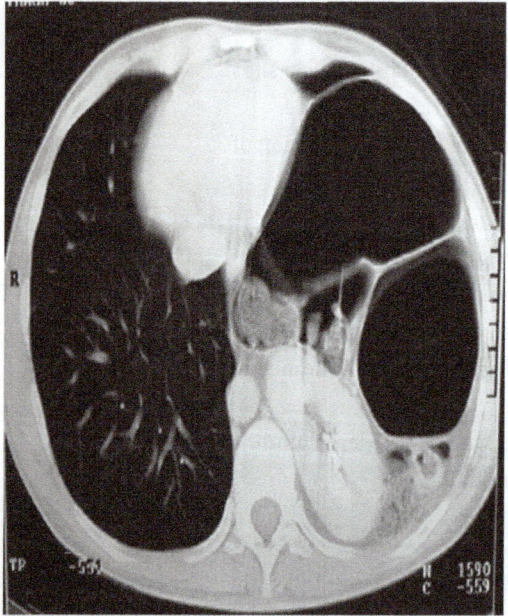

Fig. 2.2.3

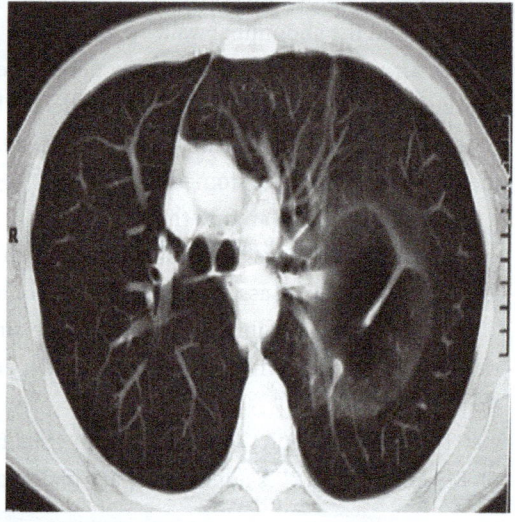

Fig. 2.2.4

A 36-year-old man referred with dyspnea and history of chest trauma.

Comments

From diaphragmatic pathology, 5 % is due to eventration. The diaphragmatic eventration is the elevation of part or all of the diaphragm or an upward displacement of the abdominal contents. It can be congenital, phrenic nerve paralysis, subphrenic abscess, for bulky right middle lobe, hepatomegaly, or trauma to the diaphragm. Usually asymptomatic and presents with loss of muscle tone of the diaphragm. It may be associated with other anomalies such as high renal ectopia and extralobar pulmonary sequestration. Also, it may be associated with alterations in the column as the kyphosis, chest deformity, or bone for pectus excavatum and pectus carinatum.

The differential diagnosis includes diaphragmatic eventration, congenital lobar emphysema and right diaphragmatic eventration cases, tumor, cyst, pleural, and/or hepatic hernia.

The chest X-ray diagnostic often many of the cases, the aid of fluoroscopy. In doubtful cases, the CT scan of upper abdomen shows hypoplastic diaphragm and liver evisceration; when the condition is right, rule out the possibility of mediastinal masses. The ability to confirm the presence of liver tomography is based on the observation of portal vessels after injection of contrast medium. The liver sections show the normal flow of the rear of the diaphragm and liver; it does not appear in its anterior portion due to its elevated position at the craniocaudal superior. It mentions the MRI as a very accurate method of third order.

Imaging Findings

CRX film (frontal and lateral) shows elevation of the left hemidiaphragm with substantial presence of bowel loops (Figs. 2.2.1 and 2.2.2). CT scan (lung window) shows left massively distended colon below the left diaphragm (Figs. 2.2.3 and 2.2.4). RNM shows left colon massively distended below the diaphragm and presence of left paravertebral mass (Figs. 2.2.5 and 2.2.6).

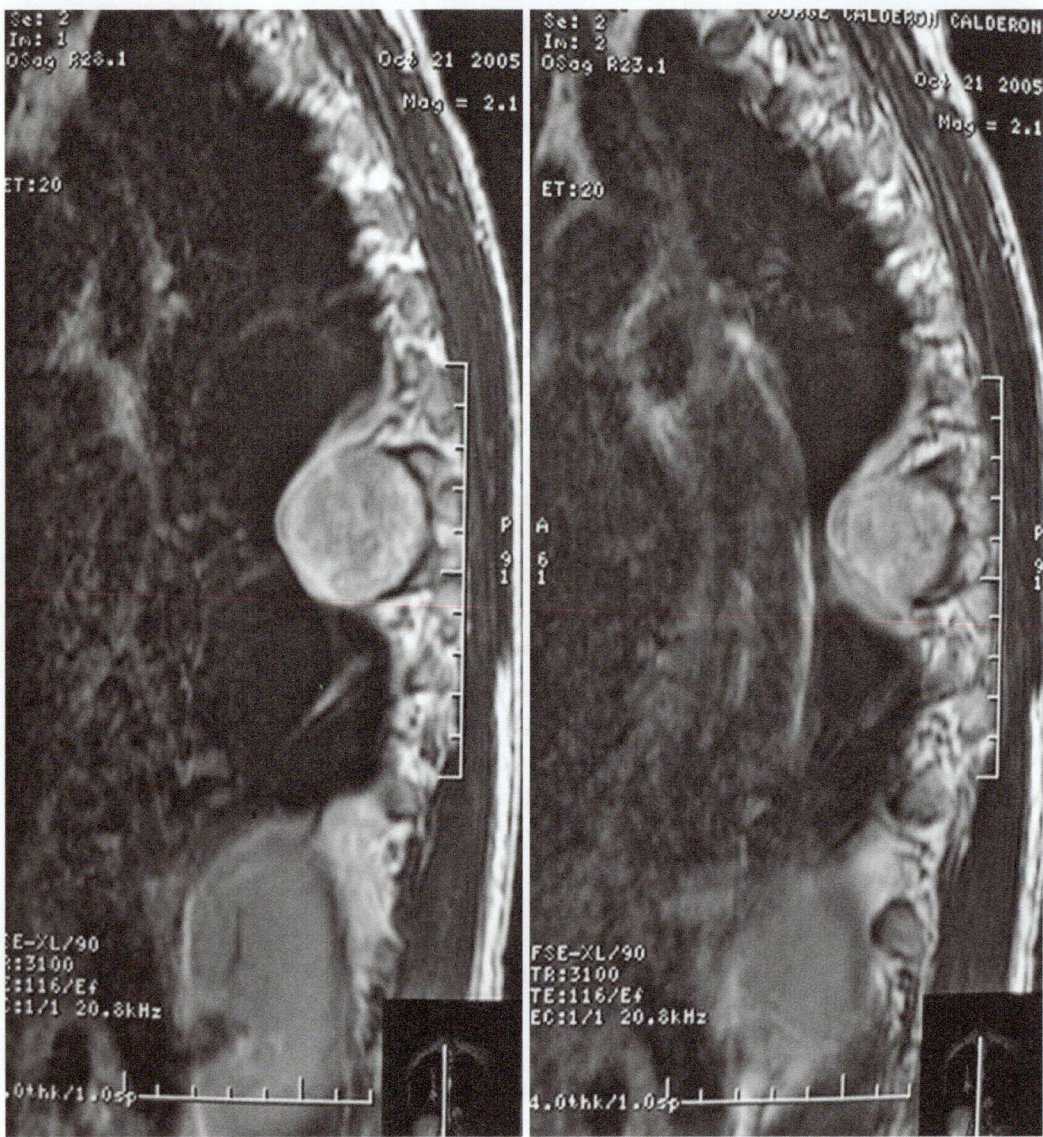

Fig. 2.2.5

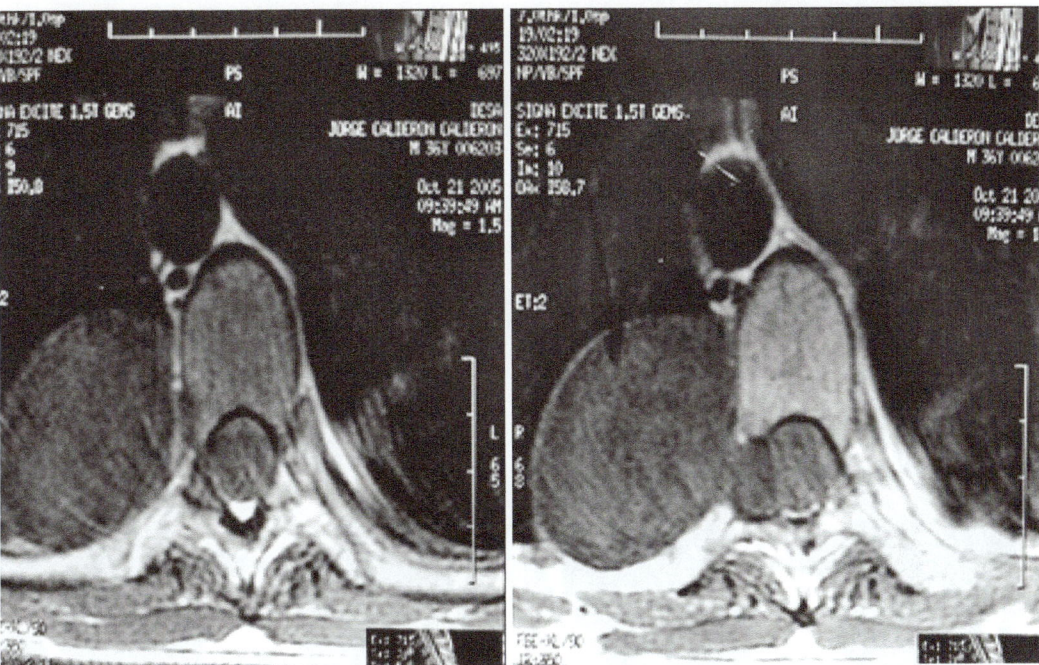

Fig. 2.2.6

Case 3: Hiatal Hernia

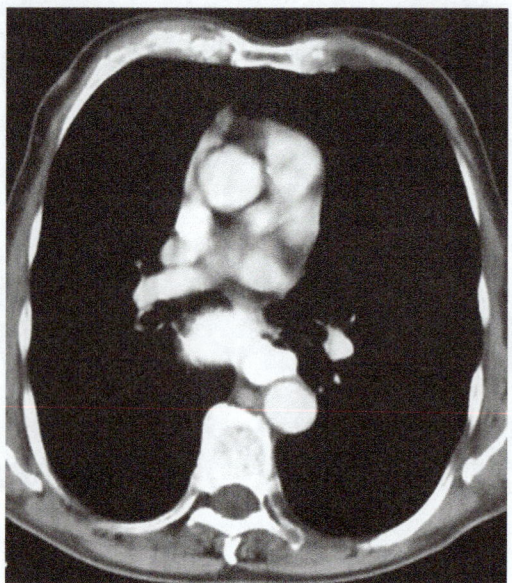

Fig. 2.3.1

Fig. 2.3.2

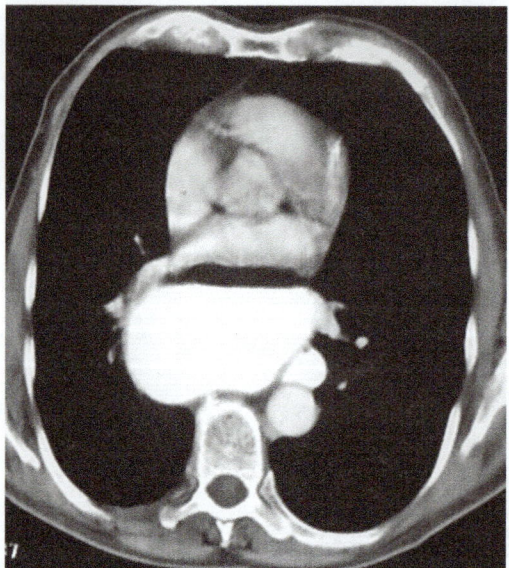

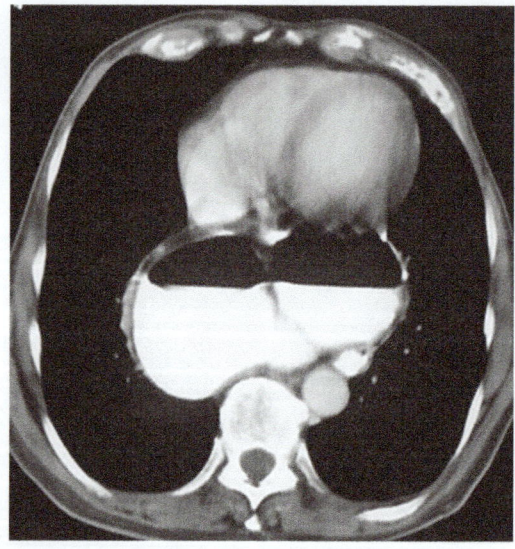

Fig. 2.3.3

Fig. 2.3.4

A 45-year-old man is referred for symptoms of a 6-month history of dry cough and frequent heartburn.

The most common type of gastric hernia is a hiatal hernia, in which weakening of the phrenoesophageal membrane and gradual enlargement of the esophageal hiatus of the diaphragm allow the gastric cardia and fundus to herniate through the diaphragm into the thorax. The prevalence of hiatal hernias increases with age; 60 % of elderly persons in the United States are found to have a hiatal hernia on barium studies.

The hiatal hernias are divided into three or four types. The intrathoracic stomach may be found in paraesophageal hiatal hernias (types 2–4). The paraesophageal hiatal hernia (types 2–4) is an uncommon disorder, representing approximately 5 % of all hernias occurring through the esophageal hiatus. An intrathoracic stomach results from a paraesophageal hiatal hernia in which a substantial portion of the stomach has herniated into the chest.

Type 1 hiatal hernia is also called the sliding or axial hernia. This type of hernia represents 95 % of all hiatal hernias. The esophagogastric junction is displaced into the chest because of diffuse weakening and stretching of the phrenicoesophageal membrane.

Type 2 hiatal hernia is called the paraesophageal or rolling hernia. This type of hernia has a focal defect in the anterior and lateral aspect of the phrenicoesophageal membrane. The gastric cardia and the esophagogastric junction remain below the diaphragm.

Type 3 hiatal hernia is called the "mixed" or "compound" hiatal hernia. This type of hernia is the most common form of paraesophageal hernias, combining the features of the type 2 and the type 1 hernias.

In type 4 hiatal hernia, with marked widening of the diaphragmatic hiatus, other organs such as the colon, omentum, small bowel, and liver can also herniate into the chest.

Radiography Findings: Hiatal hernia typically manifests radiographically as a retrocardiac mass, usually containing air or air-fluid level. A large mass may contain a double air-fluid level. In cases in which most of stomach has herniated through hiatus, the stomach may undergo volvulus.

CT Findings: Widening of esophageal hiatus allows stomach and omentum to protrude into chest. Normally, esophageal hiatus is elliptical and measures ≤15 mm in width. Multidetector CT with coronal and sagittal reformatted images is most effective and useful imaging technique in assessing diaphragmatic hernias.

CT scan (arterial phase) shows typical appearance of large hiatal hernia. There are superior displacement of the stomach, which contains oral contrast prior to the examination (Figs. 2.3.1, 2.3.2, 2.3.3, and 2.3.4).

Case 4: Morgagni Hernia

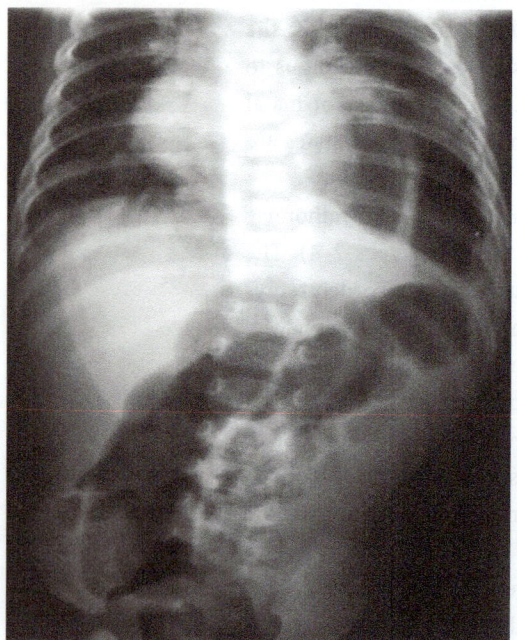

Fig. 2.4.1

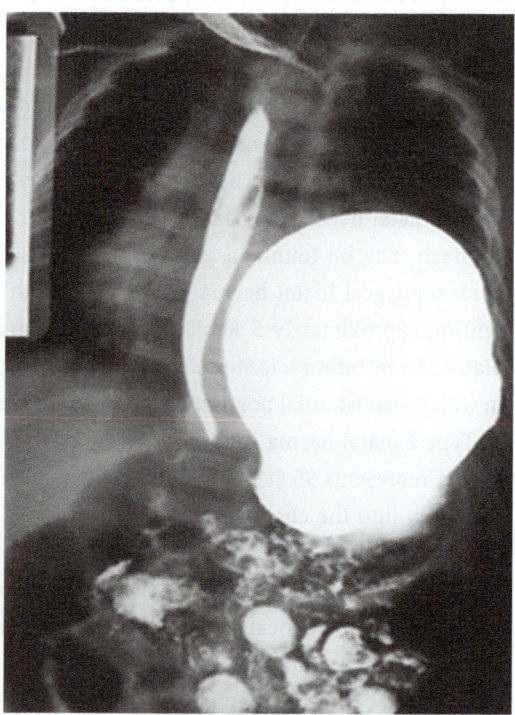

Fig. 2.4.2

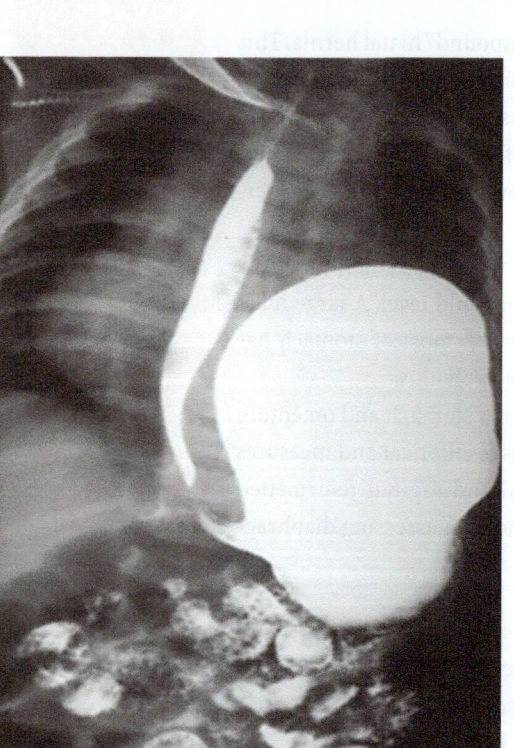

Fig. 2.4.3

An 8-month-old female child without symptoms underwent routine chest radiography.

The foramen of Morgagni is an anterior opening in the diaphragm that extends between the sternum medially and the eighth rib laterally. It is caused by failure of fusion between the transverse septum and the lateral body wall where the internal mammary artery crosses the diaphragm.

Morgagni hernia was first reported by Giovanni Battista Morgagni in 1761 that occurs in 5–10 % of CDH. It accounts for less than 2 % of all diaphragmatic hernias. Morgagni hernias are more frequently detected in women (61 %) with an average age of 58 years. They usually present in childhood with respiratory symptomatology. Incidental findings of this condition in adults are less common. These hernias are characterized by a defect between the septum transversum and the costal margin of the diaphragm, most frequently occurring on the right.

Herniated organs in Morgagni hernia may include omentum, stomach, small bowel, large bowel, and liver. In adults, protrusion of omentum is common and only rarely with bowel, stomach, or liver. Newborn patients may present with right-sided heart, decreased breath sounds on affected side, scaphoid abdomen, bowel sounds in the thorax, respiratory distress, and/or cyanosis on auscultation. Adult patients may exhibit chest mass on chest radiograph, gastric volvulus, splenic volvulus, and/or large bowel obstruction.

Radiographically, Morgagni hernia appears as a fatty mass in the right cardiophrenic angle and can be difficult to differentiate from prominent epicardial fat pad. Other fat-containing masses include lipoma, teratoma, thymoma, thymolipoma, or liposarcoma.

Ultrasonography has been shown to be useful in assessing diaphragmatic hernias, but CT is the most sensitive method by demonstration of anatomical detail on the contents of the hernia and its complications such as strangulation.

CT or MRI demonstrates displaced curvilinear omental vessels within the "mass" or coursing across the diaphragmatic defect which is characteristic for Morgagni hernia.

CRX film shows the foramen of Morgagni hernia. The contrast will intestines that are in front of the chest (Figs. 2.4.1, 2.4.2, and 2.4.3).

Case 5: Diaphragmatic Sarcoma

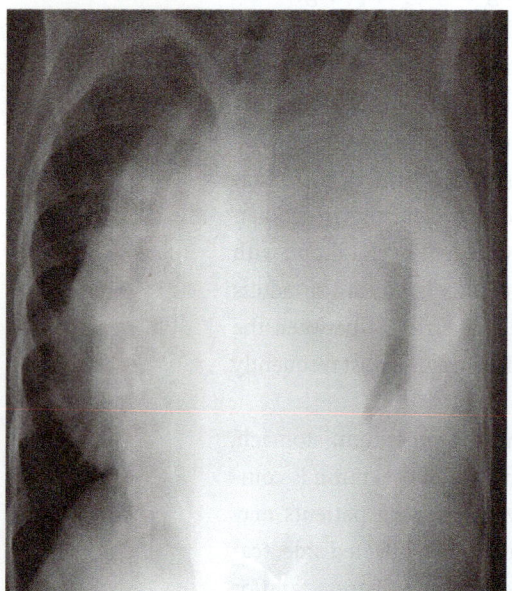

Fig. 2.5.1

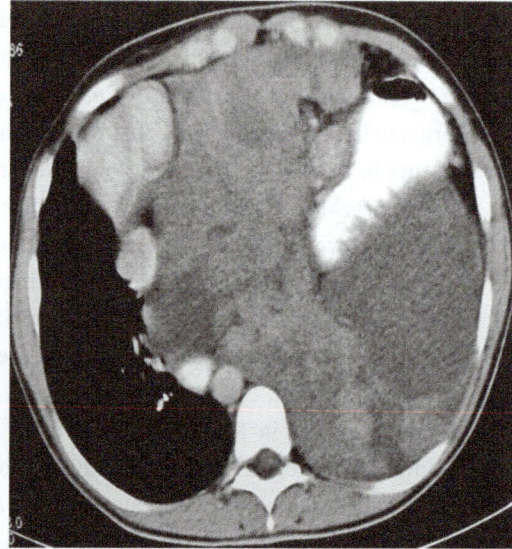

Fig. 2.5.2

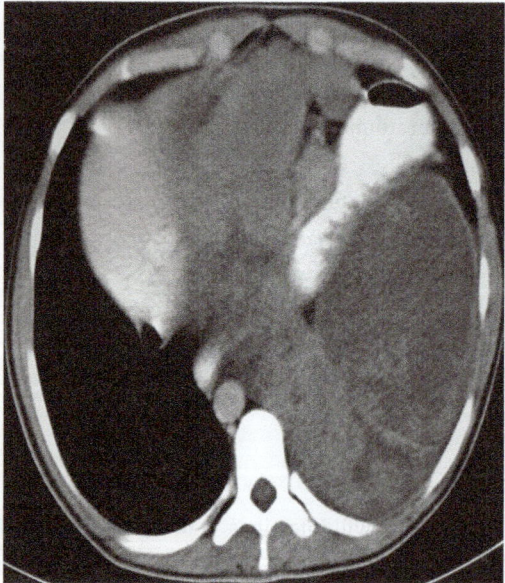

Fig. 2.5.3

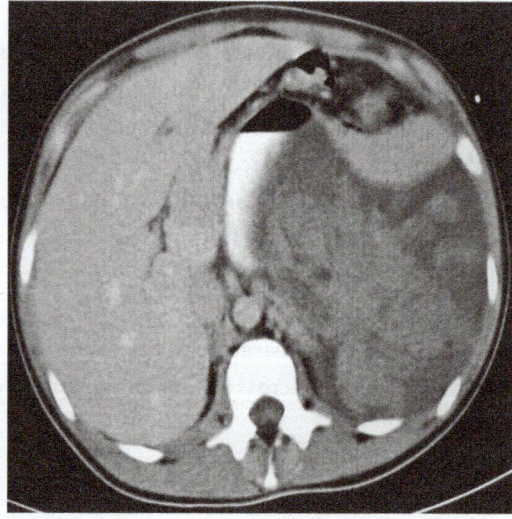

Fig. 2.5.4

A 36-year-old man was referred for dyspnea, chest pain, and weight loss of 3-month duration.

Extraskeletal Ewing's sarcoma (EES) is simply Ewing's sarcoma arising in soft tissues, which is now regarded as a member of the family of small, round cell neoplasms of bone and soft tissue, including primitive neuroectodermal tumor and neuroblastoma. The most frequent sites of occurrence are the chest wall, lower extremities, and paravertebral region. Less frequently, the tumor occurs in the pelvis and hip region, the retroperitoneum, and the upper extremities. It occurs predominantly in adolescents and young adults between the ages of 10 and 30 years. Extraskeletal Ewing's sarcoma of the diaphragm presenting with hemothorax has been reported.

Primary tumors of the diaphragm are rare. They can occur at any age, but most cases occur in the fourth and fifth decades of life. Primary tumors may be benign or malignant. Sarcomas with diaphragmatic origin are extraordinarily rare, with fibrosarcoma, rhabdomyosarcoma, and leiomyosarcoma representing the majority of cases.

CRX film shows opacity in left hemithorax displacing the mediastinum contralaterally (Fig. 2.5.1). CT scan (arterial phase) shows expansive inhomogeneous tumor mass in the left upper abdomen (Figs. 2.5.2, 2.5.3, and 2.5.4).

Case 6: Diaphragmatic Hernia

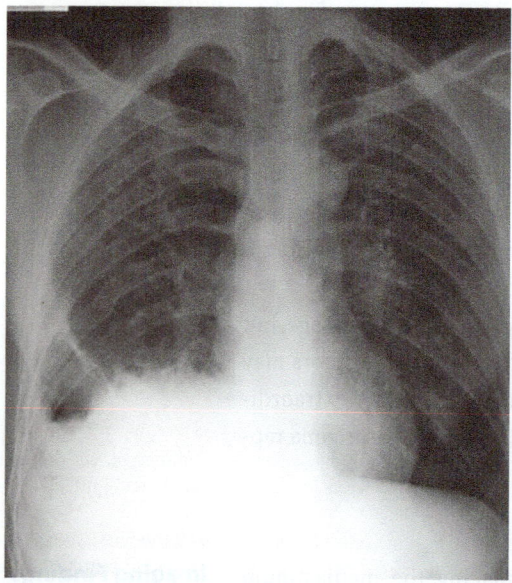

Fig. 2.6.1

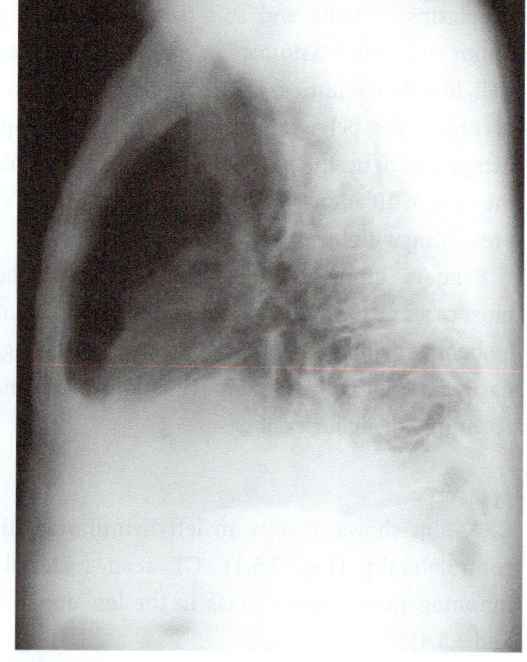

Fig. 2.6.2

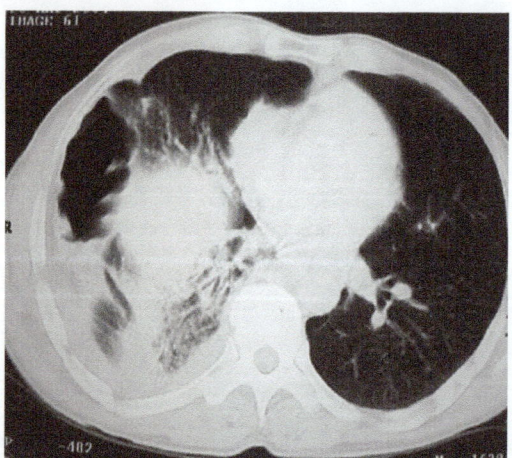

Fig. 2.6.3

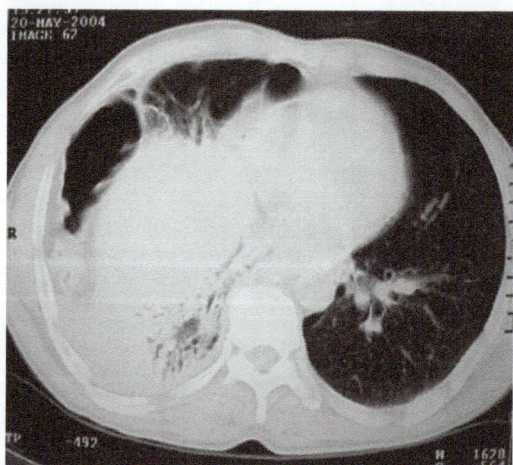

Fig. 2.6.4

A 59-year-old man presents with symptoms of right rib pain and occasional dry cough and a history of trauma.

Diaphragm injury may result from blunt and penetrating trauma. Blunt diaphragm rupture (BDR) is an uncommon injury with an overall reported incidence of 0.16–5 %. Acute diaphragm injury is associated with widely ranging mortality of 5.5–51 %, with death typically resulting from associated injuries or in-hospital complications, such as adult respiratory distress syndrome.

Chest radiography allows diagnosis of 27–60 % of left-sided injuries but only 17 % of right-sided injuries. Differentiation of a herniated liver through a diaphragmatic tear from other causes of elevated diaphragm such as atelectasis, pleural effusion, or pulmonary contusion or laceration remains difficult.

Specific diagnostic findings of diaphragmatic tears on chest radiographs include the following: (*a*) intrathoracic herniation of a hollow viscus (stomach, colon, small bowel) with or without focal constriction of the viscus at the site of the tear (collar sign) and (*b*) visualization of a nasogastric tube above the hemidiaphragm on the left side.

Computed tomography has a variable sensitivity of 14–61 % and specificity of 76–99 % in the diagnosis of diaphragmatic rupture. Helical CT has proved to be more valuable in the detection of diaphragmatic injuries with a sensitivity of 71 % (78 % for left-sided injuries and 50 % for right-sided injuries), a specificity of 100 %, and an accuracy of 88 % for left-sided injuries and 70 % for right-sided injuries.

CRX film shows right basal opacity and presence of intestinal loop (Figs. 2.6.1 and 2.6.2). CT scan (lung window) shows defect through right diaphragm, which produces upward movement of intestinal contents (Figs. 2.6.3 and 2.6.4).

Case 7: Unilateral Diaphragmatic Paralysis

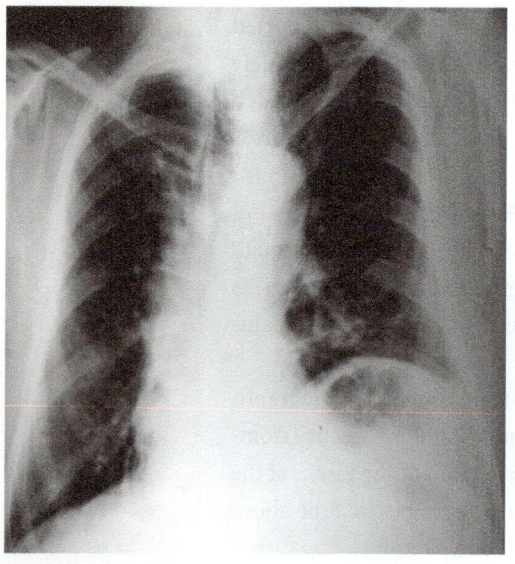

Fig. 2.7.1

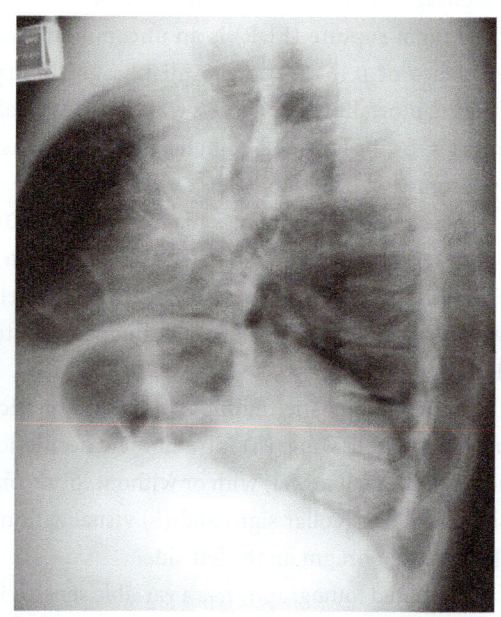

Fig. 2.7.2

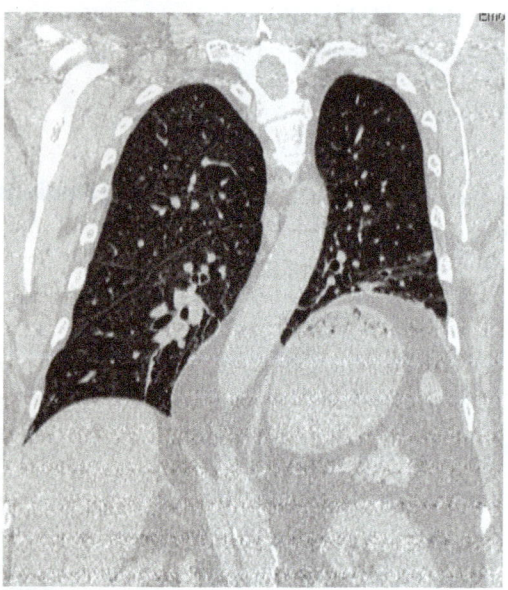

Fig. 2.7.3

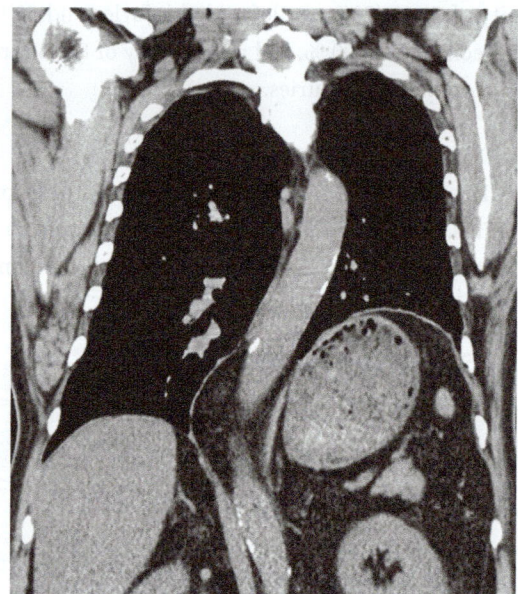

Fig. 2.7.4

A 68-year-old man is referred with dry cough, history of chronic bronchitis, and is a heavy smoker.

Diaphragmatic paralysis can occur after disruption of the phrenic nerve integrity. Idiopathic unilateral paralysis accounts for the majority of cases, followed by malignancy and surgical trauma. Outcome and prognosis differ among affected subjects, from persistent disease to complete resolution, and appear to be directly related to the underlying etiology and whether muscle dysfunction is unilateral or bilateral.

Diaphragmatic paralysis can involve either the whole diaphragm (bilateral) or only one leaflet (unilateral). The etiology remains unidentified in more than two-thirds of cases. Bilateral diaphragmatic paralysis is characterized by profound symptoms and abnormalities of pulmonary and respiratory muscle function, whereas unilateral dysfunction may present with very subtle symptoms and is often discovered incidentally in patients undergoing chest radiography. Hemidiaphragmatic paralysis results in a vital capacity decrement of 10–30 %, with the more substantial decrements seen in the supine position. Measurement of the transdiaphragmatic pressure remains the accepted standard diagnostic test for bilateral paralysis, whereas fluoroscopy with sniff test reliably confirms the diagnosis of unilateral diaphragmatic paralysis. The M mode ultrasonography has been also introduced as an accurate method to evaluate the paralyzed diaphragm.

Diaphragmatic paralysis is likely most often idiopathic and unilateral. When a cause for diaphragmatic paralysis can be identified, it may be due to: trauma or surgery causing cervical cord or phrenic nerve damage (high C-spine injuries involving C3–C5, phrenic nerve injury during cardiac surgery), mechanical ventilation, COPD and other diseases that cause lung hyperinflation, myopathies and neuropathies (myasthenia gravis, critical illness neuro-/myopathy, amyotrophic lateral sclerosis, poliomyelitis, with a 35-year delay until diaphragmatic weakness), inflammatory disorders (e.g., sepsis), and mediastinal masses.

Findings on transthoracic ultrasound of the chest include paradoxical cephalad displacement of the hemidiaphragm, muscle atrophy, and evidence of decreased contraction and shortening during inspiration, compared to the normal diaphragm.

The following criteria are part of unilateral diaphragmatic paralysis: (1) elevation of the diaphragm (about 4 cm or more above the normal position: the extent of the elevation was determined by comparison with the sound side) and (2) paradoxical movement (especially noticeable on sniffing, the sound side descends on inspiration, while the paralyzed side rises by a smaller amount). Chest X-ray is 90 % sensitive for unilateral paralysis but only 44 % specific (high false-positive rate).

CRX film shows elevation of the left hemidiaphragm (Figs. 2.7.1 and 2.7.2). CT scan (mediastinal and lung window) shows elevation of the left hemidiaphragm and basal subsegmental atelectasis (Figs. 2.7.3 and 2.7.4).

Comments

Imaging Findings

Further Reading

Pneumoperitoneum

Baker SR (1997) Unenhanced helical CT versus plain abdominal radiography: a dissenting opinion. Radiology 205(1):45–47

Balthazar EJ, Moore SL (1996) CT evaluation of infradiaphragmatic air in patients treated with mechanically assisted ventilation: a potential source of error. AJR Am J Roentgenol 167(3):731–734

Cho KC, Baker SR (1997a) Depiction of diaphragmatic muscle slips on supine plain radiographs: a sign of pneumoperitoneum. Radiology 203(2):431–433

Cho KC, Baker SR (1997b) Visualization of the extrahepatic segment of the ligamentum teres: a sign of free air on plain radiographs. Radiology 202(3):651–654

Earls JP, Dachman AH, Colon E (1993) Prevalence and duration of postoperative pneumoperitoneum: sensitivity of CT vs left lateral decubitus radiography. AJR Am J Roentgenol 161(4):781–785

Miller RE (1973) The technical approach to the acute abdomen. Semin Roentgenol 8(3):267–279

Radin R, Van Allan RJ, Rosen RS (1996) The visible gallbladder: a plain film sign of pneumoperitoneum. AJR Am J Roentgenol 167(1):69–70

Woodring JH, Heiser MJ (1995) Detection of pneumoperitoneum on chest radiographs: comparison of upright lateral and posteroanterior projections. AJR Am J Roentgenol 165(1):45–47

Diaphragmatic Eventration

Gierada DS, Slone RM, Fleishman MJ (1998) Imaging evaluation of the diaphragm. Chest Surg Clin N Am 8(2):237–280

Moinuddeen K, Blatzer JW et al (2001) Diaphragmatic eventration: an uncommon presentation of a phrenic nerve schwannoma. Chest 119(5):1615–1616

Rubinstein Z, Solomon A (1981) CT findings in partial eventration of the right diaphragm. J Comput Assist Tomogr 5(5):719–721

Watanabe S, Shimokawa S et al (1998) Large eventration of diaphragm in an elderly patient treated with emergency plication. Ann Thorac Surg 65(6):1776–1777

Worthy SA, Young KE et al (1995) Diaphragmatic rupture: CT findings in 11 patients. Radiology 194:885–888

Hiatal Hernia

Abbara S, Kalan MMH, Lewicki AM (2003) Intrathoracic stomach revisited. AJR Am J Roentgenol 181:403–414

Huang SY, Levine MS, Rubesin SE, Katzka DA, Laufer I (2007) Large hiatal hernia with floppy fundus: clinical and radiographic findings. AJR Am J Roentgenol 188:960–964

Morgagni Hernia

Minneci PC et al (2004) Foramen of Morgagni hernia: changes in diagnosis and treatment. Ann Thorac Surg 77:1956–1959

Bragg WD, Bumpers H, Flynn W (1996) Morgagni hernias: an uncommon cause of chest masses in adults. Am Fam Physician 54(6):2021–2024

Nasr A, Fecteau A (2009) Foramen of Morgagni hernia: presentation and treatment. Thorac Surg Clin 19:463–468

Sandstrom CK, Stern EJ (2011) Diaphragmatic hernias: a spectrum of radiographic appearances. Curr Probl Diagn Radiol 40(3):95–115

Horton JD, Hofmann LJ, Hetz SP (2007) Presentation and management of Morgagni hernias in adults: a review of 298 cases. Surg Endosc 22:1412–1420

Pineda V, Andreu J, Caceres J et al (2007) Lesions of the cardiophrenic space: findings at cross-sectional imaging. Radiographics 27:19–32

Diaphragmatic Sarcoma

Eustace S, Fitzgerald E (1993) Primary rhabdomyosarcoma of the diaphragm: an unusual cause of adolescent pseudo-achalasia. Pediatr Radiol 23:622–623

Raney RB, Anderson JR, Andrassy RJ, Crist WM, Donaldson SS, Maurer HM (2000) Soft-tissue sarcomas of the diaphragm: a report from the Intergroup Rhabdomyosarcoma Study Group from 1972 to 1997. J Pediatr Hematol Oncol 22:510–514

Rud NP, Reiman H, Pritchard DT, Frassica FJ, Smithson WA (1989) Extraosseous Ewing's sarcoma: a study of 42 cases. Cancer 64:1548–1553

Weksler B, Ginsberg RJ (1998) Tumors of the diaphragm. Chest Surg Clin N Am 8:441–447

Diaphragmatic Hernia

Iochum S, Ludig T et al (2002) Imaging of diaphragmatic injury: a diagnostic challenge? Radiographics 22:S103–S118

Sliker CW (2006) Imaging of diaphragm injuries. Radiol Clin North Am 44:199–211

Unilateral Diaphragmatic Paralysis

Dernaika TA, Younis WG, Carlile PV (2008) Spontaneous recovery in idiopathic unilateral diaphragmatic paralysis. Respir Care 53(3):351–354

Freedman B (1950) Unilateral paralysis of the diaphragm and larynx associated with inflammatory lung disease. Thorax 5:169

Kara M et al (2006) Unilateral diaphragm paralysis possibly due to cervical spine involvement in multiple myeloma. Med Princ Pract 15:242–244

McCool FD, Tzelepis GE (2012) Dysfunction of the diaphragm. N Engl J Med 366:932–942

Stowasser M, Cameron J, Oliver WA (1990) Diaphragmatic paralysis following cervical herpes zoster. Med J Aust 153(9):555–556

Mediastinum and Pulmonary Circulation   3

John C. Pedrozo Pupo, Diego Pardo Pinzón, Alfonso Uriza Carrasco, Elida Laurens Meza, Eliana Amaya Lacouture, and Beatriz Aldana Jaramillo

Contents

J.C. Pedrozo Pupo (ed.), *Learning Chest Imaging*, Learning Imaging,
DOI 10.1007/978-3-642-34147-2_3, © Springer-Verlag Berlin Heidelberg 2013

Case 1: Massive Pulmonary Embolism

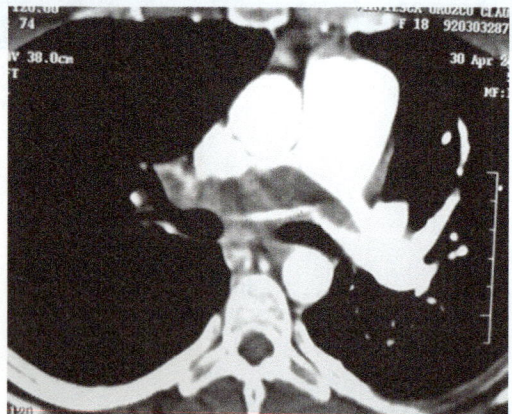

Fig. 3.1.1

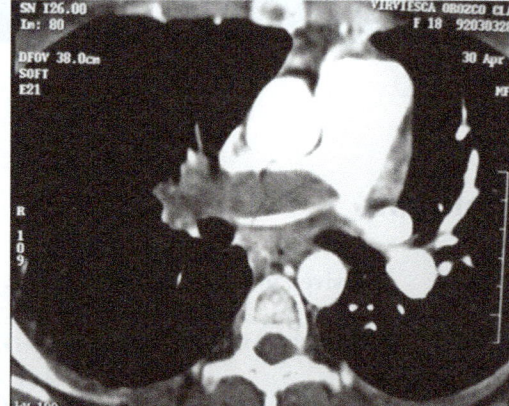

Fig. 3.1.2

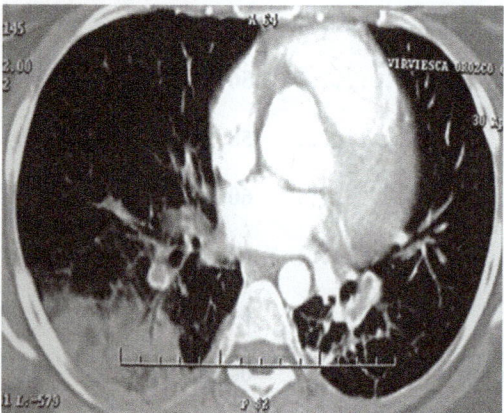

Fig. 3.1.3

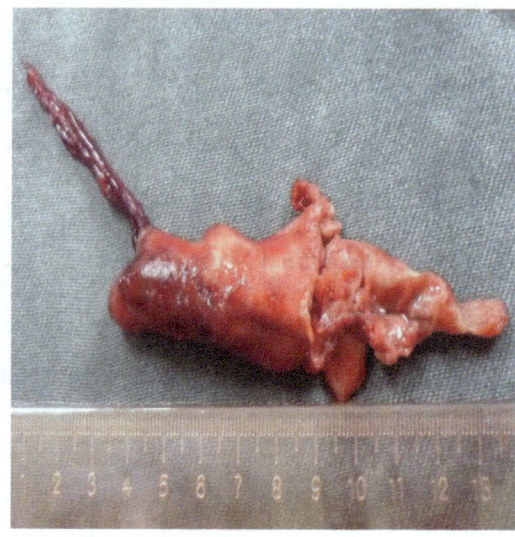

Fig. 3.1.4

A 24-year-old woman diagnosed with postpartum massive pulmonary embolism. She received anticoagulation therapy and thromboembolectomy.

Comments Massive pulmonary embolism is associated with an increased mortality. It is secondary to migration of a venous thrombus to the right atrium or ventricle (thrombus in transit) towards the pulmonary circulation. The hemodynamic performance depends on the baseline cardiopulmonary status of the patient and the extent of obstruction.

The chest radiograph is usually nonspecific in PE. Significant hypoxemia, particularly in the setting of hypotension and a relatively clear chest radiograph, should lead to suspicion of PE. However, PE may also be superimposed upon preexisting radiographic abnormalities due to pneumonia or acute respiratory distress syndrome. Certain radiographic findings, such as focal hyperlucency of the lung parenchyma and enlargement of the descending pulmonary arteries, may serve as important clues, but they are not diagnostic. Classic Findings: Atelectasis, pleural effusion, parenchymal opacification, elevation of hemidiaphragm, Hampton's Hump (wedge shaped pleural-based triangular opacity with apex pointing toward hilus), Westermark's sign (decreased vascularity).

Ventilation-perfusion scanning—Ventilation-perfusion lung scanning is the focal point for the diagnosis of PE. Combining ventilation-perfusion scanning with the level of clinical suspicion of PE is crucial.

Echocardiography—Echocardiography can be obtained rapidly and may reveal findings suggestive of hemodynamically significant PE. The following findings are more impressive and more common with massive PE.

More than 80 percent of patients with documented PE have imaging abnormalities of right ventricular size or function, or Doppler abnormalities of tricuspid regurgitant flow velocity. The accuracy of echocardiography may be even greater in cases of massive PE.

Helical CT scanning may also prove useful in rapidly identifying central emboli causing hemodynamic compromise.

Pulmonary arteriography remains the gold standard for the diagnosis of PE. It is necessary less often with massive PE than with smaller emboli, but may be useful, particularly if it can be rapidly performed.

Open pulmonary embolectomy is an immediate and definitive form of treatment for AMPE (Acute massive pulmonary embolism), with excellent long-term results. CPB is a vital component for the early resuscitation of these patients that increases the likelihood of a successful outcome. Open embolectomy before right ventricular ischemia and cardiac arrest ensues is imperative because preoperative cardiac arrest is associated with the highest mortality in patients with AMPE.

Imaging Findings

CT scan (arterial phase) shows a intravascular filling defects, sharp interface surrounded by contrast. Eccentric or peripheral intraluminal defects form acute angles with the vessel wall. Total cutoff of vascular enhancement for arterial occlusion may enlarge vessels caliber. We can see dilatacion of right ventricule, leftward bowing of interventricular septum, dilated IVC with reflux of contrast into hepatic veins for right ventricular failure. The pulmonary findings are subsegmental atelectasis and infarcts. Those are pleural based wedge shaped opacities with no contrast enhancement that may cavitate. Chronic PE shows mural based or crescent shaped intraluminal defects with obtuse angles with vessel wall. There is stenotic vessels, intimal irregularities, recanalization, webs, bands, flaps or occlusion. The lung shows mosaic perfusion pattern. (Figs. 3.1.1, 3.1.2, and 3.1.3). Anatomical piece show thrombus molded thromboembolectomy (Fig. 3.1.4).

Case 2: Interlobar Artery Aneurysm

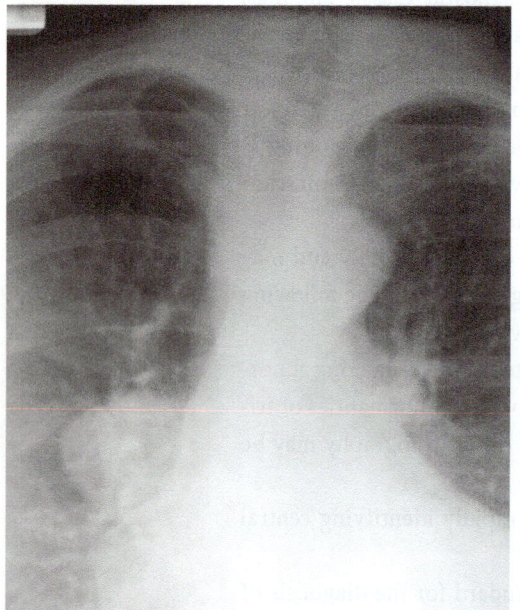

Fig. 3.2.1

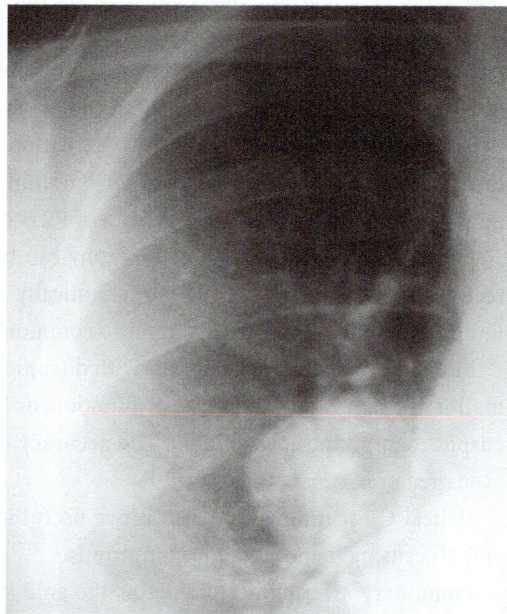

Fig. 3.2.2

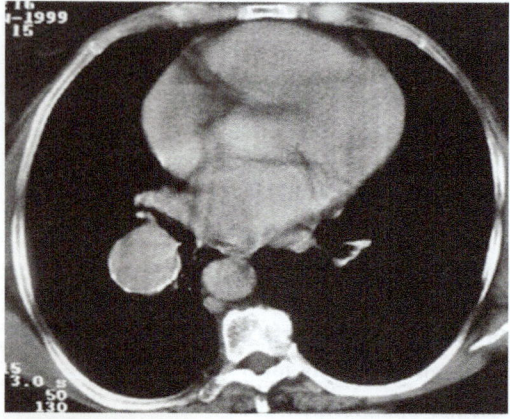

Fig. 3.2.3

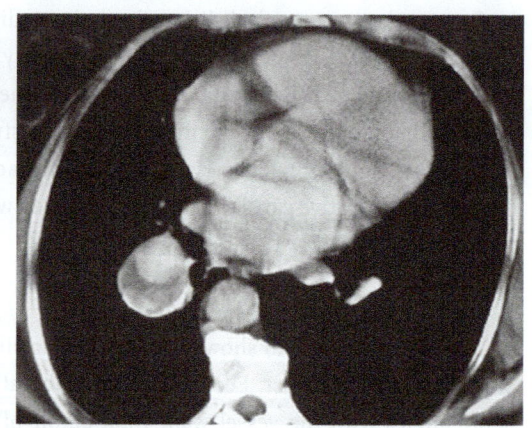

Fig. 3.2.4

A 35-year-old man consulted for grade 2 dyspnea and chest pain.

Comments

In the normal adult anatomy, the pulmonary trunk, or main pulmonary artery, may have a diameter as great as 28 mm. The main, left, and right pulmonary arteries are intrapericardial. The right pulmonary artery has a longer mediastinal course than the left, and it divides into two lobar branches at the root of the right lung. The left pulmonary artery courses over the left main bronchus and penetrates the root of the left lung, where the artery divides into two lobar branches. The right and left pulmonary arteries should be of approximately equal size, although the left pulmonary artery appears slightly larger in most subjects. The segmental arteries are always seen near the accompanying branches of the bronchial tree, and the subsegmental arteries are easily recognized as dichotomous divisions of the corresponding segmental artery.

Pulmonary arteries (main, lobar, segmental, and subsegmental) with a diameter greater than 0.5 mm are referred to as elastic pulmonary arteries. They course downward along the bronchi to the subsegmental level, and their diameters are similar to those of the adjacent airways. Beyond the subsegmental bronchi, these vessels transition to muscular arteries, which accompany the peripheral airways downward to the level of the terminal bronchioles. As the smooth-muscle layer progressively thins, these arteries become arterioles (0.15–0.015 mm in diameter), which proceed along the respiratory bronchioles and alveolar ducts to eventually form a capillary network in the alveolar walls.

Focal dilatation of the pulmonary arteries can be congenital or acquired. Common causes include vasculitis, infection, neoplasm, and trauma, often iatrogenic. On radiographs, aneurysms may appear as hilar enlargement or a lung nodule. The diagnosis is usually confirmed with contrast-enhanced CT.

CT provides useful information regarding the size, number, location, and extent of aneurysms and pseudoaneurysms. MRI also can show arterial wall thickening in connective tissue disease and provide information regarding blood flow direction in cases of poststenotic dilatation due to disease of the pulmonary valve. Early recognition and treatment are important for reducing morbidity and preventing mortality.

Most congenital anomalies of the pulmonary arteries can be detected with chest radiography, and a definitive diagnosis can be reached with CT or MR imaging. CT has an important role to play in the noninvasive assessment of patients suspected of having pulmonary hypertension; not only can it help to detect the condition but it also can indicate the possible causes. Radiologists should be aware that pulmonary hypertension and acute pulmonary embolism may secondarily affect the heart. It is important to recognize the CT signs of these conditions because their presence has implications for the prognosis.

Some of the entities, whether congenital in origin or acquired, result in decreased pulmonary flow and, thus, cause the development of systemic collateral vessels, mainly from the bronchial arteries.

Imaging Findings

CRX film shows radiodense image of round right pulmonary hilum (Figs. 3.2.1 and 3.2.2). CT scan (arterial phase) shows tubular structure, hilar, with homogeneous enhancement by interlobar artery aneurysm on the right (Figs. 3.2.3 and 3.2.4).

Case 3: Small Cell Lung Cancer

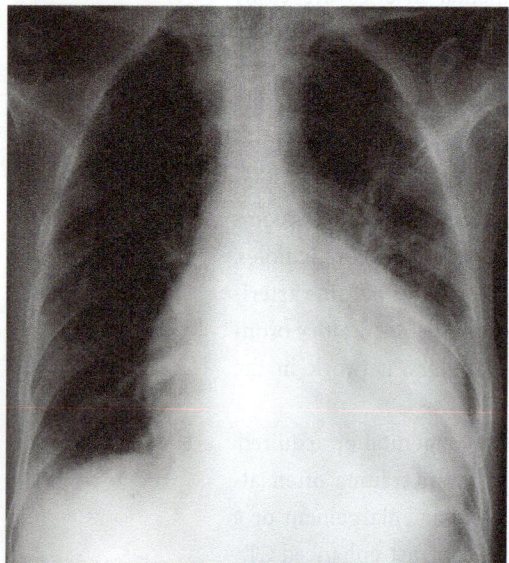

Fig. 3.3.1

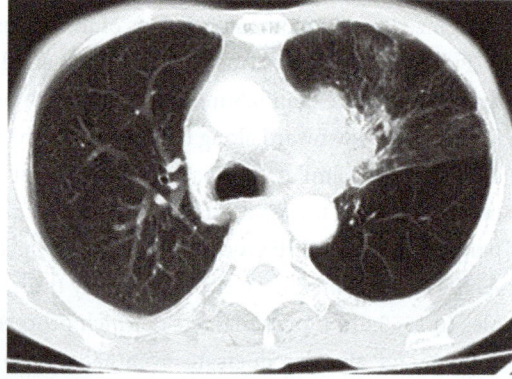

Fig. 3.3.2

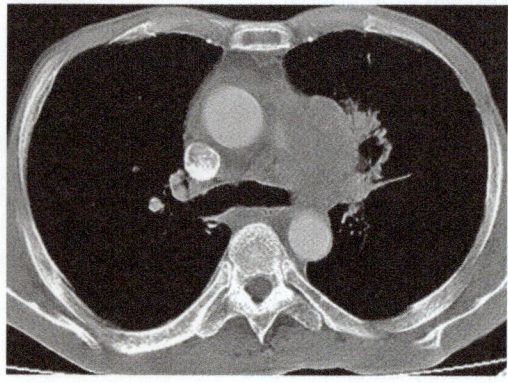

Fig. 3.3.3

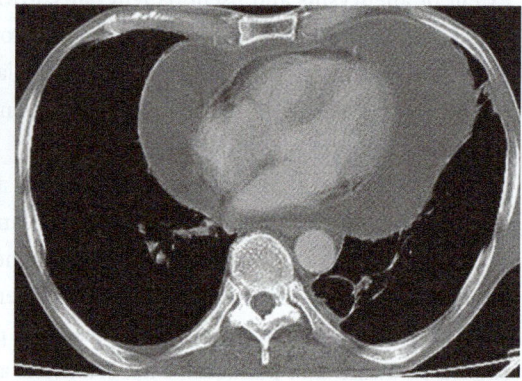

Fig. 3.3.4

A 55-year-old man consulted for symptoms of 9-month history of chest pain, fatigue, weakness, dyspnea, and weight loss and smoking history of 30 packs/year.

Comments

Small cell lung cancer occurs almost exclusively in smokers, particularly heavy smokers, and tends to grow and spread quickly. Because of this, surgery is considered less often in patients with small cell lung cancer than with non-small-cell lung cancer. Small cell lung cancer (SCLC) makes up about 15 % of all lung cancers. The majority of lung cancers, 75–85 %, are called non-small-cell lung cancers, and they behave differently from small cell lung cancers.

Chest radiographs may show unilateral hilar enlargement, increased hilar opacity, a perihilar mass, mediastinal mass, or a combination of these. Less commonly, small cell lung cancer (SCLC) may appear as a solitary pulmonary nodule.

Compression of the bronchi is relatively common in SCLC because of the central location of the tumor in most cases. About 30–50 % of SCLCs show evidence of obstructive pneumonitis on the initial presentation. SCLC can appear as segmental or lobar atelectasis with or without an obvious hilar mass. The S sign of Golden is seen when a collapsed upper lobe forms a meniscus concave toward the hilum and when an enlarged hilar mass forms the convex meniscus of the S. Occasionally, endobronchial growth or bronchial compression may be appreciated as a bronchial cutoff or filling defect.

Thickening of the right paratracheal stripe may be an indication of right paratracheal lymphadenopathy. With massive subcarinal lymphadenopathy, widening of the carinal angle may occasionally be observed. Subtle changes of hilar asymmetry, increased opacity, a convex or lobulated outer hilar border, or any change from a previous radiograph should be viewed with suspicion.

Involvement of pleura or pericardium may result in pleural or pericardial effusions. Rarely, involvement of a pulmonary artery may result in compression of the artery with oligemia in the area of distribution. Invasion of pulmonary artery may result in pulmonary metastatic lesions. Large mediastinal masses may lead to lymphatic obstruction, which may result in reticulonodular opacities in the lung. Lateral views are complementary to the frontal views and help in assessing the mediastinal abnormalities, especially in the retrosternal and hilar regions. Paratracheal masses and thickening of the posterior wall of the bronchus intermedius may be seen on the lateral view.

CT is used to assess the size or volume of the tumor, mediastinal involvement, pathologically enlarged lymph nodes, and vascular invasion. It is also sensitive in detecting pleural and pericardial effusion or thickening. Nodularity of pleura or pericardium is the hallmark of metastatic involvement. Contrast-enhanced CT can sometimes be used to differentiate a tumor mass from the adjacent collapsed lung or pneumonitis, which usually enhances more than the tumor.

CT of the chest routinely includes imaging of the adrenal glands, which are common sites for of small cell lung cancer metastases. A lesion with an attenuation value less than 10 HU (Hounsfield units) on a nonenhanced CT scan most likely represents an adenoma (90 % accuracy). CT of the abdomen and pelvis is also generally indicated in staging of small cell lung cancer to rule out metastases to the liver, nodes, or other organs.

MRI is not routinely used for detecting the primary tumor or for staging.

PET is one of the most rapidly emerging modalities for the evaluation, staging, and posttherapeutic follow-up of cancer. PET combines the functional and anatomic aspects of the lesions. PET primarily depends on the metabolism of glucose, which is usually high in tumor cells.

Imaging Findings

CRX shows infiltrated around the left pulmonary hilum, and enlargement of heart chambers (Fig. 3.3.1). CT scan (lung window) show soft tissue mass with perilesional infiltrates in the left hilum (Fig. 3.3.2). CT scan (arterial phase) show left hilar mass with giant pericardial effusion (Figs. 3.3.3 and 3.3.4).

Case 4: Mediastinitis

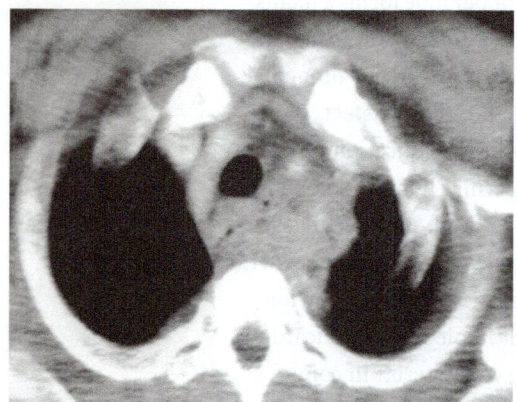

Fig. 3.4.1

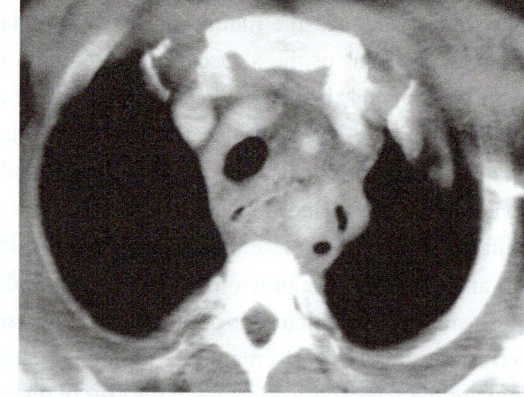

Fig. 3.4.2

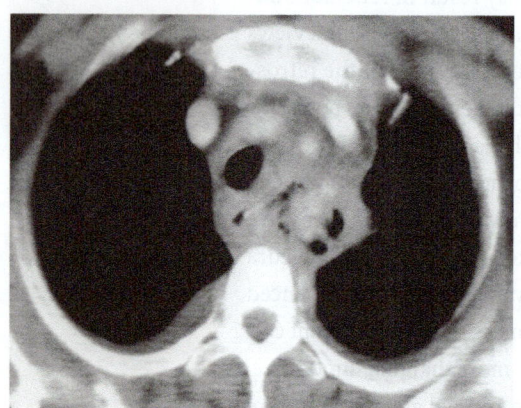

Fig. 3.4.3

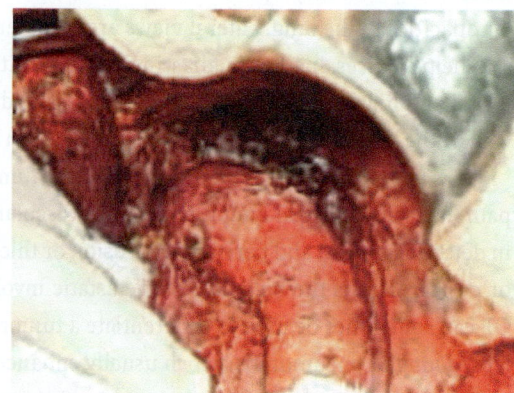

Fig. 3.4.4

A 42-year-old woman with mediastinitis and perforation of the subclavian artery by thorn. Drainage and rebuilding of the esophagus and the left subclavian artery ligation.

Mediastinitis refers to inflammation of the tissues located in the middle chest cavity. It can be secondary to infectious or noninfectious causes and depending on the etiology may be acute or chronic. The majority of cases of acute mediastinitis are secondary to esophageal perforation and open chest surgery. Less common causes include tracheal, bronchial perforation, or direct extension of infection from adjacent tissues. Chronic or slowly developing mediastinitis mostly arise from tuberculosis, histoplasmosis, other fungal infections, cancer, or sarcoidosis. In a minority of cases, the etiology is lymphatic obstruction or an autoimmune disease.

Radiological imaging plays an essential role in the diagnosis and therapeutic approach to mediastinitis. Generally, the initial radiological work-up includes radiographic studies either with or without contrast material. However, conventional chest radiography may be misleading in the diagnosis of mediastinitis. Cross-sectional imaging techniques are generally required for diagnosis and evaluation of the site and extent of mediastinal involvement. Radiography findings: Widening and poor definition of margins of superior mediastinum, air may also be seen in soft tissues of neck (subcutaneous emphysema), and pneumomediastinum: visualization of pleura as white line adjacent to mediastinum, linear streaks of radiolucency in mediastinum, cervical soft tissues, focal retrosternal air collections, "continuous diaphragm," and V sign of Naclerio.

Computed tomography and magnetic resonance imaging may also guide the choice of the optimal therapeutic approach. CT finding soft tissue infiltration of mediastinal fat, obliteration of fat planes, localized fluid collections, mediastinal widening, lymphadenopathy, and gas bubbles.

CT scan (arterial phase) shows increased density and striation of mediastinal fat, with poor definition of the left subclavian artery and extravasation of contrast medium for vascular injury. Additionally, pneumomediastinum observed esophageal perforation. Posterior to the esophagus is a hyperdense image, corresponding to linear fishbone (Figs. 3.4.1, 3.4.2, and 3.4.3). Intraoperative view shows mediastinal infection (Fig. 3.4.4).

Case 5: Hodgkin Lymphoma

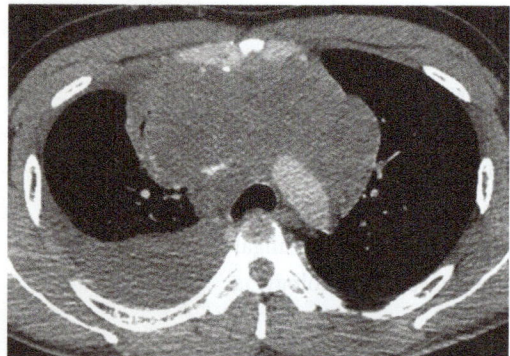

Fig. 3.5.1

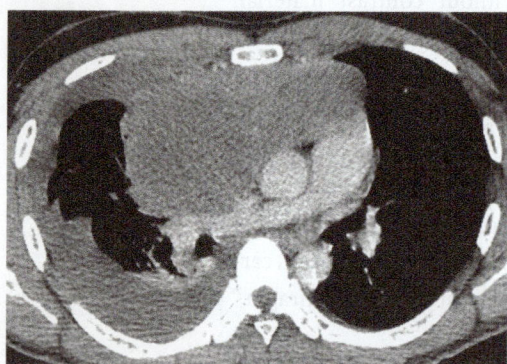

Fig. 3.5.2

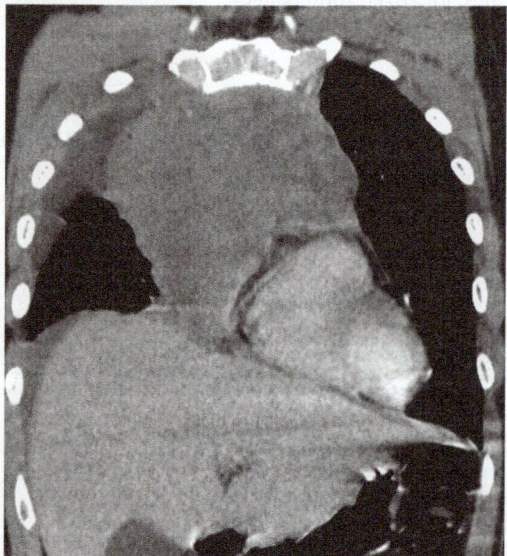

Fig. 3.5.3

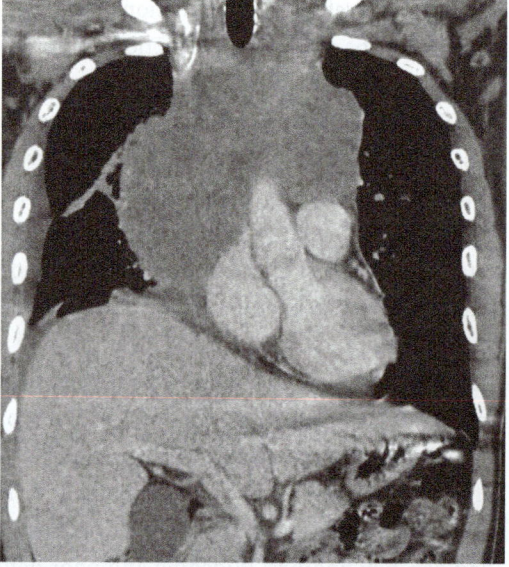

Fig. 3.5.4

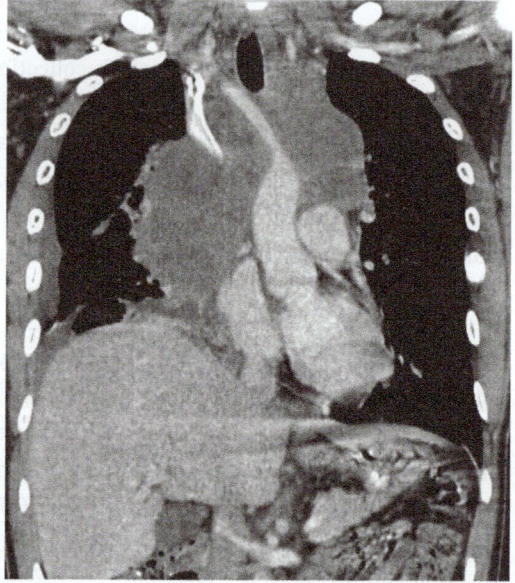

Fig. 3.5.5

A 35-year-old man with history of dyspnea, dry cough, chest pain, and weight loss.

Lymphomas are a diverse group of neoplastic disorders. They are divided into Hodgkin lymphoma (HL) and non-Hodgkin lymphoma (NHL) and further subdivisions depend on the histologic types.

Intrathoracic involvement is commoner in HL than NHL. Although HL represents only 10–15 % of all cases of lymphomas, approximately 85 % of patients with HL have intrathoracic disease at presentation. NHL represents about 85–90 % of all cases of lymphoma, and approximately 40–45 % of patients with NHL have intrathoracic disease at the initial presentation. However, at onset, nodal and splenic involvements are more common in Hodgkin disease, whereas extranodal involvement is more frequent in non-Hodgkin lymphomas.

HL is the most common lymphoma presenting with mediastinal lymphadenopathy and most frequently involves lymph nodes in anterior mediastinal and paratracheal areas in a contiguous manner and thus involves in decreasing order of frequency the nodes in the hilar, subcarinal, peridiaphragmatic, paraesophageal, and internal mammary areas.

Pulmonary involvement is identified more often in HL than in NHL. The lung is more frequently involved in disseminated or recurrent disease than in primary disease. Pulmonary parenchymal involvement may present with variable patterns. The commonest feature of pulmonary involvement is a direct extension from hilar or mediastinal nodes toward the lungs; very few cases of primary pulmonary Hodgkin disease with no hilar or mediastinal node disease have been reported.

Imaging Findings

On CT, HL is characterized by the presence of an anterior mediastinal mass with a lobulated contour. The tumor most commonly demonstrates homogeneous soft-tissue attenuation, although large lymph node masses may demonstrate heterogeneity with complex low attenuation representing necrosis, hemorrhage, or cystic degeneration.

CT is superior to conventional radiography in assessing chest disease, although MR imaging is more sensitive than CT in detecting chest wall involvement (Figs. 3.5.1, 3.5.2, 3.5.3, 3.5.4, and 3.5.5).

Case 6: Thymoma

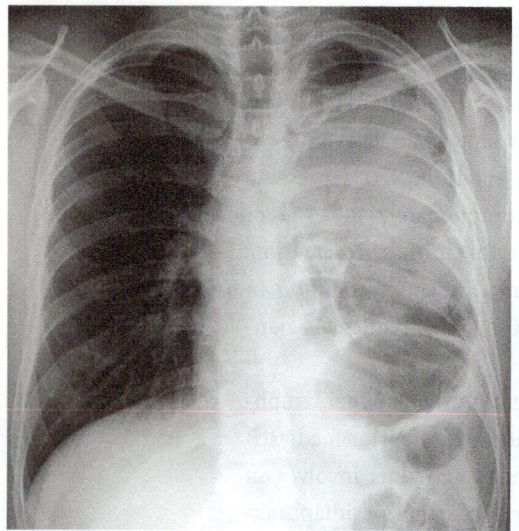

Fig. 3.6.1

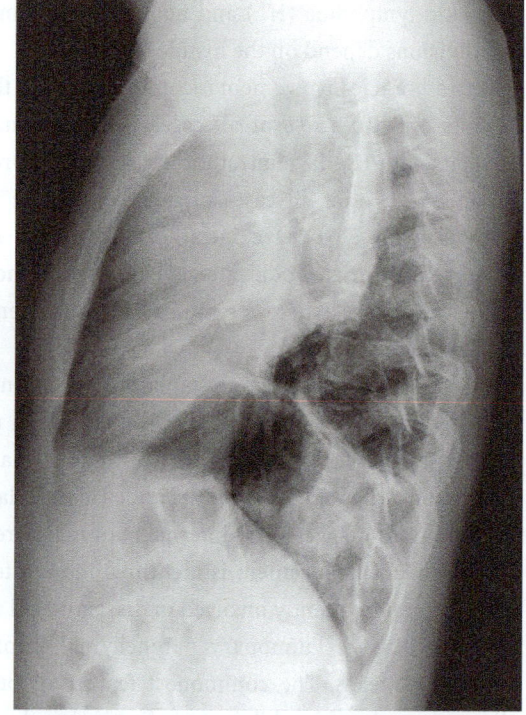

Fig. 3.6.2

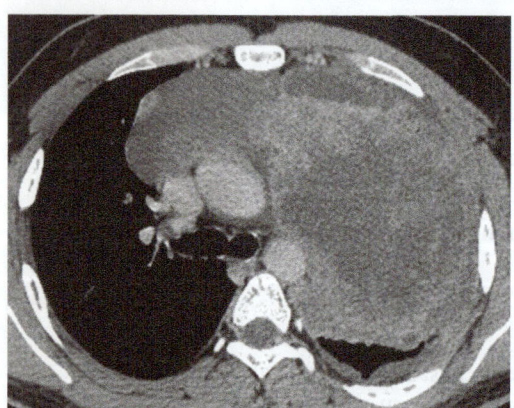

Fig. 3.6.3

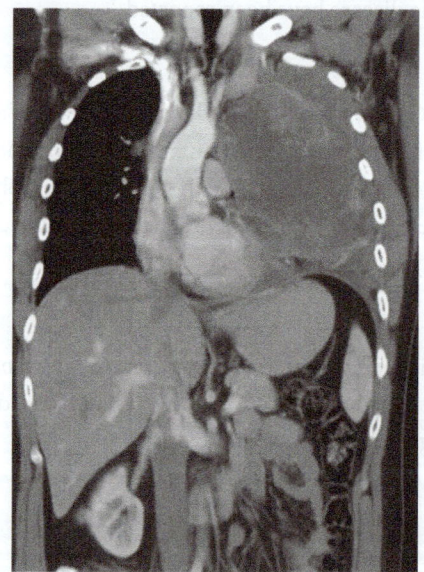

Fig. 3.6.4

A 45-year-old man referred for dry cough and dyspnea.

Comments

The thymus is a lymphatic organ that plays a vital role in the development and maturation of the immune system during childhood, specifically T cells, which are instrumental in regulating cellular immunity, and B cells, which are instrumental in regulating humoral immunity. The thymus arises bilaterally from the third and fourth branchial pouches and contains elements derived from all three germinal layers.

The thymus is located in the anterior mediastinum. It overlies the pericardium, aortic arch, left innominate vein, and trachea. The thymus may extend superiorly to the lower pole of the thyroid and inferiorly to the diaphragm.

Thymic neoplasms are rare tumors that account for less than 1 % of all adult malignancies. Tumors of the thymus are classified into epithelial tumors including thymoma and thymic carcinoma, lymphomas including Hodgkin and non-Hodgkin lymphomas, Langerhans cell histiocytosis, thymolipoma, carcinoid tumor, germ cell tumors, sarcoma, and metastatic tumors. In adults, thymoma is the most frequent primary tumor of the thymus.

Thymomas typically occur in patients older than 40 years of age, are rare in children, and affect men and women equally.

Patients with thymoma are frequently asymptomatic; however, 20–30 % of patients have pressure-induced symptoms such as cough, chest pain, dyspnea, dysphagia, hoarseness, or superior vena cava syndrome. One-third to one-half of thymoma patients develop myasthenia gravis.

Imaging Findings

At radiography, thymomas typically appear as sharply marginated retrosternal areas of increased opacity with smooth or lobulated borders. Thymomas may project to either side of the mediastinum and obscure the heart border (Figs. 3.6.1 and 3.6.2). On CT scans, thymomas usually appear as homogeneous solid masses with soft-tissue attenuation and well-demarcated borders. Thymomas may be oval, round, or lobulated and usually do not conform to the shape of the thymus. Large thymomas may show areas of cystic or necrotic degeneration. Calcification may be present in the capsule or throughout the mass. Well-defined fat planes between the thymoma and adjacent structures generally indicate absence of extensive local invasion. However, minimal invasion may escape detection at imaging. Certain findings, such as encasement of mediastinal structures, infiltration of fat planes, and an irregular interface between the mass and lung parenchyma, are highly suggestive of invasion. Pleural thickening, nodularity, or effusion generally indicates pleural invasion by the thymoma (Fig. 3.6.3). At MR imaging, thymomas commonly appear as homogeneous or heterogeneous masses with low signal intensity on T1-weighted images and high signal intensity on T2-weighted images (Fig. 3.6.4).

Case 7: Mediastinal Mature Teratoma

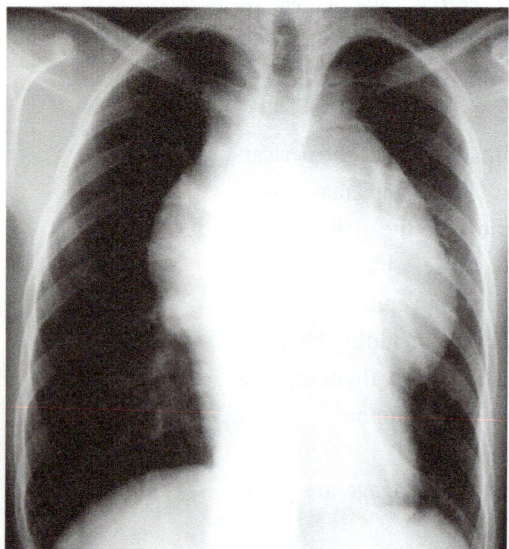

Fig. 3.7.1

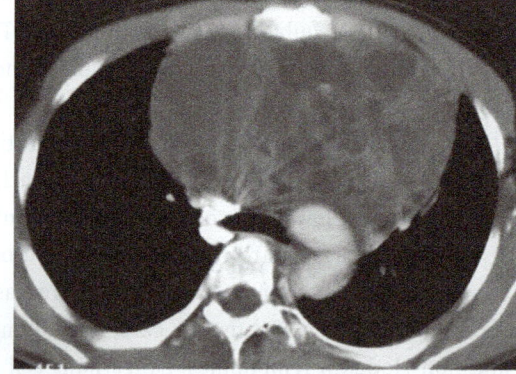

Fig. 3.7.2

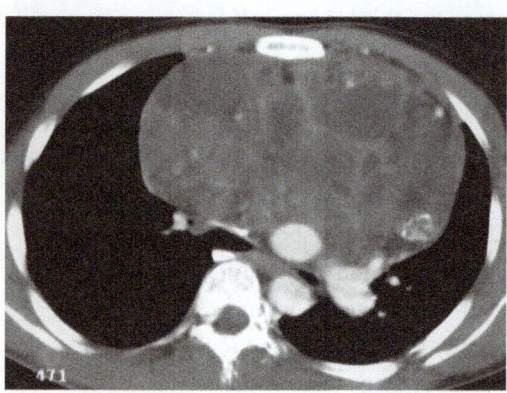

Fig. 3.7.3

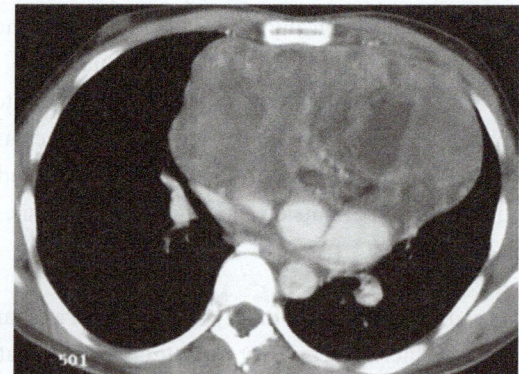

Fig. 3.7.4

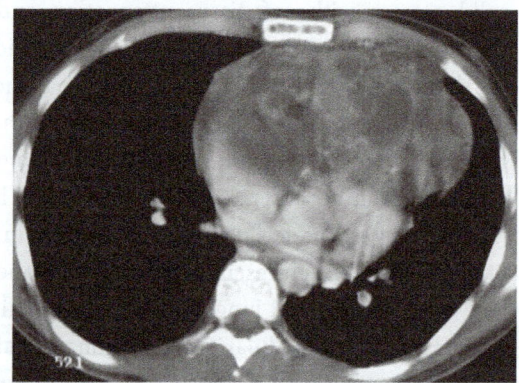

Fig. 3.7.5

A 22-year-old man with symptoms of 2 years of chest pain and dyspnea.

Mediastinal mature teratoma is a rare primary germ cell neoplasm composed of well-differentiated tissues derived from more than one of the three embryonic germ cell layers. The anterior mediastinum is the most common location of extragonadal germ cell tumors. Mediastinal mature teratoma is a rare, benign, slow-growing neoplasm that usually occurs within or near the thymus gland and accounts for up to 75 % of primary germ cell tumors of the mediastinum.

Chest radiography typically reveals a mediastinal mass, but in rare cases (8 %), particularly in the pediatric population, opacities, consolidations, mediastinal widening, and cardiomegaly are initially revealed.

CT is the imaging technique of choice in the evaluation of the abnormal mediastinum. On CT, these tumors are heterogeneous, sharply marginated, spherical, or lobulated anterior mediastinal masses with cystic components. The cystic areas are frequently compartmentalized by thin-tissue septa (85 %), but nodular soft-tissue elements (67 %) are also seen. Soft tissue is always visualized and is rarely the dominant component of the tumor; fluid is common (89 %) and the dominant component in 80 % of masses. Fat, calcification, or both are present in 85 % of tumors. Cystic lesions without fat or calcification account for 15 % of lesions. The most frequent combination of CT alienuations is soft tissue, fluid, fat, and calcium, seen in 39 % of masses. Fat-fluid levels are visualized in 11 % of masses. CT is useful for suggesting the correct diagnosis in most patients, based on the high frequency of cystic areas and fat seen in mature teratomas.

MR imaging revealed masses of heterogeneous signal intensity consistent with fluid in 88 % of tumors and with fat in 63 % of tumors. However, MR imaging and sonography did not contribute additional information in any case.

The differential diagnosis of fat-containing mediastinal masses includes mediastinal fat pad, mediastinal lipomatosis, lipoma, omental herniation, thymolipoma, and liposarcoma. However, mature teratomas are easily distinguished from these lesions by their cystic appearance with predominance of fluid elements and high frequency of calcification, findings readily seen on CT scans.

CRX film shows a giant mediastinal mass with well-defined edges (Fig. 3.7.1). CT scan (arterial phase) shows lobulated anterior mediastinal masses with cystic components and calcification inside (Figs. 3.7.2, 3.7.3, 3.7.4, and 3.7.5).

Case 8: Intrathoracic Goiter

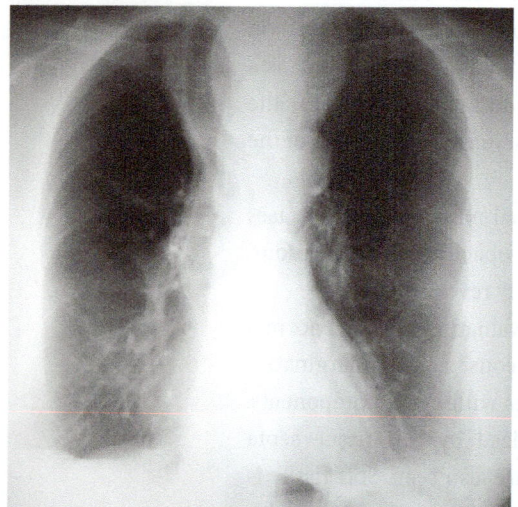

Fig. 3.8.1

Fig. 3.8.2

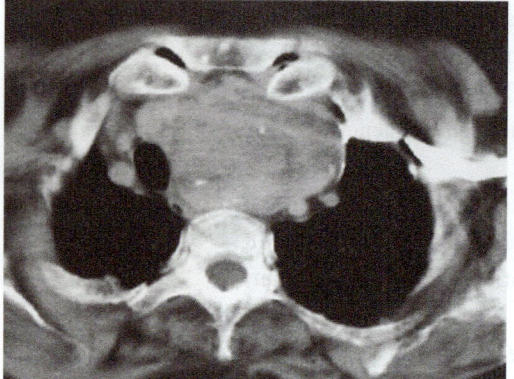

Fig. 3.8.3

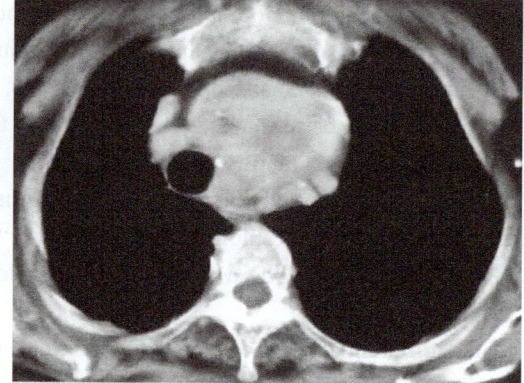

Fig. 3.8.4

A 63-year-old man referred by findings on chest radiography. Respiratory asymptomatic.

Intrathoracic goiter is one of the major diagnostic considerations in the evaluation of superior mediastinal masses. They generally represent intrathoracic extensions of cervical thyroid tissue, although, rarely, a completely intrathoracic goiter arising from ectopic thyroid tissue can occur.

Substernal goiter, usually in the anterior mediastinum, is generally due to massive enlargement of a cervical goiter and is seen in 1–10 % of all thyroidectomies. Less than 10 % of substernal goiters are located in the posterior mediastinum between the trachea and esophagus or even behind the esophagus, cephalad or caudal to the body of the 4th thoracic vertebra, behind the subclavian, innominate vessels, and azygos vein.

The radiographic features of intrathoracic thyroid glands include contralateral displacement of the hyoid, trachea, and larynx; movement of the mass with swallowing; flecks of calcification; and compression of the trachea or esophagus. However, these findings apply mostly to typical anterior mediastinal or ipsilateral posterior mediastinal extensions. The contralateral retroesophageal or retrotracheal goiter produces deviation of the trachea and esophagus to the same side on which the mass presents on the chest film.

A CT scan and the patterns of anterior or posterior compression of the esophagus from barium esophagographic study usually permit the anatomic location of the mass to be characterized with great accuracy.

99m Tc SPECT/CT is a valuable method for correct discrimination between mediastinal metastases/tumors and intrathoracic goiter, and biopsy may be unnecessary. SPECT/CT had 100 % sensitivity and specificity.

The differential diagnosis for a middle mediastinal mass can be broadly divided in malignant and nonmalignant lesions. Malignant masses include lymphoma, lymphatic metastases, and tracheal tumors. Nonmalignant masses can be further categorized infectious (lymphadenopathy due to tuberculosis or fungal infections), inflammatory (sarcoidosis, silicosis, pneumoconiosis), vascular (aortic aneurysm, ectatic azygos vein), or congenital (esophageal or bronchial-related foregut cysts).

CRX show superior mediastinal mass, which displaces the trachea to the right (Figs. 3.8.1 and 3.8.2). CT scan (arterial phase) show goiter is introduced in the upper mediastinum (Figs. 3.8.3 and 3.8.4).

Case 9: Mediastinal Neurofibroma

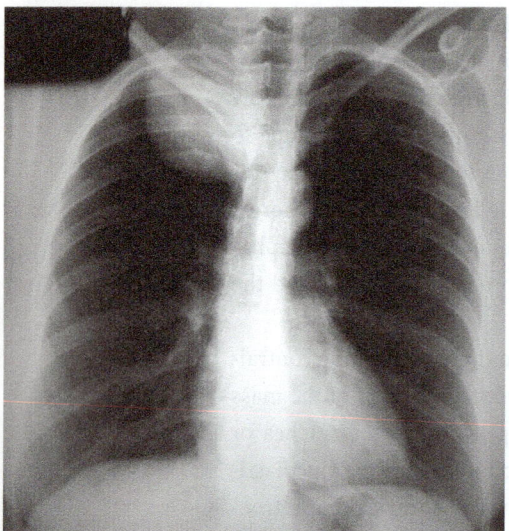

Fig. 3.9.1

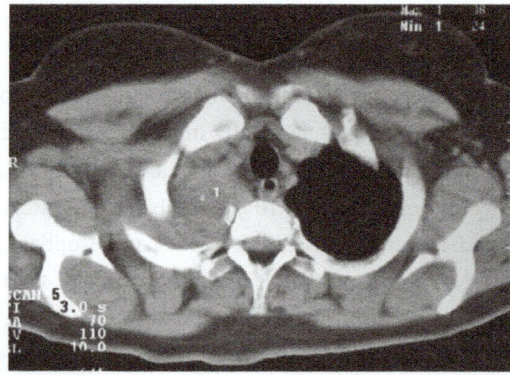

Fig. 3.9.2

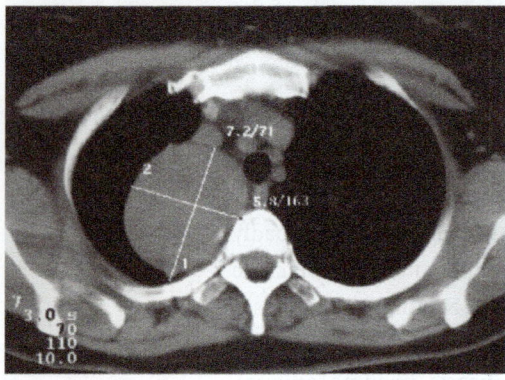

Fig. 3.9.3

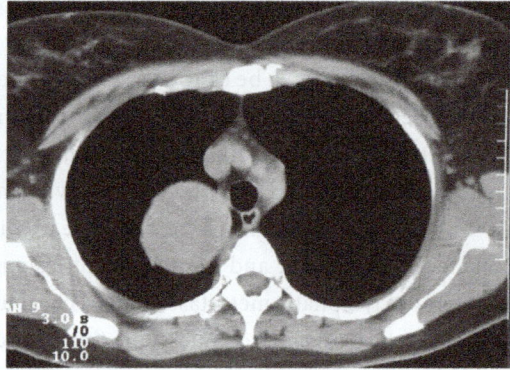

Fig. 3.9.4

A 37-year-old woman with chest pain and dry cough.

Comments

Neurogenic tumors are one of the most commonly encountered mediastinal tumor. They constitute almost 15–25 % of mediastinal tumors and are located predominantly in the posterior mediastinal compartment. Nerve sheath tumors, including neurilemmomas and neurofibromas, appear as an encapsulated spherical mass, and they can extend through a spinal foramen and grow into a dumbbell shape in both the spinal canal and the paravertebral region. Neurofibromas account for approximately 20 % of mediastinal neurogenic tumors. The peak age of occurrence is 20–30 years. Localized neurofibromas have a true capsule or pseudocapsule.

On CT, they manifest as a sharply marginated, smooth, or lobulated mass of soft-tissue density. Approximately 50 % of cases are associated with bony abnormalities, such as expansion of a neural foramen and erosion of the vertebral body or rib.

MRI has become the best imaging modality for evaluating the widening of the intervertebral foramen and any spinal cord involvement. Findings of low attenuation areas within the tumor, destruction of the adjacent bony structures, pleural effusion, or pleural nodules are also suggestive of malignancy.

CT and MR could not reliably distinguish benign from malignant lesions, although mass inhomogeneities, infiltrative margins, or bone destruction are more common in malignant lesions.

Imaging Findings

CRX show well demarcated mass located in the superior mediastinum (Fig. 3.9.1). CT scan show homogeneous density mass in the superior mediastinum (Figs. 3.9.2, 3.9.3 and 3.9.4).

Case 10: Neurofibrosarcoma

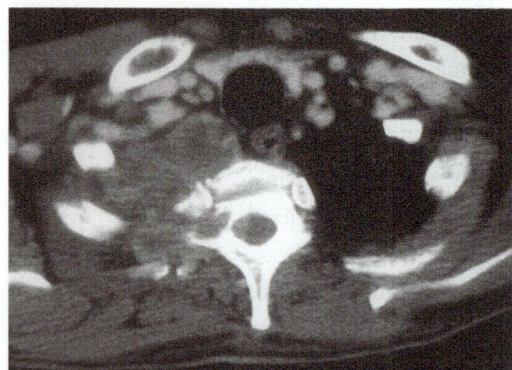

Fig. 3.10.1

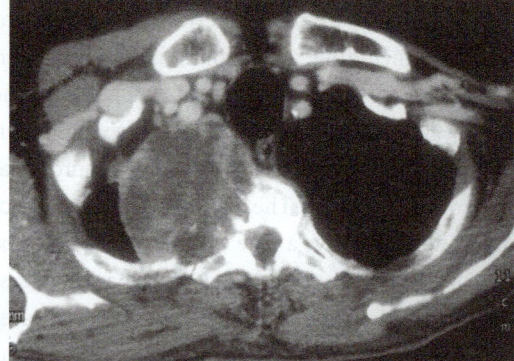

Fig. 3.10.2

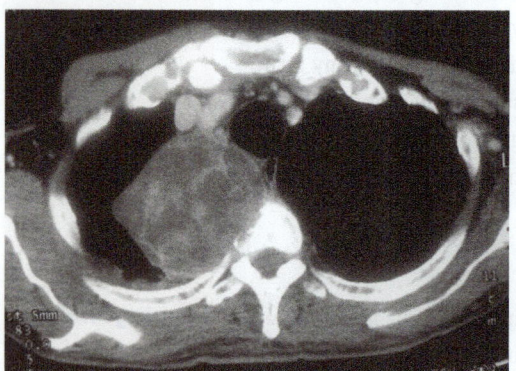

Fig. 3.10.3

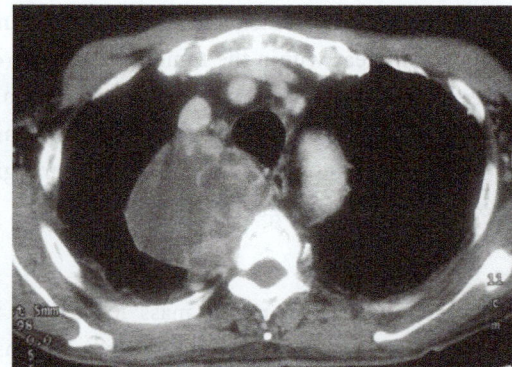

Fig. 3.10.4

A 41-year-old man with chest pain, dry cough, weight loss, fatigue, and weakness of 2 months duration.

Thoracic neurofibrosarcomas (also called *malignant peripheral nerve sheath tumors* or *malignant schwannomas*) usually arise in preexisting neurofibromas of the intercostal nerves or spinal nerve roots or in the brachial plexus. Occasionally, neurofibrosarcomas have been associated with radiation therapy. About half of these tumors are associated with type 1 neurofibromatosis and have been reported to occur in up to 29 % of these patients. The tumors mostly occur in adults and present as an enlarging, painful mass.

Neurofibrosarcomas are usually of variable signal intensity on T1- and T2-weighted MR images. Imaging features suggestive of malignant degeneration of a benign neurogenic tumor to neurofibrosarcoma include a sudden increase in size or development of heterogeneous attenuation at CT due to internal necrosis and hemorrhage. The development of heterogeneous signal intensity on T2-weighted MR images with loss of the peripherally hyperintense and centrally hypointense appearance (target sign) that is characteristic of neurofibromas is indicative of malignant transformation.

Neurofibrosarcomas are treated with resection and radiation therapy, if possible. The overall 5-year survival rate is approximately 50 % in patients with resectable tumors.

Comments

CT scan (arterial phase) show heterogeneous density mass located in superior mediastinum (Figs. 3.10.1, 3.10.2, 3.10.3 and 3.10.4).

Imaging Findings

Case 11: Primary Anterior Mediastinal Seminoma

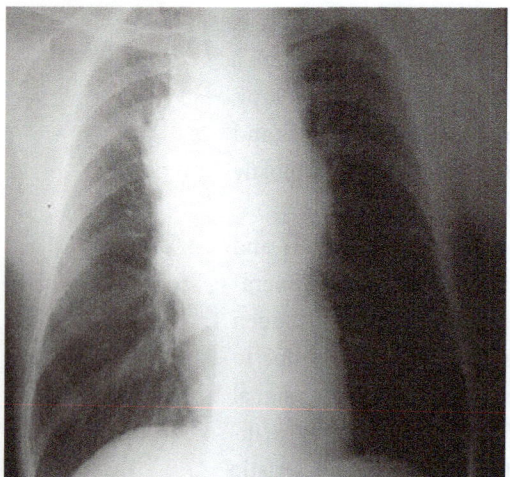

Fig. 3.11.1

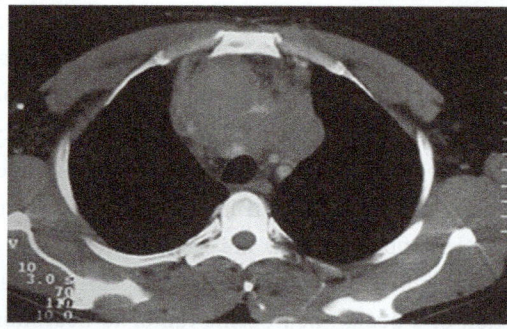

Fig. 3.11.2

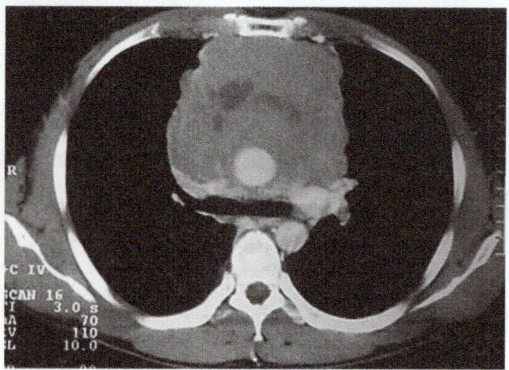

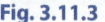

Fig. 3.11.3

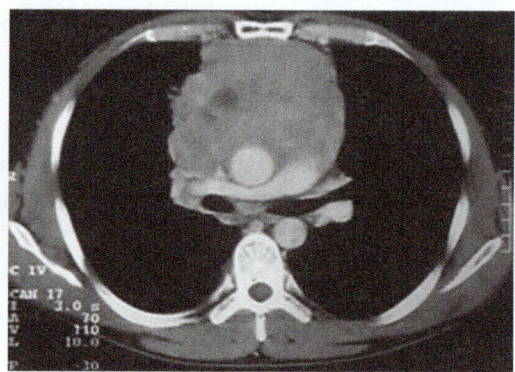

Fig. 3.11.4

A 41-year-old man consulted for weight loss, dyspnea, headache, flushing, and clinical signs of superior vena cava syndrome.

Primary mediastinal germ cell tumors are rare lesions accounting for only 10–15 % of mediastinal masses. Most of these tumors are benign lesions; however, up to one-third may be malignant, and seminoma is the most common histologic subtype. Most of these tumors arise in the anterior mediastinum, although rarely these lesions may be centered in other locations.

Occurring most frequently in men ages 20–40 years. Patients present with dyspnea, substernal pain, weakness, cough, fever, gynecomastia, or weight loss. Because of the tumor location, about 10 % of patients present with superior vena cava syndrome. However, tumors can grow 20–30 cm before symptoms develop.

Radiographically, seminomas are bulky, lobulated, homogenous masses. Local invasion is rare, but metastasis to lymph nodes and bone does occur.

On CT, mediastinal seminomas present as bulky, lobular anterior mediastinal masses that may encase or invade local structures. Calcification is distinctly unusual, but regions of cyst formation or cystic degeneration may be present. CT and gallium scanning is used to evaluate the extent of disease.

CRX film shows anterior mediastinal mass (Fig. 3.11.1). CT scan (arterial phase) shows voluminous anterior mediastinal mass of heterogeneous density. Necrosis inside (Figs. 3.11.2, 3.11.3 and 3.11.4).

Case 12: Bronchogenic Cyst

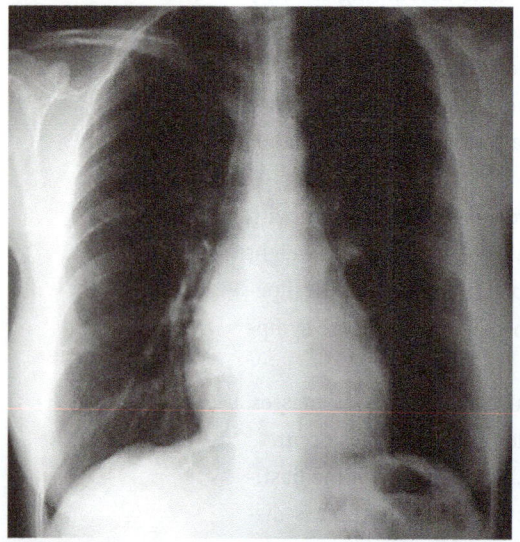

Fig. 3.12.1

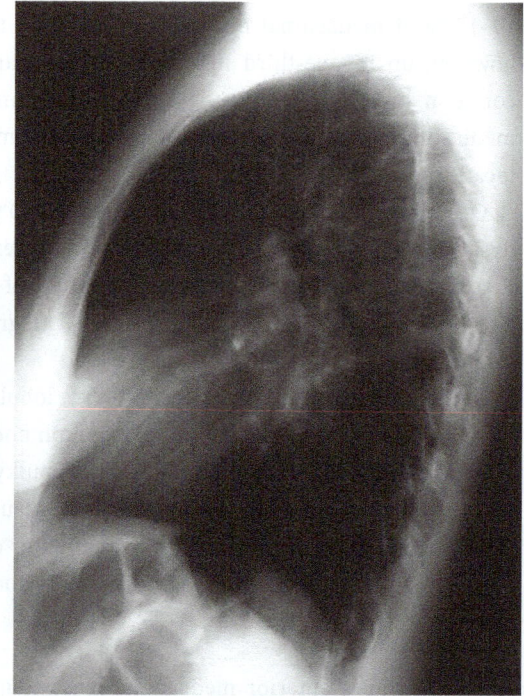

Fig. 3.12.2

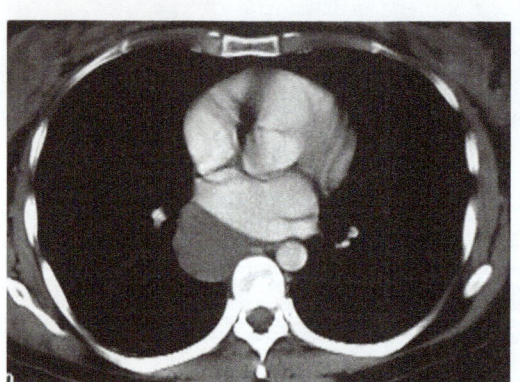

Fig. 3.12.3

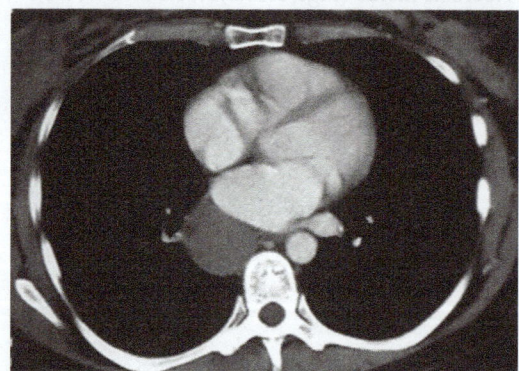

Fig. 3.12.4

A 21-year-old man consulted for flu; CRX was requested for medical evaluation.

Comments

Bronchogenic cysts are congenital lesions arising from the abnormal budding of the ventral foregut that occurs between the 26th and 40th days of gestation. The cysts are lined by ciliated columnar or cuboidal epithelium and are surrounded by tissues similar to those of the normal bronchus, including cartilage, smooth muscle, elastic tissue, and mucous glands. Most of the cysts are located in the mediastinum along the tracheobronchial tree, but they can also be found in the lung parenchyma or may extend to or below the diaphragm as dumbbell cysts.

The most common location is the middle mediastinum (65–90 %). The distribution of locations can be quite varied: mediastinal, 70 %, usually does not communicate with the tracheobronchial tree, subcarinal, right paratracheal, and hilar locations; most common approximate incidence includes carinal area 50 %, paratracheal area 20 %, orophageal wall 15 %, and retrocardiac area 10 %.

Parenchymal (intrapulmonary) typically perihilar, predilection for lower lobes.

Other uncommon locations are neck, skin, pericardium, extending across the diaphragm and appearing dumbbell shaped and retroperitoneally.

Radiologic findings of mediastinal bronchogenic cysts are well known. The CT findings show the cyst as a well-defined spherical mass either with or without mass effect with the attenuation of water or soft tissue. When bronchogenic cysts manifest as water-attenuation masses on CT scans, differentiation from other mediastinal processes such as lymphadenopathy or neoplasia is not difficult. However, when bronchogenic cysts manifest as soft-tissue attenuation masses on CT scans, differentiation from solid lesions can be more problematic. Variable fluid composition explains the different CT attenuations observed. Approximately 50 % are fluid density (0–20 HU); however, a significant proportion are of soft-tissue density (>30 HU) or even hyperdense to surrounding mediastinal soft tissues. CT is better able to detect calcium oxalate (milk of calcium) layering dependently.

Differential diagnosis: congenital cysts and malformations, pericardial cyst, cystic hygroma/lymphangioma, neurenteric cyst, anterior or lateral meningocele, esophageal duplication cyst, thyroid colloid cyst, and thymic cyst.

Imaging Findings

CRX film shows ill-defined lesion in the posterior mediastinum (Figs. 3.12.1 and 3.12.2). CT scan (arterial phase) shows cystic lesion in the posterior mediastinum (Figs. 3.12.3 and 3.12.4).

Further Reading

Massive Pulmonary Embolism

Bergqvist D, Lindblad B (1985) A 30-year survey of pulmonary embolism verified at autopsy: an analysis of 1274 surgical patients. Br J Surg 72:105

Come PC (1992) Echocardiographic evaluation of pulmonary embolism and its response to therapeutic interventions. Chest 101:151S

Coon WW, Willis PW (1959) Deep venous thrombosis and pulmonary embolism: prediction, prevention and treatment. Am J Cardiol 4:611

Dauphine C (2005) Pulmonary embolectomy for acute massive pulmonary embolism. Ann Thorac Surg 79:1240–1244

Garg K (2002) CT of pulmonary thromboembolic disease. Radiol Clin North Am 40(1):111–122

Goldhaber SZ, Hennekens CH, Evans DA et al (1982) Factors associated with correct antemortem diagnosis of major pulmonary embolism. Am J Med 73:822

Grifoni S, Olivotto I, Cecchini P et al (1998) Utility of an integrated clinical, echocardiographic, and venous ultrasonographic approach for triage of patients with suspected pulmonary embolism. Am J Cardiol 82:1230

Guidelines on diagnosis and management of acute pulmonary embolism (2000) Task Force on Pulmonary Embolism, European Society of Cardiology. Eur Heart J 21:1301

Kasper W, Meinertz MD, Henkel B et al (1986) Echocardiographic findings in patients with proved pulmonary embolism. Am Heart J 112:1284

Kucher N, Goldhaber SZ (2005) Management of massive pulmonary embolism. Circulation 112:e28

PIOPED Investigators: value of the ventilation/perfusion scan in acute pulmonary embolism (1990) JAMA 263:2753

Soloff LA, Rodman T (1967) Acute pulmonary embolism. II. Clinical. Am Heart J 74:829

Interlobar Artery Aneurysm

Castañer E et al (2006) Congenital and acquired pulmonary artery anomalies in the adult: radiologic overview. Radiographics 26:349–371

de Lima Bastos A, Alves de Brito IL (2011) Pulmonary artery aneurysms in Behçet's disease: case report. Radiol Bras 44(6):396–398

Deffebach ME, Charan NB, Lakshminarayan S, Butler J (1987) The bronchial circulation: small, but a vital attribute of the lung. Am Rev Respir Dis 135:463–481

Frazier AA, Galvin JR, Franks TJ, Rosado-de-Christenson ML (2000) From the archives of the AFIP: pulmonary vasculature–hypertension and infarction. Radiographics 20:491–524

Morgan PW, Foley DW, Erickson SJ (1991) Proximal interruption of a main pulmonary artery with transpleural collateral vessels: CT and MR appearances. J Comput Assist Tomogr 15:311–313

Nguyen ET, Silva CIS, Seely JM, Chong S, Lee KO, Müller NL (2007) Pulmonary artery aneurysms and pseudoaneurysms in adults: findings at CT and radiography. AJR Am J Roentgenol 188:W126–W134

Remy-Jardin M, Remy J, Mayo JR, Müller NL (2001) Anatomy and normal variants. In: CT angiography of the chest. Lippincott Williams & Wilkins, Philadelphia, pp 15–17

Small Cell Lung Cancer

Boland GW, Lee MJ, Gazelle GS (1998) Characterization of adrenal masses using unenhanced CT: an analysis of the CT literature. AJR Am J Roentgenol 171(1):201–204

Decker RH, Wilson LD (2008) Advances in radiotherapy for lung cancer. Semin Respir Crit Care Med 29(3):285–290

Kreisman H, Wolkove N, Quoix E (1992) Small cell lung cancer presenting as a solitary pulmonary nodule. Chest 101(1):225–231

Mediastinitis and Perforation of the Subclavian Artery

Akman C, Kantarci F, Cetinkaya S (2004) Imaging in mediastinitis: a systematic review based on aetiology. Clin Radiol 59:573–585

Carrol CL, Jeffrey RB Jr, Federle MP et al (1987) CT evaluation of mediastinal infections. J Comput Assist Tomogr 11:449–454

Exarhos DN, Malagari K et al (2005) Acute mediastinitis: spectrum of computed tomography findings. Eur Radiol 15:1569–1574

Jeung MY, Gangi A, Gasser B et al (1999a) Imaging of chest wall disorders. Radiographics 19:617–637

Hodgkin Lymphoma

Bae YA, Lee KS (2010) Cross-sectional evaluation of thoracic lymphoma. Thorac Surg Clin 20:175–186

Guermazi A, Brice P, Kerviler E, Fermé C, Hennequin C, Meignin V, Frija J (2001) Extranodal Hodgkin disease: spectrum of disease. Radiographics 21:161–179

Toma P, Granata C, Rossi A, Garaventa A (2007) Multimodality imaging of Hodgkin disease and non-Hodgkin lymphomas in children. Radiographics 27:1335–1354

Thymoma

Benveniste M, Rosado-de-Christenson M, Sabloff B, Moran C, Swisher S, Marom E (2011) Role of imaging in the diagnosis, staging, and treatment of thymoma. Radiographics 31:1847–1861

Nasseri F, Eftekhari F (2011) Clinical and radiologic review of the normal and abnormal thymus: pearls and pitfalls. Radiographics 30:413–428

Nishino M, Ashiku S, Kocher O, Thurer R, Boiselle P, Hatabu H (2006) The thymus: a comprehensive review. Radiographics 26:335–348

Mediastinal Mature Teratoma

Jeung MY et al (2002) Imaging of cystic masses of the mediastinum. Radiographics 22:S79–S93

Moeller KH, Rosado-de-Christenson ML, Templeton PA (1997) Mediastinal mature teratoma: imaging features. AJR Am J Roentgenol 169:985–990

Wu TT et al (2002) Mature mediastinal teratoma sonographic imaging patterns and pathologic correlation. J Ultrasound Med 21:759–765

Intrathoracic Goiter

Ahmadzadehfar H et al (2012) The utility of 99mTc pertechnetate SPECT/CT in the diagnosis of intrathoracic masses. J Nucl Med 53(Suppl 1):2044

Bashist B, Ellis K, Gold RP (1983) Computed tomography of intrathoracic goiters. AJR Am J Roentgenol 140: 455–460

Dhaliwal RS et al (1999) Posterior mediastinal goiters: literature review and report of three cases. Asian Cardiovasc Thorac Ann 7:228–232

Shahian DM et al (1988) Posterior mediastinal goiter. Chest 94:599–602

Mediastinal Neurofibroma

Ikezoe J, Sone S (1986) Higashihara T CT of intrathoracic neurogenic tumours. Eur J Radiol 6:266–269

Lonergan GJ, Schwab CM, Suarez ES, Carlson CL (2002) Neuroblastoma, ganglioneuroblastoma, and ganglioneuroma: radiologic-pathologic correlation. Radiographics 22:911–934

Strollo DC, Rosado-de-Christenson ML, Jett JR (1997) Primary mediastinal tumors. Part II. Tumors of the middle and posterior mediastinum. Chest 112:1344–1357

Topcu S, Alper A, Gulhan E, Kocyigit O, Tastepe I, Cetin G (2000) Neurogenic tumours of the mediastinum: a report of 60 cases. Can Respir J 7:261–265

Woo OH, Yong HS et al (2008) Wide spectrum of thoracic neurogenic tumours: a pictorial review of CT and pathological findings. Br J Radiol 81:668–676

Neurofibrosarcoma

Aughenbaugh GL (1984) Thoracic manifestations of neurocutaneous diseases. Radiol Clin North Am 22:741–756

Gladish GW et al (2002) Primary thoracic sarcomas. Radiographics 22:621–637

Jeung MY, Gangi A, Gasser B et al (1999b) Imaging of chest wall disorders. Radiographics 19:617–637

Lee J, Sohn SK, Ahn BC, Chun KA, Lee K, Kim CK (1997) Sarcomatous transformation of neurofibromas: comparative imaging with Ga-67, Tl-201, Tc-99m pentavalent DMSA and Tc-99m MIBI. Clin Nucl Med 22:610–614

Primary Anterior Mediastinal Seminoma

Duwe BV, Sterman DH, Musani AI (2005) Tumors of the mediastinum. Chest 128:2893–2909

Ravenel JG, Gordon LL, Block MI, Chaudhary U (2004) Primary posterior mediastinal seminoma. AJR Am J Roentgenol 183:1835–1837

Slawson R et al (1983) Primary mediastinal seminoma. Radiographics 3(1):100–106

Bronchogenic Cyst

Lyon RD, Mcadams HP (1993) Mediastinal bronchogenic cyst: demonstration of a fluid-fluid level at MR imaging. Radiology 186(2):427–428

McAdams HP et al (2000) Bronchogenic cyst: imaging features with clinical and histopathologic correlation. Radiology 217:441–446

Naidich DP, Srichai MB, Krinsky GA (2007) Computed tomography and magnetic resonance of the thorax. Lippincott Williams & Wilkins, Philadelphia. ISBN 0781757657

Yoon YC et al (2002) Intrapulmonary bronchogenic cyst: CT and pathologic findings in five adult patients. AJR Am J Roentgenol 179:167–170

Air Space and Bronchi – I

4

John C. Pedrozo Pupo, Diego M. Celis Mejía, Claudia Patricia García Calderón, Victoria Eugenia Murillo, Bernardo J. Muñoz Palacio, and Carlos de la Rosa Pérez

Contents

J.C. Pedrozo Pupo (ed.), *Learning Chest Imaging*, Learning Imaging,
DOI 10.1007/978-3-642-34147-2_4, © Springer-Verlag Berlin Heidelberg 2013

Case 1: Pulmonary Epithelioid Hemangioendothelioma

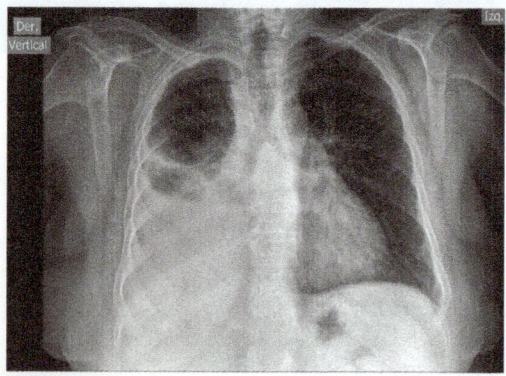

Fig. 4.1.1

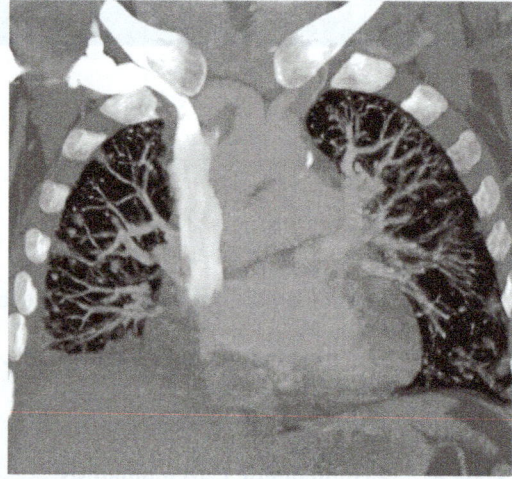

Fig. 4.1.3

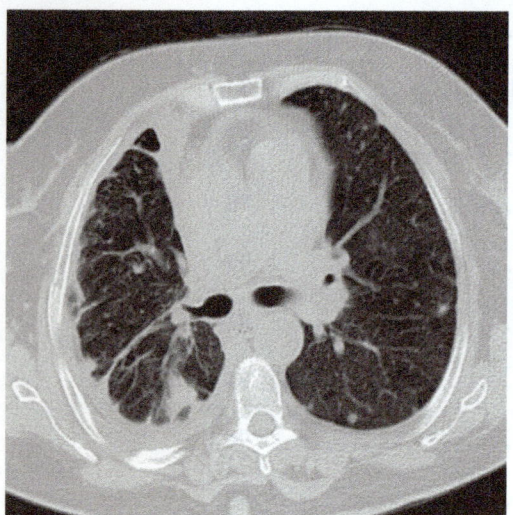

Fig. 4.1.2

A 57-year-old housewife with a past history of systemic arterial hypertension and type 2 diabetes of recent onset. She has no past history of smoking but cooked with wood for over 10 years. She comes to the emergency room with symptoms that started in January of 2012 with dyspnea on exertion that has progressed in the last 4 months to dyspnea with minimal effort associated with cough with sputum, weight loss (approximately 5 kg), and pleuritic chest pain on the right side.

Due to the absence of infectious disease, the patient is submitted to thoracoscopy with biopsies, and because of the thyroid enlargement, a possibility of a thyroid metastasis was considered, so a biopsy of this organ was also performed revealing only hyperplasic nodules.

Pleural biopsy showed fibrosis with mild to moderate infiltration of lymphocytes and neutrophils. No granulomas or malignant cells were seen.

Comments

The *epithelioid hemangioendothelioma* is a tumor of low frequency and therefore a rare disease. It was first described by Weiss and Enzinger. In the past, it was classified as an intravascular bronchoalveolar tumor. This tumor appears as a primary disease of the blood vessels that can affect the lungs, pleura, liver, brain, or the bones either primarily or simultaneously. There is a tendency to affect more females.

The characteristic of this tumor in the lung is the presence of multiple nodules that have a random distribution, which are usually slow growing as it has been reported in several series and clinical case presentations. The clinical symptomatology is diverse and ranges from asymptomatic patients who have an incidental finding on a chest radiograph performed as part of a medical work-up or presenting with symptoms such as dry cough, chest pain, and dyspnea that may or may not be associated with the presence of pleural effusion.

This tumor arises in the blood vessels where the presence of Weibel-Palade bodies demonstrated by electron microscopy allows the determination of their endothelial lineage. Accumulation of cells or cell nests is seen within the vessel wall. These tumors have low mitotic activity. Growth is centrifugal from the vessel wall but can destroy the elastic and muscular tunic and fill the inside of the vessels with an eosinophilic amorphous substance.

The findings in the images (chest X-ray and CT scan) are the presence of nodules of various sizes but overall with an average of 0.5–2 cm. Due to their random distribution on chest X-ray, it is necessary to make a differential diagnosis with other causes of pulmonary nodules such as alveolar microlithiasis, carcinomatosis, metastases, lymphangitic spread of leukemia, multiple myeloma, tuberculosis, histoplasmosis, or nocardiosis.

Fig. 4.1.4

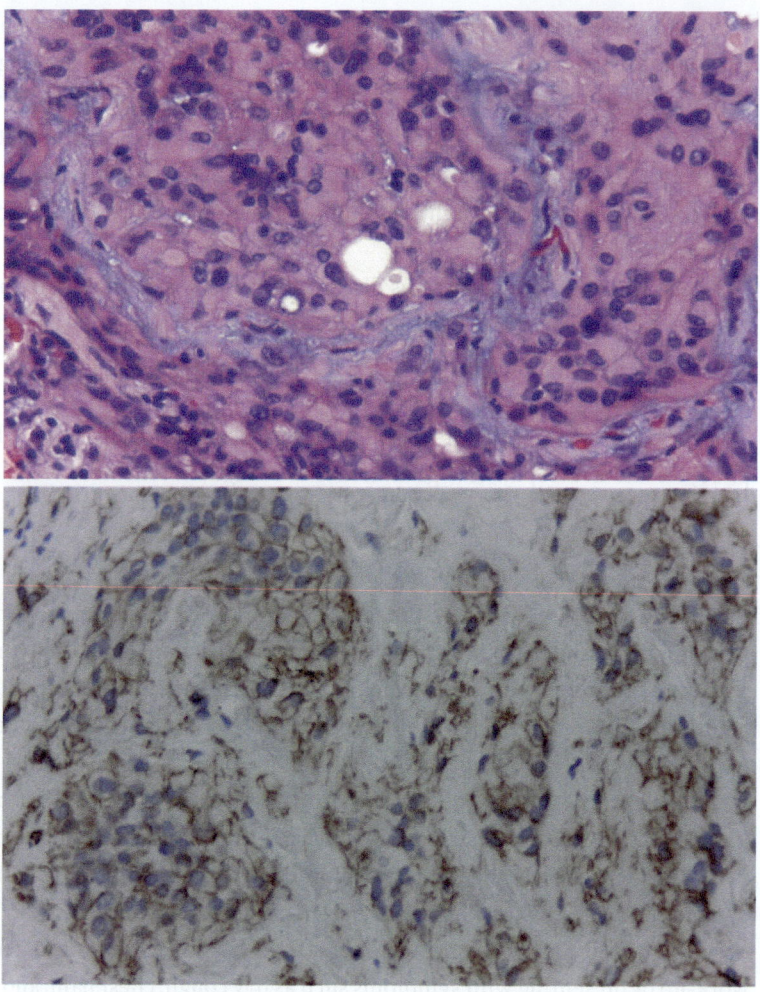

Chest X-ray revealed an opacity on the right lung field compatible with a pleural effusion, but on the lung fields, small nodules were also visible on the chest X-ray. The finding suggested the presence of pleural disease with parenchymal nodular disease (Fig. 4.1.1). Chest CT shows thyroid gland with nodular and heterogeneous enlargement of both lobes, right pleural thickening and pleural fluid with a density of 20 HU and air on its interior, and subcutaneous emphysema in the lateral thoracic right wall. In the lung window, multiple random pulmonary nodules with diameters between 5 and 10 mm are not calcified and without cavitation. No tree in bud pattern is seen. Laminar atelectasis in the right lower lung field is present (Figs. 4.1.2 and 4.1.3). The lung biopsy revealed multiple nodules formed by cells with uniform regular nucleus, some with cytoplasmic intranuclear inclusions with dense eosinophilic cytoplasm with intracytoplasmic vacuoles forming nests, in filtrating myxoid stroma with areas of collagen deposits, and many of them located in the adventitia of blood vessels or within their lumens and also in the alveoli (Fig. 4.1.4). Immunohistochemical analysis demonstrated a negative TTF-1, tiroglobulina, CK, CK7, CK 20, AML, CD56, synaptophysin, and S100. And it was CD31 positive compatible with the vascular origin (Fig. 4.1.4).

Case 2: Calcified Pulmonary Nodules

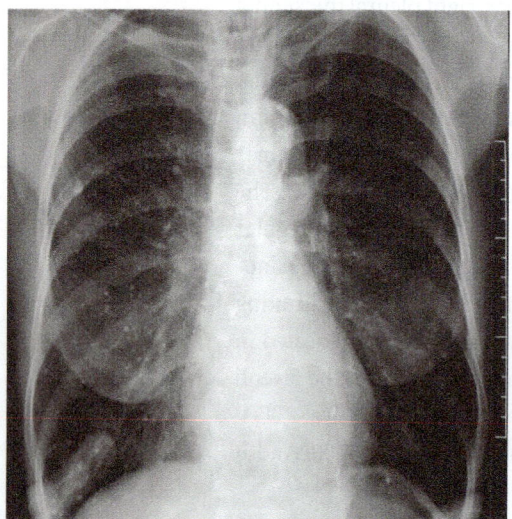

Fig. 4.2.1

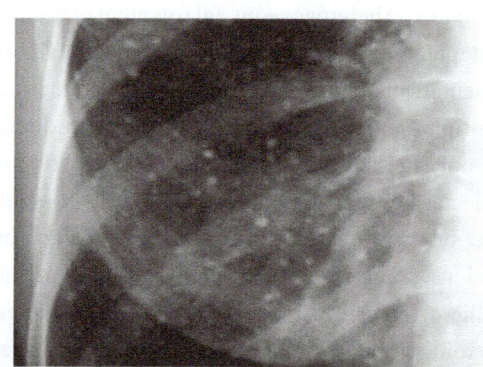

Fig. 4.2.3

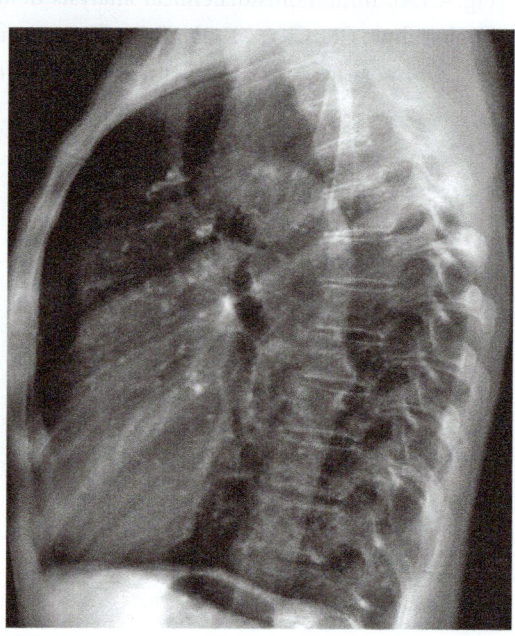

Fig. 4.2.4

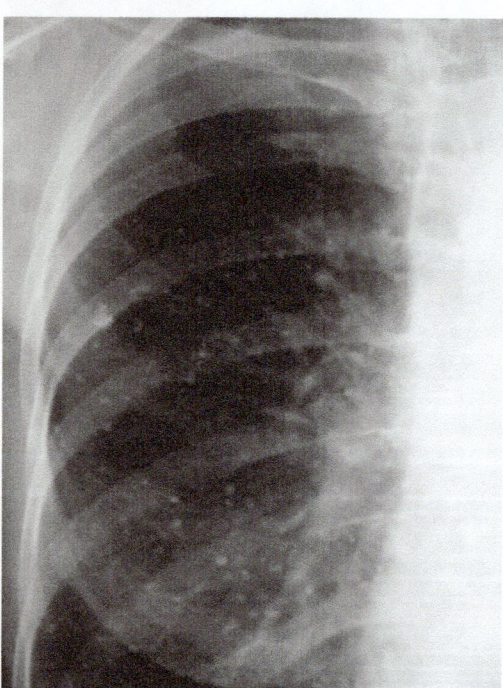

Fig. 4.2.2

A 75-year-old woman came to the clinic for cough in recent days. She has a history of varicella pneumonia in childhood.

Pulmonary involvement in adults by the varicella-zoster virus (VZV) is a
serious complication that affects 15 % of those infected.

The conventional chest imaging studies usually show an interstitial infiltrate
and, less frequently, alveolar infiltrate, which usually disappears a week after
solving the cutaneous picture. Nodules sometimes remain for weeks and may
calcify and persist for years, which is more often in smokers. On CT, the lesions
appear as nodules of 1–10 mm, well defined, and infrequently as a coalescence
of nodules. The finding of multiple calcified pulmonary micronodules in
asymptomatic patients should make us think about the possibility of lung disease varicella, thus enabling the realization of others remove additional diagnostic studies such as those mentioned above.

Calcified pulmonary nodules are a subset of hyperdense pulmonary nodules and a group of nodules with a relatively narrow differential. The commonest cause of nodule calcification is granuloma formation, usually in
response to healed infection.

- Healed infection
  - Calcified granulomata, e.g., histoplasmosis and recovered miliary tuber-
    culosis (rare)
  - Healed varicella pneumonia
- Occupational disease: pneumoconioses
  - Silicosis
    - Associated with nodal egg-shell calcification
    - Multiple small densely calcified nodules in mid and upper zones
  - Coal worker's pneumoconiosis
- Metastatic calcification
  - Typically, nodules are poorly defined and larger (3–10 mm)
  - Calcium and phosphate metabolism abnormalities (Sarcoidosis, Chronic
    renal failure, Multiple myeloma, Secondary hyperparathyroidism,
    Massive osteolysis caused by metastases, IV calcium therapy)
- Pulmonary hemosiderosis
  - Idiopathic pulmonary hemosiderosis
  - Mitral stenosis
  - Goodpasture's syndrome
- Pulmonary alveolar microlithiasis
  - Tiny micronodules
  - Apparent calcification of interlobular septa
  - Small subpleural cysts

The chest radiograph in the PA and lateral projections shows diffuse calcified
micronodules randomly distributed, all measuring less than 4 mm (Figs. 4.2.1,
4.2.2, 4.2.3, and 4.2.4).

Case 3: Pulmonary Metastasis

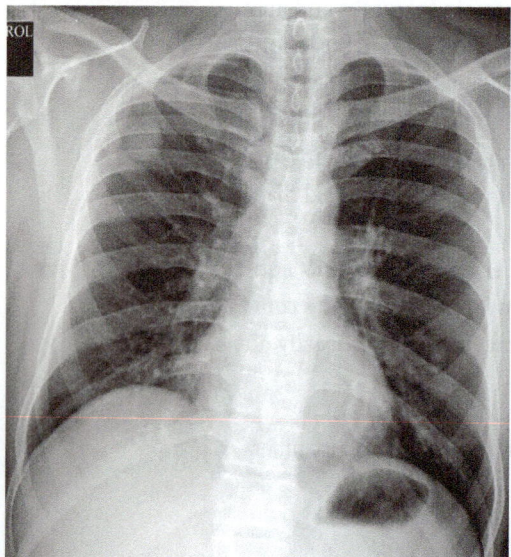

Fig. 4.3.1

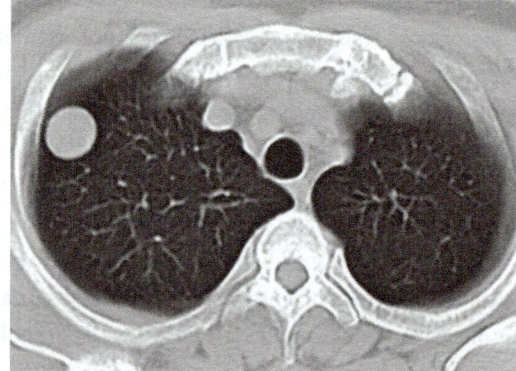

Fig. 4.3.2

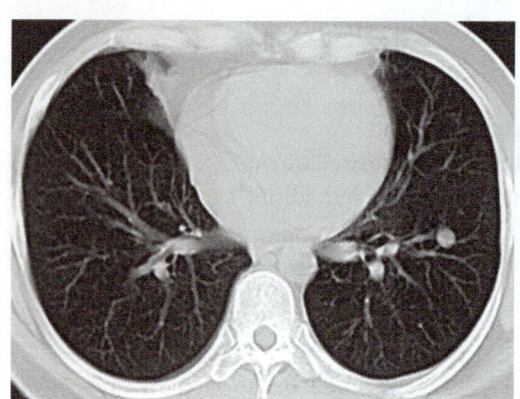

Fig. 4.3.3

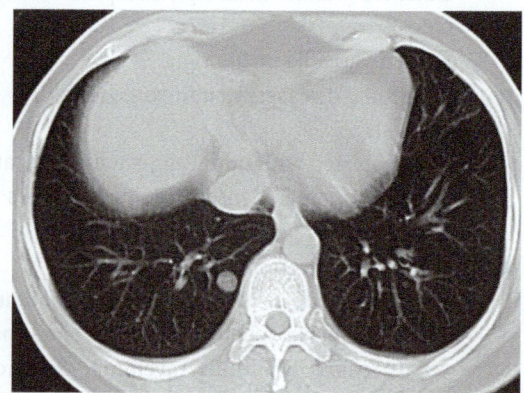

Fig. 4.3.4

A 33-year-old man presents with dyspnea grade 2, dry cough, fatigue, weakness, and weight loss. He had sarcoma.

Comments

The lung is the most common site of metastatic disease commitment, after the lymph nodes and liver. The most common manifestation of pulmonary metastatic disease is the presence of multiple nodules. Large series of autopsies of patients with extrathoracic malignancies reveal malignant pulmonary metastases in 20–50 % of patients. Among the autopsy cases, breast, colon, uterus, kidney, and head and neck are the most common primary sites with pulmonary metastases. Early diagnosis of pulmonary metastases in patients with known malignancy may be critical in planning effective therapy.

Computed tomography (CT) is now accepted as the diagnostic modality of choice for detection of possible pulmonary metastases above the chest radiograph because of its higher sensitivity.

The vast majority of pulmonary metastases reach the lungs via the pulmonary artery system. The most common manifestation of pulmonary metastatic disease is the presence of multiple nodules, which are found predominantly in the outer third of lung and subpleural, with predilection for the bases, suggesting the interaction of gravity.

Metastases are identified typically as multiple nodules with rounded, soft tissue density that captures the intravenous contrast medium, usually bilateral and of variable size.

Although metastases are usually multiple in number, some tumors are more likely to manifest as a solitary metastasis; these include primary tumors of the colon and kidney, melanoma, and sarcoma.

Atypical radiological or unusual features of metastases are frequently found; this causes the differentiation from other malignant lung diseases difficult. These characteristics include:

- Nodules with cavitation, especially in primary squamous cell type
- Calcified nodules in primary tumors of osteogenic origin
- Bleeding around the metastatic nodules, especially in choriocarcinomas and melanomas
- Appearance of pneumothorax in subpleural nodules secondary sarcomas
- Pattern of occupation of the airspace in lymphomas and adenocarcinomas
- Miscellaneous, tumor embolism, metastatic endobronchial mass, solitary dilated vessels in a metastatic mass and sterilized

Imaging Findings

CRX film shows multiple nodular lesions in both lungs (Fig. 4.3.1). CT scan (lung window) shows nodular lesions, randomly distributed in different shapes and sizes and density of soft tissue by hematogenous metastases (Figs. 4.3.2, 4.3.3, and 4.3.4).

Case 4: Lymphangitic Carcinomatosis

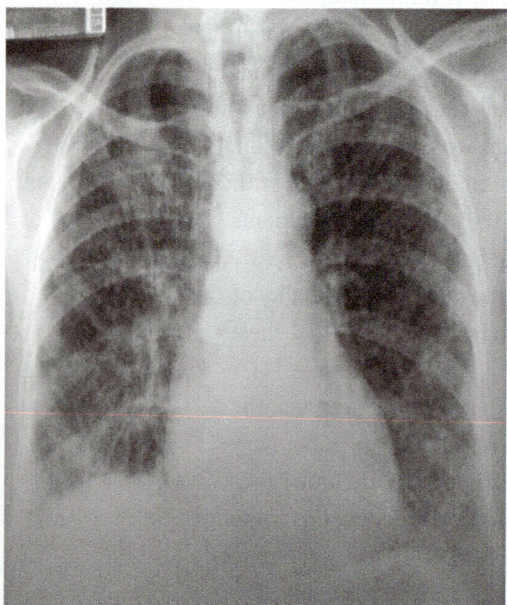

Fig. 4.4.1

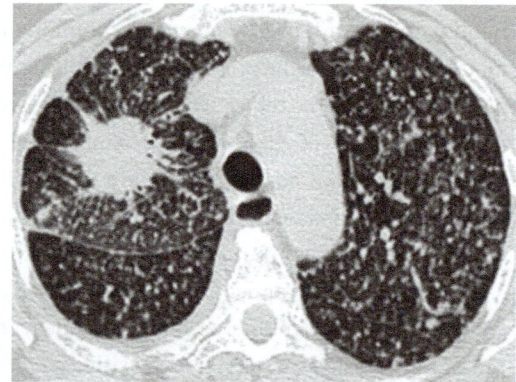

Fig. 4.4.2

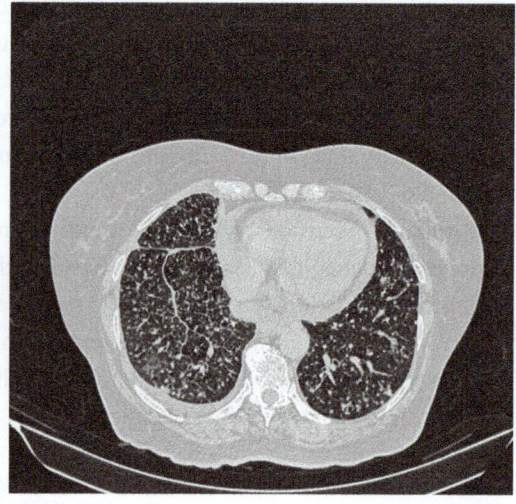

Fig. 4.4.4

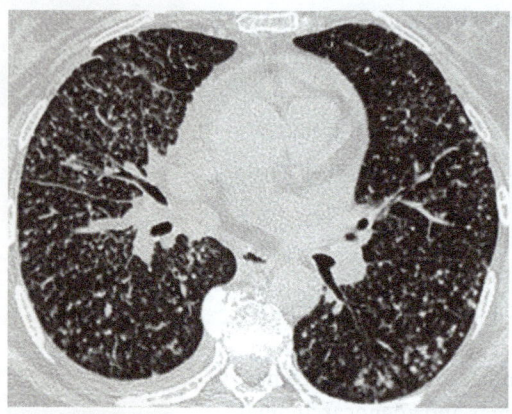

Fig. 4.4.3

A 71-year-old woman came by with dyspnea grade 1, dry cough, chest pain, and weakness. She had asthma from childhood, is a nonsmoker, and with non-small cell carcinoma-type micropapillary adenocarcinoma stage IV.

Also known as "lymphangitic spread of tumors," "lymphangitis carcinomatosa," or "lymphangiosis carcinomatosa," LC refers to the infiltration of pulmonary parenchymal lymphatic channels by tumor cells. Usually, spread to lungs is hematogenous, while spread within, lungs is lymphangitic. Unilateral (primary lung cancer and breast carcinoma) involvement is less common than bilateral (stomach, pancreas, prostate, cervical, thyroid, colon, or adenocarcinoma from an unknown site). Eighty percent of the metastases are adenocarcinomas.

On radiographs, LC appears as reticular or reticulonodular opacification, often with associated septal lines (Kerley A and B lines), peribronchial cuffing, pleural effusions, and mediastinal and/or hilar lymphadenopathy (20–50 % of cases).

The mainstay of LC detection is HRCT scanning. Although HRCT scanning is a sensitive technique, the findings may not be diagnostic. HRCT scan findings include the following:

- Irregular, nodular, and/or smooth, interlobular septal thickening
- Thickening of the fissures as a result of the involvement of the lymphatics concentrated in the subpleural interstitium
- Preservation of normal parenchymal architecture at the level of the secondary pulmonary lobule
- Peribronchovascular thickening
- Centrilobular peribronchovascular thickening, which predominates over interlobular septal thickening in a minority of patients
- Polygonal arcades or polygons with prominence of the centrilobular bronchovascular bundle in association with interlobular septal thickening (50 %)
- Mediastinal and/or hilar lymphadenopathy (30–50 %)
- Pleural effusions (30–50 %)

Findings may be unilateral or bilateral, focal or diffuse, and symmetrical or asymmetrical. Focal, unilateral disease accounts for 50 % of cases. This pattern is associated in particular with underlying bronchogenic carcinoma. All of the changes described above are often associated with nodular opacities.

- Sarcoidosis
- Silicosis
- Coal worker's pneumoconiosis
- Extrinsic allergic alveolitis (hypersensitivity pneumonitis)
- Unilateral pulmonary edema
- Lymphoma and Kaposi sarcoma

CRX film shows diffuse reticulonodular infiltrates and presence of right apical mass (Fig. 4.4.1). CT scan (lung window) shows multiple nodes along the interlobular septa which form the sign of "beads" and associated randomly subpleural nodules under 3 mm. Right apical mass was evident (Figs. 4.4.2, 4.4.3, and 4.4.4).

Comments

Differential Diagnosis

Imaging Findings

Case 5: Pulmonary Leukemic Infiltrates (PLI)

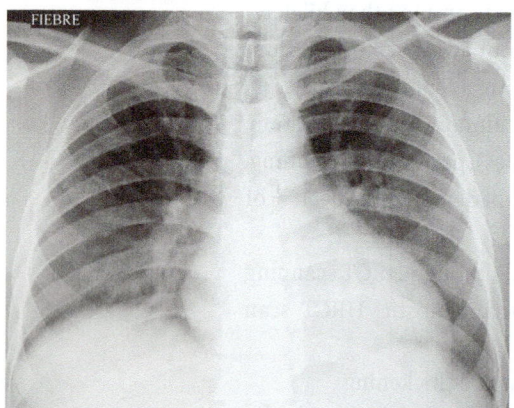

Fig. 4.5.1

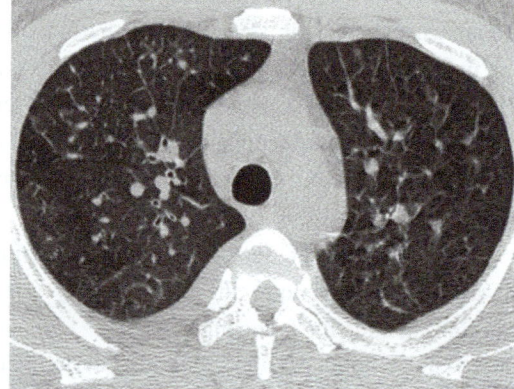

Fig. 4.5.2

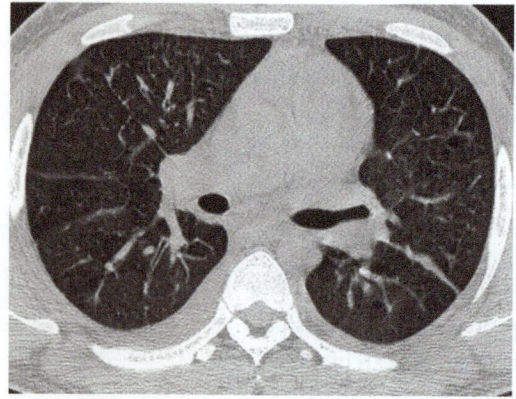

Fig. 4.5.3

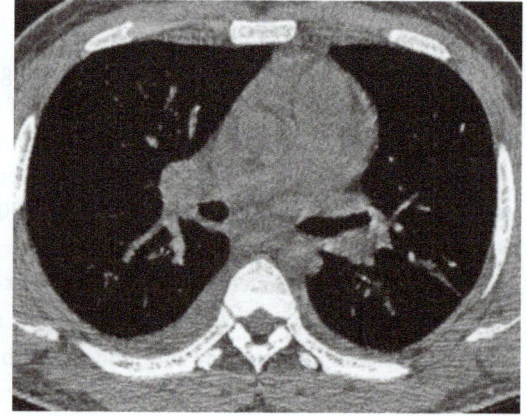

Fig. 4.5.4

A 29-year-old man, came for a clinical consultation for 5 days of fever, fatigue, weakness, dry cough, and dyspnea in the last 2 weeks. Chronic myelogenous (or myeloid) leukemia (CML) diagnosed almost 2 years ago, treated with imatinib 400 mg/day. CBC: WBC, 80,000; neutrophil, 10 %; lymphocytes, 40 %; immature cells, 50 %; hemoglobin, 7.9; hematocrit, 18 %. It is currently in blast crisis.

Comments

Chronic myeloid leukemia (CML) was the first malignancy associated with a genetic lesion and is the primary form of leukemia defined as a distinct entity. It is a chronic myeloproliferative syndrome (SMPC) of clonal nature, originating in a pluripotent stem cell (CMP) common to all 3 hematopoietic series. It accounts for 15–20 % of leukemias, and their impact in Western countries is estimated at 1.5 cases per 100,000 population per year. The median age of onset is around 53 years, and the peak incidence is between 30 and 40. It is lightly predominant in males, with a ratio of 1.3:1.

The disease is characterized by a biphasic or triphasic course and passes through different phases. A chronic phase (CP) is characterized by an expansion of myeloid cells with a normal maturation; 90 % of patients are diagnosed at this stage, and these 15 or 20 % are asymptomatic at diagnosis. The chronic phase progresses to a more aggressive stage, two large patterns following clinical tests: the accelerated phase (AP) and blast crisis (BC). In the later stages, the leukemic cells lose the capacity for terminal differentiation and results in acute leukemia, which is highly resistant to chemotherapy.

Patients with leukemia will encounter various pulmonary complications: infections (bacterial, fungal, viral, and so on), leukemia involvement (pulmonary leukostasis, pulmonary leukemic infiltration, and leukemic cell lysis pneumopathy), and alveolar proteinosis (drug/radiation toxicity, hemorrhage, transfusion-related acute lung injury – TRALI).

All leukemia subtypes can involve the lung, but acute myeloid leukemia, acute lymphoblastic leukemia, and

CLL/SLL are most often seen. Infiltrates are predominantly restricted to the pulmonary lymphatic distribution and rarely form micronodules. Leukemic counts greater than 200,000/μm cause capillary leukostasis with resultant thrombosis. Pulmonary edema, infarct, and diffuse alveolar damage may result.

The X-ray features of PLI are nonspecific and can be normal or show focal homogeneous opacities, diffuse reticulonodular infiltration, or ground glass-like alveolar-type filling opacities. These findings would resemble those of progressive opportunistic infection or severe pulmonary edema. A chest CT is one of the most useful, noninvasive tools for evaluating PLI. In particular, a high-resolution CT (HRCT) is superior to a conventional CT in generating detailed images of the lung parenchyma.

A diagnosis of PLI would be considerably more complicated by chronic graft versus host diseases of the lung (late-onset noninfectious pulmonary complications) such as bronchiolitis obliterans (BO) and organizing pneumonia (OP) in patients after hematopoietic stem cell transplantation (HSCT). Bronchial dilation, centrilobular opacities, tree-inbud appearance, and a mosaic pattern are typical CT findings of BO. Characteristic CT findings of OP are GGO or airspace consolidation distributed along the peribronchial and subpleural regions.

Imaging Findings

CRX film shows interstitial infiltrate, predominantly perihilar (Fig. 4.5.1). CT scan (lung and mediastinal window) shows nodules and nodular thickening of interlobular septa and bilateral pleural effusion (Figs. 4.5.2, 4.5.3, and 4.5.4).

Case 6: Lung Cystic

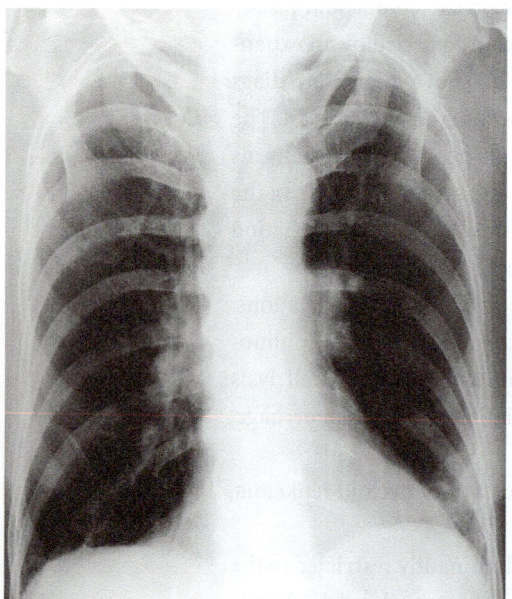

Fig. 4.6.1

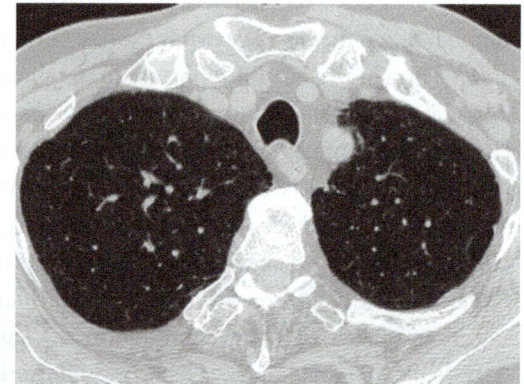

Fig. 4.6.2

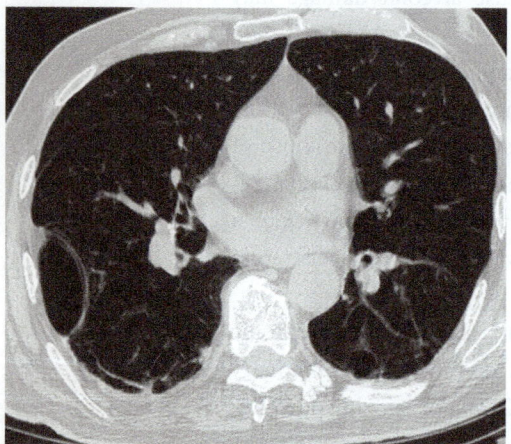

Fig. 4.6.3

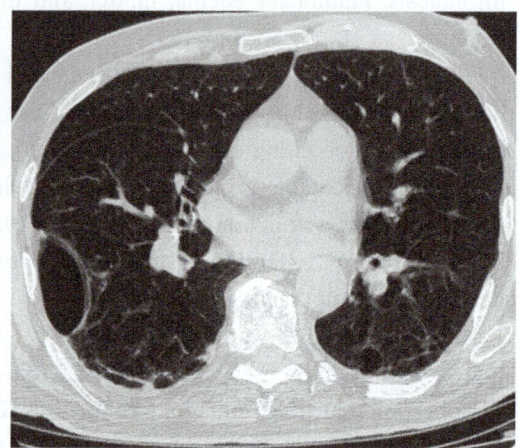

Fig. 4.6.4

A 73-year-old man with diagnosis of COPD, type bullous.

Comments

A lung cyst is defined as a well-circumscribed, air-filled structure that is localized within the lung parenchyma, is >1 cm in diameter, and has a definable epithelial or fibrous wall that is usually <1 mm thick but that may be up to 2 or 3 mm thick. Pulmonary cysts may occur as an isolated abnormality but may also be present in a multifocal distribution or even involve the lung parenchyma diffusely.

Cystic lung diseases are rare entities characterized by multiple intrapulmonary cysts. The more common of these rare disorders are Langerhans cell histiocytosis (LCH) and lymphangioleiomyomatosis (LAM). Less common ones include *Pneumocystis jiroveci* pneumonia, Birt-Hogg-Dubé syndrome (BHDS), lymphocytic interstitial pneumonia (LIP), and amyloidosis.

Air-filled lucencies within the lung parenchyma are frequently detected on routine chest CT. These lucent areas may represent pulmonary cysts, but other causes include cavities, emphysema, bronchiectasis, and honeycombing. These entities can mimic a lung cyst on both chest radiograph and chest CT and should be excluded before labeling a patient as having cystic lung disease. Additional imaging findings, clinical data, and laboratory data help narrow the differential diagnosis.

Causes of focal or multifocal cystic lung:

Bullae

Blebs

Pneumatoceles

Congenital cystic lesions (bronchogenic cyst, congenital adenomatoid malformation)

Infections (coccidioidomycosis, *Pneumocystis jiroveci*, hydatid disease)

Traumatic cysts

Causes of diffuse cystic lung:

Pulmonary lymphangioleiomyomatosis

Pulmonary Langerhans cell histiocytosis

Honeycomb lung (idiopathic pulmonary fibrosis, connective tissue disease-related pulmonary fibrosis, asbestosis, chronic hypersensitivity pneumonitis)

Advanced sarcoidosis

Bronchiectasis, diffuse

Metastatic disease (rare)

Imaging Findings

CRX film shows signs of pulmonary overexpansion and presence of air density image in the right lower lobe in intimate contact with the pleura (Fig. 4.6.1). CT scan (lung window) shows presence of air density image, thin walls (1–2 mm), the largest in the right lower lobe in intimate contact with the pleura (Figs. 4.6.2, 4.6.3, and 4.6.4).

Case 7: Atelectasis

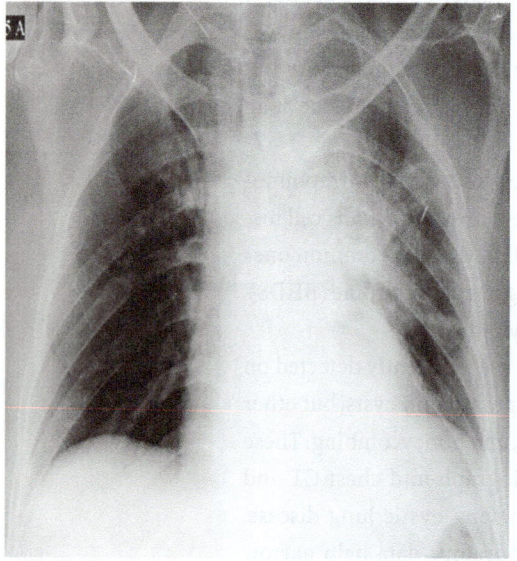

Fig. 4.7.1

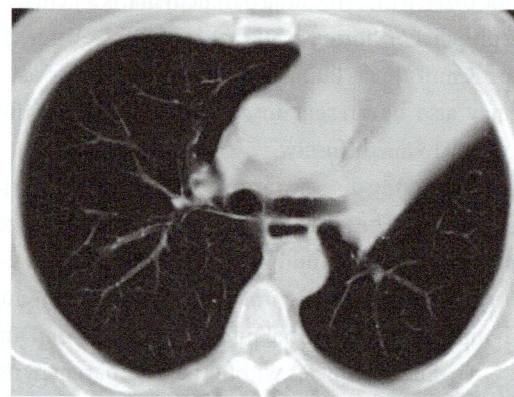

Fig. 4.7.2

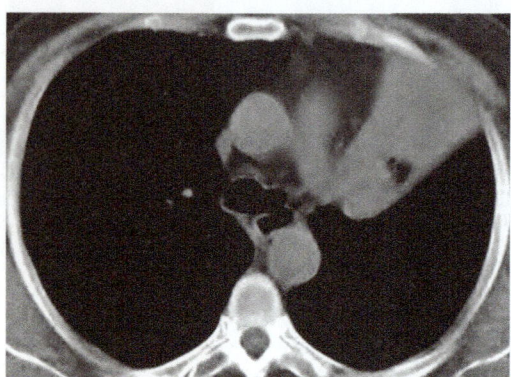

Fig. 4.7.3

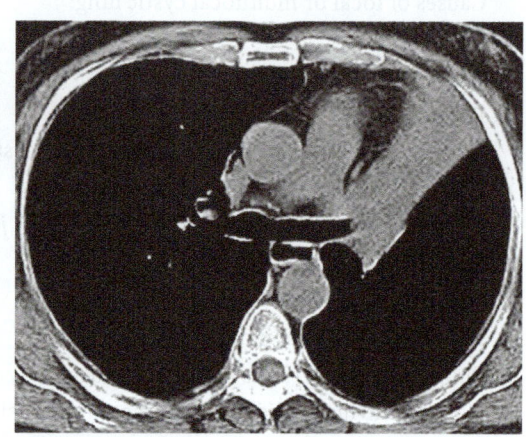

Fig. 4.7.4

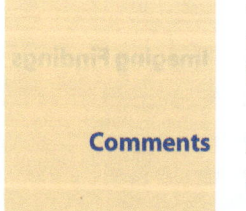

A 55-year-old man refers dry cough and chest pain. History of carcinoma of the penis. Bronchoscopy shows endobronchial lesion obstructing 90 % at the bifurcation of the left upper lobe.

Comments   Atelectasis is reduced inflation of all or part of the lung. The synonym *collapse* is often used interchangeably with *atelectasis*, particularly when it is severe or accompanied by obvious increase in lung opacity.

Chest radiographs and CT scans show direct and indirect signs of lobar collapse. Direct signs include displacement of fissures and opacification of the collapsed lobe. Indirect signs include the following: displacement of the hilum, mediastinal shift toward the side of collapse, loss of volume in the ipsilateral hemithorax, elevation of the ipsilateral diaphragm, crowding of the ribs, compensatory hyperlucency of the remaining lobes, and silhouetting of the diaphragm or heart border.

Right upper lobe collapse: The RUL is bordered medially by the mediastinum, superiorly by the chest wall, inferiorly by the minor fissure, and posteroinferiorly by the superior portion of the oblique fissure. On CT scanning, RUL collapse appears as a right paratracheal opacity, and the minor fissure appears concave laterally. The RUL collapses against the mediastinum, and this is identified as a wedge of uniform attenuation extending along the mediastinum to the anterior chest wall.

Right middle lobe collapse: The RML is bounded medially by the right heart border, anteriorly and laterally by the chest wall, posteriorly by the major fissure, and superiorly by the minor fissure. As the RML collapses, the minor fissure shifts downward, and the oblique fissure is displaced forward. With a progressive loss of volume, the middle lobe collapses medially against the right heart border. The collapsed middle lobe is a wedge-shaped opacity that extends laterally from the hilum toward the lateral chest wall. It is bounded posteriorly by the RLL and anteriorly by the hyperinflated RUL. On CT scans, a triangular opacity along the right heart border, with the apex pointing laterally, is a characteristic finding. This appearance resembles a tilted ice-cream cone.

Right lower lobe collapse: The RLL is bordered inferiorly by the hemidiaphragm, posteriorly and laterally by the chest wall, medially by the heart and mediastinum, and anteriorly by the major fissure. The RLL generally collapses in a posteromedial direction against the posterior mediastinum and spine. An endobronchial lesion may result in a convex lateral contour of the collapsed RLL. The major fissure is displaced posteromedially.

Left upper lobe collapse: The LUL is bounded medially by the mediastinum, inferiorly by the left heart border, superiorly and laterally by the chest wall, and posteriorly by the major fissure. CT scanning shows the inferior location of the collapsed lobe and the shift of the RUL across the midline. LUL collapse occurs anterosuperiorly. As opposed to the RUL, the collapsed LUL maintains more contact with the anterior and lateral chest wall. Hyperaeration of the superior segment of the LLL may cause displacement and superior movement; these changes may account for periaortic lucency or the *Luftsichel* sign on PA images.

Left lower lobe collapse: The LLL is bordered inferiorly by the hemidiaphragm, posteriorly and laterally by the chest wall, medially by the heart and mediastinum, and anteriorly by the major fissure. The LLL collapses medially toward the mediastinum and maintains contact with the hemidiaphragms.

Imaging Findings

CRX film shows pulmonary opacity and decreased left lung volume, with consequent elevation of the left hemidiaphragm (Fig. 4.7.1). CT scan (lung and mediastinal window) shows image attenuating associated left upper lobe bronchus abrupt discontinuation (Figs. 4.7.2, 4.7.3, and 4.7.4).

Case 8: Cavitary Lung

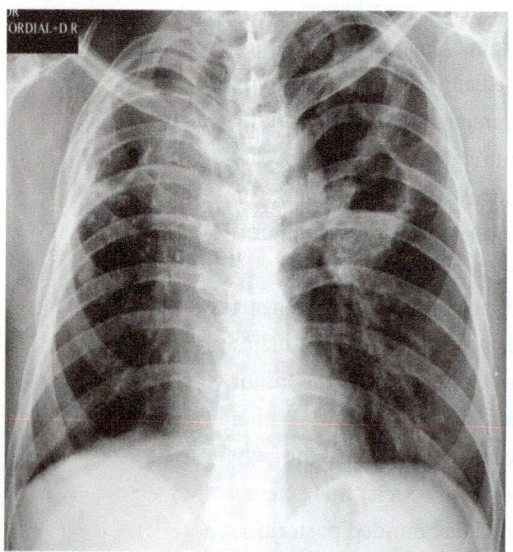

Fig. 4.8.1

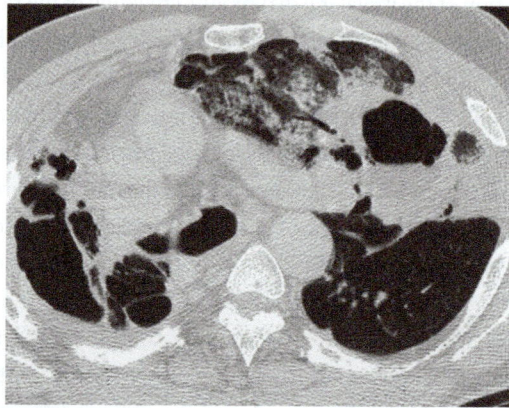

Fig. 4.8.2

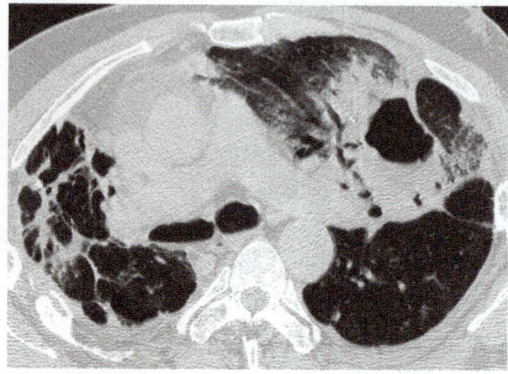

Fig. 4.8.3

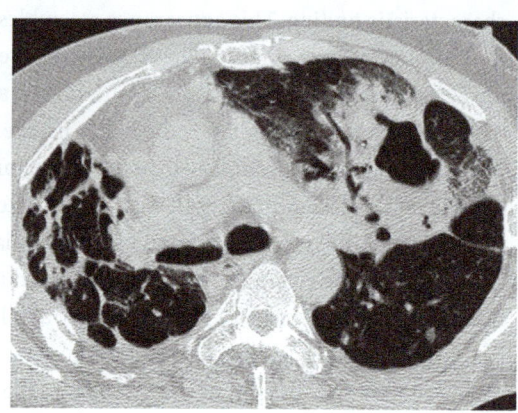

Fig. 4.8.4

A 51-year-old man with diagnosis of tuberculosis.

Comments   Cavities are air-filled spaces within the pulmonary parenchyma with definable walls that are thicker than the ones seen in lung cysts (usually >4 mm). The distinction between lung cysts and cavities is mainly based on this difference in wall thickness.

Causes of focal or multifocal cavitary lung:

Neoplastic: bronchogenic carcinomas, metastases, lymphomas

Infections: bacteria (*Staphylococcus aureus*, gram-negative bacteria, pneumococcus, mycobacteria, melioidosis, anaerobes, actinomycosis, nocardiosis), fungi (histoplasmosis, coccidioidomycosis, blastomycosis, aspergillosis, mucormycosis, cryptococcosis, *P. jiroveci*, sporotrichosis), parasites (hydatid disease, paragonimiasis, amebiasis)

Immunologic: Wegener's granulomatosis, rheumatoid nodule

Thromboembolism or septic embolism

Progressive massive fibrosis (pneumoconiosis)

Bronchiectasis, localized

Congenital lesions (sequestration, congenital adenomatoid malformation)

The differential diagnosis of cavitary lesions is broader. Most isolated cavitary lung lesions are bronchogenic carcinomas. Cavitation in primary lung cancer is not rare. Cavitation detected on plain chest radiographs has been reported in 2–16 % of primary lung cancers, and it is detected with computed tomography (CT) in 22 % of primary lung cancers. Squamous cell carcinoma is the most common histological type of lung cancer to cavitate (82 % of cavitary primary lung cancer).

Metastatic lung lesions also can cavitate, but this occurs less frequently than in primary lung cancers. The frequency of cavitation in metastatic tumor detected by plain radiograph is 4 %.

Cavitary lesions in patients with lymphoma are infrequent; however, pulmonary lymphoma can cavitate. These cavities are usually multiple with thick walls and have an upper lobe predominance. However, in lymphoma patients with human immunodeficiency virus (HIV) infection, cavitation is not rare, and ≤25 % of patients can have a cavitary lesion detected on CT images.

Pulmonary embolism causes infarction in less than 15 % of cases, and only about 5 % of infarctions cavitate.

Causes of diffuse cavitary lung:

Pulmonary lymphangioleiomyomatosis

Pulmonary Langerhans cell histiocytosis

Honeycomb lung (idiopathic pulmonary fibrosis, connective tissue disease-related pulmonary fibrosis, asbestosis, chronic hypersensitivity pneumonitis)

Advanced sarcoidosis

Bronchiectasis, diffuse

Metastatic disease (rare)

Imaging Findings

CRX film shows right apical lung opacity, resulting in decreased volume and displacement of the trachea, with thick-walled fluid level (greater than 4 mm) in the left upper lobe (Fig. 4.8.1). CT scan (lung window) shows image with hydro-air level of apical dominance that is associated with areas of atelectasis, fibrotic bands, pleural thickening, and ground-glass opacity in the left lung (Figs. 4.8.2, 4.8.3, and 4.8.4).

Case 9: Pneumonia *P. jiroveci*

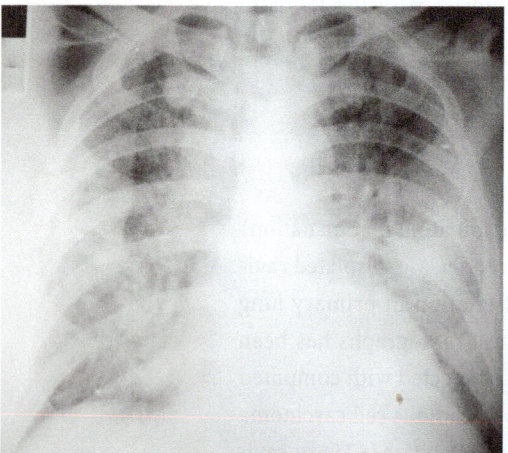

Fig. 4.9.1

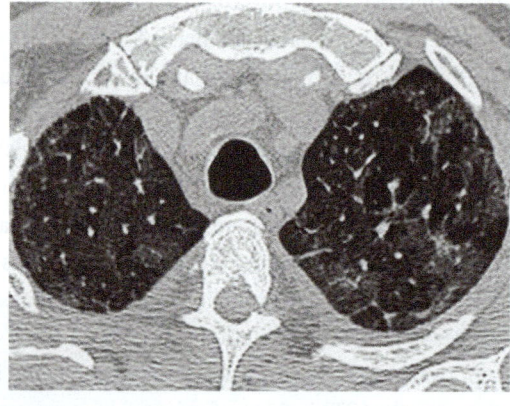

Fig. 4.9.2

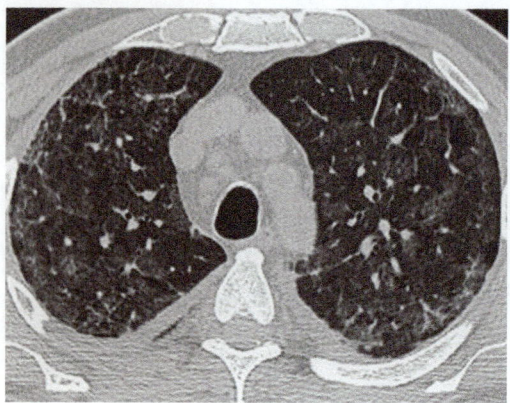

Fig. 4.9.3

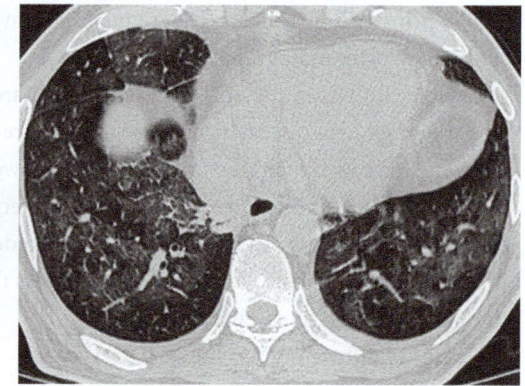

Fig. 4.9.4

A 63-year-old man with history of cough, fever, and weight loss. HIV-positive serology and Western blot indeterminate.

Comments

The disease known as Pneumocystis carinii pneumonia (PCP) is one of the entities that cause disease and death in people with immunodeficiency, including malnourished children. The PCP has long been the most common opportunistic infection in AIDS patients. The introduction of antiretroviral therapy highly active (HAART – highly active antiretroviral therapy) has been accompanied by a substantial reduction in mortality and the incidence of opportunistic infections, including PCP.

Chest radiographs should be included in the initial evaluation for PCP. Frequently, these are the only images required. High-resolution computed tomography (HRCT) scanning and, occasionally, gallium-67 (^{67}Ga) scanning are useful in symptomatic patients in whom chest radiograph findings are normal or equivocal. Chest radiograph findings may be normal in 10–39 % of patients with PCP. With CT and ^{67}Ga scanning, the appearance of PCP is nonspecific.

HRCT scanning is more sensitive than chest radiography for the detection and exclusion of *Pneumocystis pneumonia* (PCP), and the results may be positive when chest radiograph findings are normal.

The hallmark finding of PCP on HRCT scans is ground-glass attenuation, which is present in more than 90 % of patients and represents an exudative alveolitis. This usually occurs in a bilateral, symmetrical, predominantly perihilar distribution and may be geographic or mosaic in appearance (56 %), with areas of normal lung adjacent to areas of affected lung.

Thickening of interlobular septa (due to edema) and foci of consolidation may be associated. Septal thickening in the subacute stage is usually more extensive and represents organizing inflammatory infiltrate.

Differential diagnosis of *Pneumocystis pneumonia* (PCP):

The presence of ground-glass attenuation on HRCT scans in patients with AIDS is virtually diagnostic of PCP, with a diagnostic accuracy of approximately 94 %. Normal HRCT findings virtually exclude the possibility of PCP. Ground-glass attenuation is highly suggestive of PCP, but cytomegalovirus (CMV), pneumonitis, and lymphoid interstitial pneumonia can (albeit infrequently) give rise to a similar appearance.

However, CMV pneumonitis is rare in patients with CD4 counts of greater than 50 cells/mm^3.

Ground-glass opacification can also be seen in conditions such as pulmonary edema, pulmonary hemorrhage, drug toxicity, other infections, and hypersensitivity pneumonitis. Clinical correlation usually allows the exclusion of most of these differential diagnoses.

Hilar lymphadenopathy may occur in patients with tuberculosis, *Mycobacterium avium-intracellulare* (MAI or MAC) infection, fungal infection, Kaposi's sarcoma, and AIDS-related lymphoma, but this condition is rare in patients with PCP.

Imaging Findings

CRX film shows bilateral opacities predominantly peripheral which produce blurring of bronchovascular contours (Fig. 4.9.1). CT scan (lung window) shows bilateral ground-glass opacity (Figs. 4.9.2, 4.9.3, and 4.9.4).

Case 10: Radiation Pneumonitis

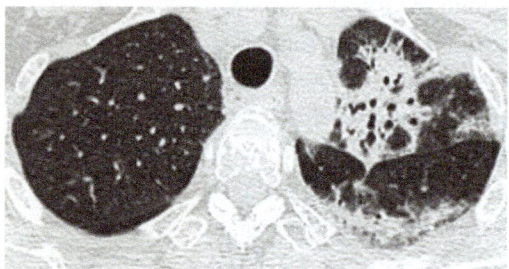

Fig. 4.10.1

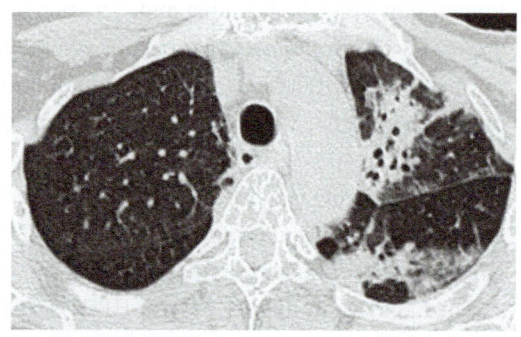

Fig. 4.10.2

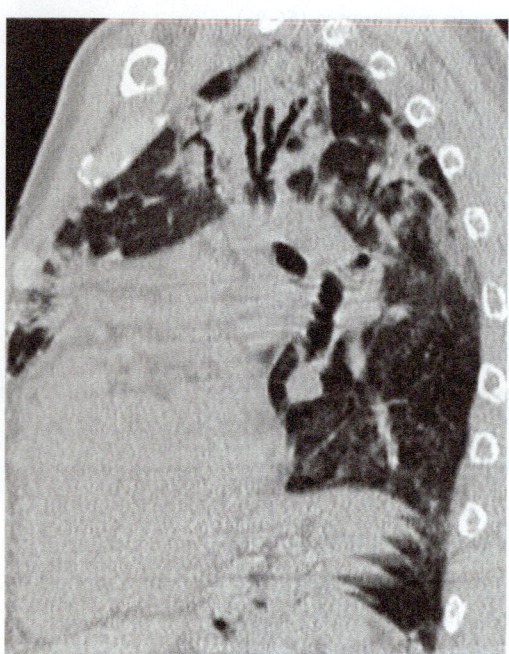

Fig. 4.10.3

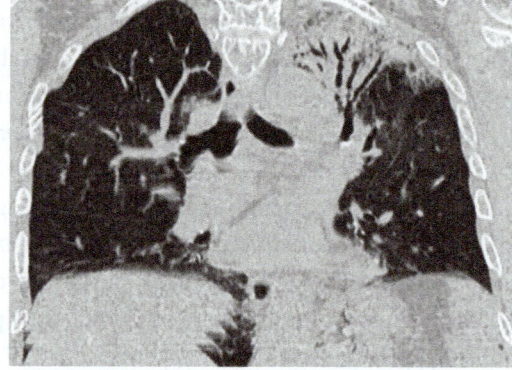

Fig. 4.10.4

A 55-year-old woman with a history of persistent dry cough. Radiation pneumonitis after radiotherapy for breast cancer.

Comments   Pneumonitis and radiation fibrosis are complications of radiation treatment affecting approximately 40 % of cancer patients undergoing this therapy, although the clinical manifestations occur in less than 7 % of cases. Radiation pneumonitis is a well-described complication of chest radiotherapy administered to patients for mediastinal, breast, and lung tumors.

Many factors fuel-induced lung damage rays among which is the lung volume irradiated, the dose received and the time it was administered, the withdrawal of corticosteroids, previous history of radiotherapy, association with cytostatic agents such as bleomycin, the existence of prior lung disease (chronic obstructive pulmonary disease: COPD) and individual susceptibility.

The harmful effects often occur when the dose varies between 3,000 and 4,000 cGy, but at higher doses, they are invariably present.

Changes are shown from 4 weeks in the methods of diagnostic imaging. As early as radiation pneumonitis, one can see areas of parenchymal consolidation, ground-glass opacities, loss of lung volume, increased radiolucency, pulmonary bullae formation, and signs of pulmonary embolism, and radiation therapy can produce an obliterative vasculitis. At the stage of fibrosis (beyond 6 months) obliteration of lung architecture, parenchymal opacities, and peripheral dense bands that radiate from the hilum to the periphery were found which require the differential diagnosis lymphangitis carcinomatosa.

Tomography of the chest with high-resolution technique (HRCT) is much more sensitive and specific than chest radiography to detect changes in patients with normal plates and also shows signs of relapse or recurrence of the underlying disease.

HRCT is sensitive and highly useful for the detection of this pathology, not only showing signs of lung injury but also pleural, pericardial, and mediastinal, allowing the diagnosis differential with a recurrence of the underlying disease whose clinical manifestations can be similar.

Acute Radiation Pneumonitis

- CT findings of acute radiation pneumonitis
  - Homogeneous slight increase in attenuation (2–4 months after therapy)
  - Patchy consolidation (1–12 months after therapy)
  - Nonuniform discrete consolidation (most commonly 3 months to 10 years after therapy)

Chronic Radiation Damage

- CT Findings
  - Solid consolidation (radiation fibrosis) + bronchiectasis (stabilized by 1 year after therapy)

Imaging Findings

CT scan (lung window) shows opacified apex projected on the left lung, causing decrease in volume and pleural thickening and traction bronchiectasis (Figs. 4.10.1, 4.10.2, 4.10.3, and 4.10.4).

Case 11: Intralobar Sequestration

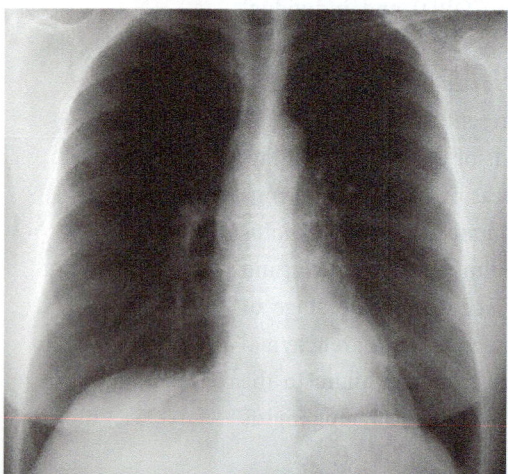

Fig. 4.11.1

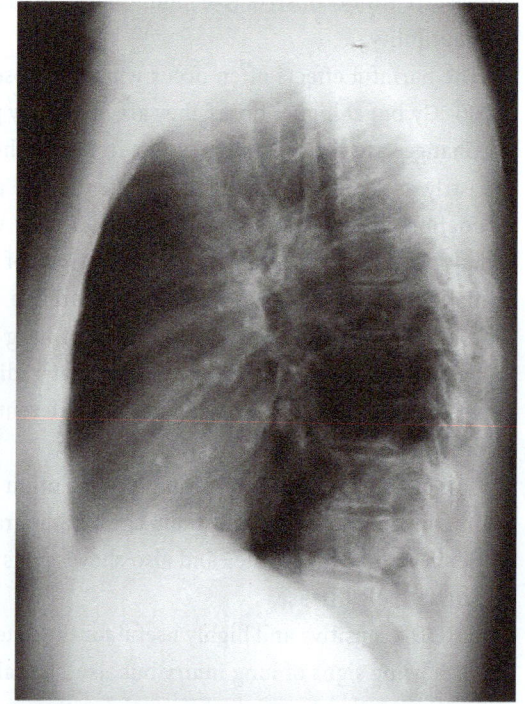

Fig. 4.11.2

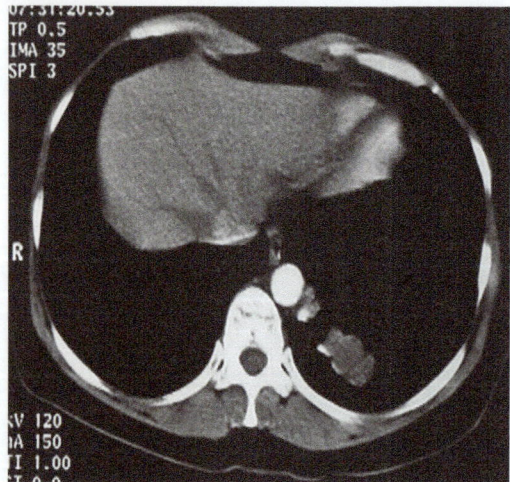

Fig. 4.11.3

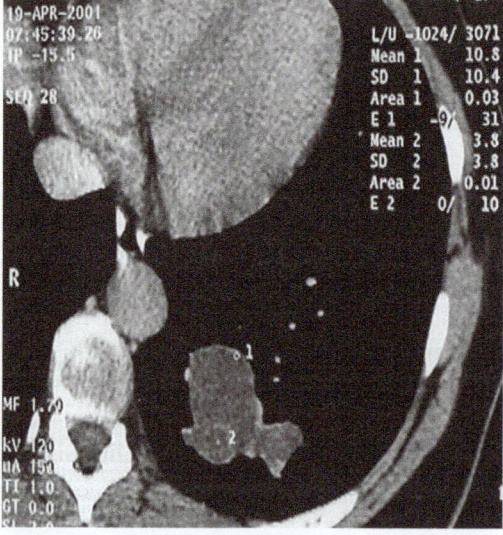

Fig. 4.11.4

A 19-year-old woman with histories of recurrent pulmonary infections.

Comments

Bronchopulmonary sequestration (BPS), sometimes referred to simply as pulmonary sequestration, is a rare congenital malformation of the lower respiratory tract. It consists of a nonfunctioning mass of lung tissue that lacks normal communication with the tracheobronchial tree and that receives its arterial blood supply from the systemic circulation.

Sequestrations are classified anatomically as follows:

Intralobar pulmonary sequestration (ILS, also known as intrapulmonary sequestration) is a relatively uncommon pulmonary disorder that is characterized by nonfunctioning lung tissue that lacks normal connection with the tracheobronchial tree and has a systemic arterial blood supply. Patients with an intralobar sequestration typically present before the age of 20 years with histories of recurrent pulmonary infections.

At radiography, intralobar sequestrations can manifest as an area of increased opacity simulating pneumonia, as a mass with or without air-fluid levels or as cysts. The lower lobes (98 %) are the most common site, particularly the left (60 %). Upper lobe or bilateral involvement is rare (2 %). Brochiectasis, subsegmental atelectasis, mediastinal shift, and prominence of the ipsilateral hilum are additional radiographic findings.

CT scans show a homogeneous or inhomogeneous solid mass, with or without definable cystic changes. It may also manifest as an aggregate of multiple small cystic lesions with air or fluid content, a well-defined cystic mass, or a large cavitary lesion with air-fluid level. Emphysematous changes at the margins are characteristic CT finding of bronchopulmonary sequestration produced by collateral air drift. Occasionally, bronchopulmonary sequestration manifests as focal emphysema generated by markedly hyperinflated alveoli. The pseudotumorous bronchopulmonary sequestration form may appear as a speculated mass mimicking a malignant tumor.

Classically, the diagnosis of pulmonary sequestration hinges on the identification of an anomalous arterial feeding vessel from the aorta. Although CT and CTA continue to be the primary means for diagnosing bronchopulmonary sequestrations, the use of MR and Gd-enhanced MRA can serve as a suitable alternative, especially in patients in which the use of iodinated contrast agents is contraindicated such as those with known allergy to iodinated contrast agents or renal insufficiency.

The radiologic differential diagnosis of pulmonary sequestration is extensive, but the main considerations include bronchial atresia, cystic adenomatoid malformation, lobar emphysema, intrapulmonary bronchogenic cyst, bronchiectasis, pneumonia, abscess, arteriovenous fistula or malformation, and systemic arterial supply to nonsequestered lung.

Imaging Findings

CRX film shows opacity in the left lung base causing slight displacement of the mediastinum (Figs. 4.11.1 and 4.11.2). CT scan (arterial phase) shows soft tissue density lesion with sharp outlines that are in contact with glass coming from the aorta (Figs. 4.11.3 and 4.11.4).

Case 12: Lipoid Pneumonia

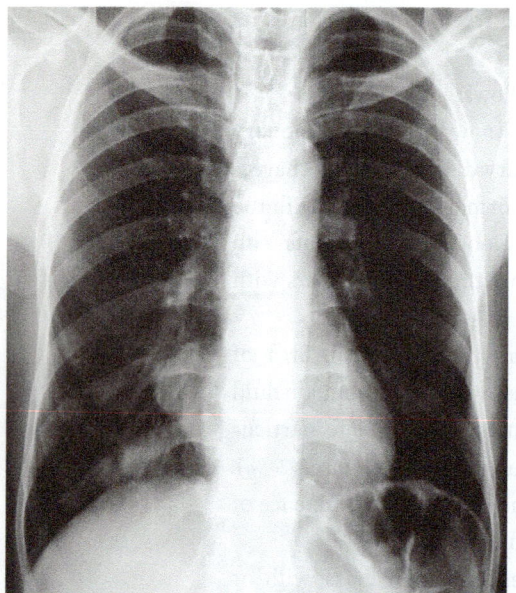

Fig. 4.12.1

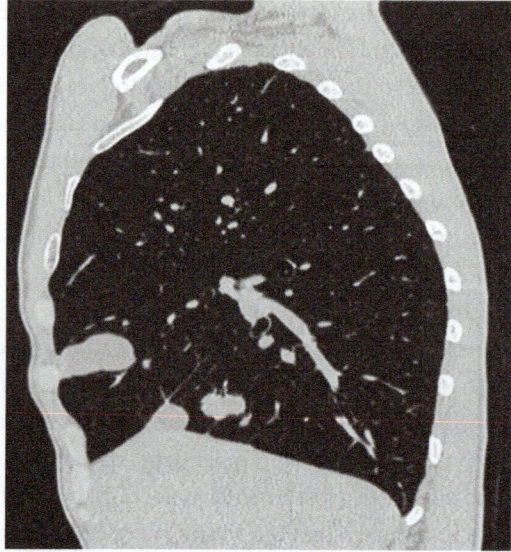

Fig. 4.12.2

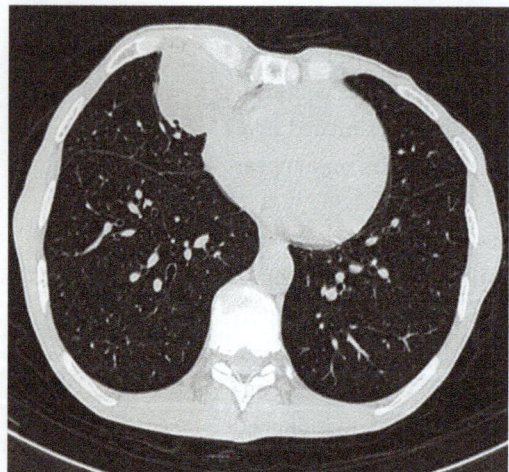

Fig. 4.12.3

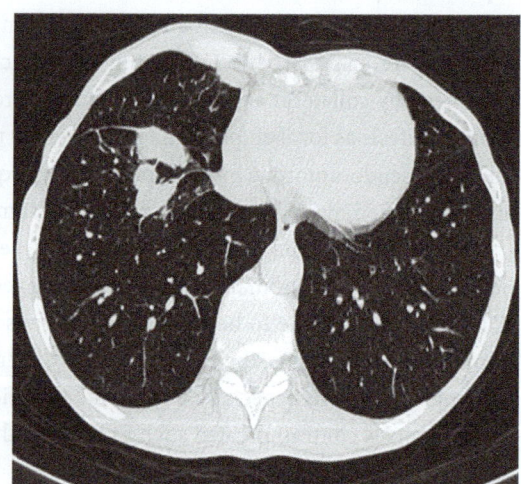

Fig. 4.12.4

A 51-year-old man with 1-month history of dry cough, fever, dyspnea, and weight loss. Hydrocarbon aspiration was by accident. Percutaneous lung biopsy is consistent with lipoid pneumonia.

Lipoid pneumonia can be either exogenous or endogenous in cause based on the source of the lipid. Exogenous lipoid pneumonia usually occurs when animal fats or mineral or vegetable oils are aspirated or inhaled, whereas endogenous lipoid pneumonia results from lipid accumulation within intra-alveolar macrophages in the setting of bronchial obstruction, chronic pulmonary infection, pulmonary alveolar proteinosis, or fat storage diseases. Unfortunately, lipoid pneumonia can mimic the clinical and radiologic features of other diseases including primary lung carcinoma, and histopathologic confirmation of the diagnosis may be necessary.

Acute exogenous lipoid pneumonia is uncommon and typically is caused by an episode of aspiration of a large quantity of a petroleum-based product. Although acute pneumonitis after aspiration of petroleum-based products typically occurs in children due to accidental poisoning, acute exogenous lipoid pneumonia also occurs in performers (fire-eaters) who use liquid hydrocarbons for flame blowing.

Chronic exogenous lipoid pneumonia usually results from repeated episodes of aspiration or inhalation of animal fat or mineral or vegetable oils over an extended period. Although chronic exogenous lipoid pneumonia typically occurs in older patients, it also has been reported in children, especially those with a predisposition to aspiration, including mental retardation and cleft palate, as well as in infants when mineral oil is used as a lubricant to facilitate feeding.

Acute exogenous lipoid pneumonia can manifest radiologically within 30 min of the episode of aspiration or inhalation, and pulmonary opacities can be seen in most patients within 24 h. The opacities are typically ground-glass or consolidative, bilateral, and segmental or lobar in distribution and predominantly involve the middle and lower lobes. Other manifestations include poorly marginated nodules, pneumatoceles, pneumomediastinum, pneumothorax, and pleural effusions.

Pneumatoceles usually occur within regions of ground-glass or consolidative opacities, typically manifest radiologically within 2–30 days after aspiration or inhalation, and are more common in patients who have aspirated or inhaled a large amount of mineral oils or petroleum-based products. Pneumothorax and pneumomediastinum are rare and have been reported to occur within 4 days after hydrocarbon aspiration.

CT scan reveals areas of fat attenuation as low as −30 HU within the consolidative opacities and nodules, a finding diagnostic of lipoid pneumonia. The radiologic manifestations of acute exogenous lipoid pneumonia typically improve or resolve over time. Resolution of opacities is variable and usually

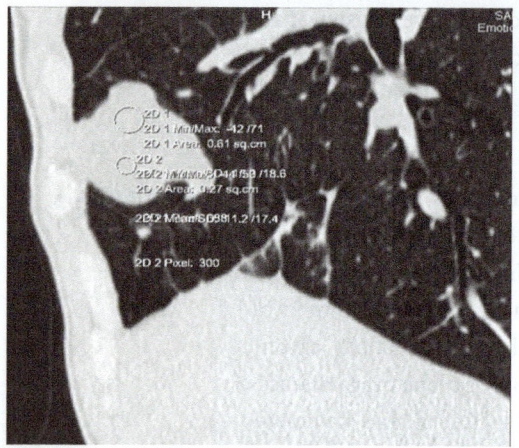

Fig. 4.12.5

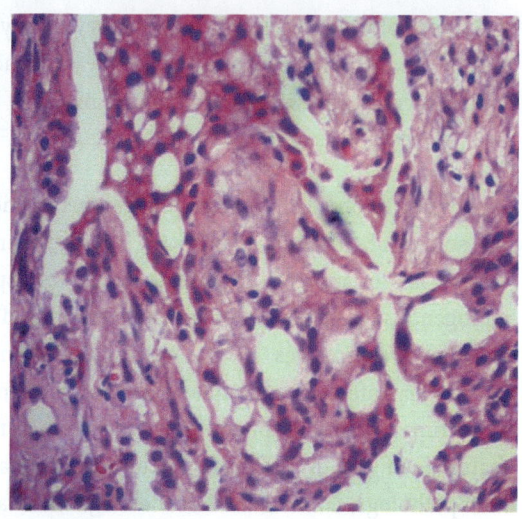

Fig. 4.12.6

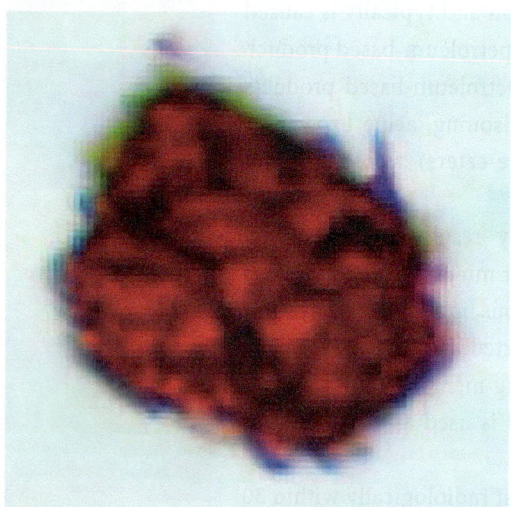

Fig. 4.12.7

occurs within 2 weeks to 8 months. Typically, resolution is complete, although minimal scarring can occur.

Chronic exogenous lipoid pneumonia most frequently manifests as ground-glass or consolidative opacities involving one or more segments, typically with a peribronchovascular distribution and predominant involvement of the lower lobes.

Architectural distortion associated with the consolidative opacities has been reported, and thickening of the interlobular septa or fibrosis in the adjacent lungs can occur in the later stages due to the transportation of oils from the alveoli into the lung interstitium. Additionally, ground-glass opacities with associated interlobular septal thickening (crazy-paving pattern) with a basilar predominance have also been described.

Characteristically, chronic exogenous lipoid pneumonia manifests as an adipose-containing mass. Although the mass is typically irregular or spiculated as a result of chronic inflammation and secondary fibrosis, the presence of fat in the mass is, with a few exceptions, a diagnostic feature of exogenous lipoid pneumonia.

Cavitation and calcification of the mass occasionally can occur. Other manifestations of chronic exogenous lipoid pneumonia are single or multiple nodules or masses that may or may not contain fat.

Imaging Findings

CRX film shows occupation of the airspace in the basal and anterior segment of the right lower lobe (Fig. 4.12.1). CT scan (lung window) shows opacity of fat density, well-defined edges, and lobed appearance in the middle lobe and right lower lobe (Figs. 4.12.2, 4.12.3, 4.12.4, and 4.12.5). Lung biopsy, HE staining and staining sudan granulomatous foreign body reaction in relation to fat, septal thickening by cellular proliferation of lymphocytes, histiocytes and fibroblasts; pneumocytes hyperplasia (Figs. 4.12.6, and 4.12.7).

Further Reading

Pulmonary Epithelioid Hemangioendothelioma

Azcárate L, Oliveros E et al (2009) Hemangioendothelioma pulmonary. Arch Bronconeumol 45(9):466–468

Cronin P, Arenberg D (2004) Pulmonary epithelioid hemangioendothelioma: an unusual case and a review of the literature. Chest 125:789–792

Gill R, O'Donnell RJ, Horvai A (2009) Utility of immunohistochemistry for endothelial markers in distinguishing epithelioid hemangioendothelioma from carcinoma metastatic to bone. Arch Pathol Lab Med 133:967–972

Jang KY, Jin GY et al (2003) Pulmonary epithelioid hemangioendothelioma: a tumor presented as a single cavitary mass. J Korean Med Sci 18:599–602

Kim EA, Lele SM, Lackner RP (2011) Primary pleural epithelioid hemangioendothelioma. Ann Thorac Surg 91:301–302

Moran C, Suster S (2010) Tumors and tumor-like conditions of the lung and pleura, 1st edn. Saunders/Elsevier, Philadelphia

Okamura K, Ohshima T, Nakano R et al (2010) Hemangioendothelioma surviving 10 years without treatment. Ann Thorac Cardiovasc Surg 16(6):432–435

Verbeken E, Beyls J, Moerman P et al (1985) Lung metastasis of malignant epithelioid hemangioendothelioma mimicking a primary intravascular bronchioalveolar tumor. A histologic, ultrastructural, and immunohistochemical study. Cancer 55:1741–1746

Weiss SW, Enziger FM (1982) Epithelioid hemangioendothelioma: a vascular tumor often mistaken for a carcinoma. Cancer 1982(50):970–981

Calcified PulmMonary Nodules

Badoual C, Cadranel J, Riquet M, Meatchi T, Danel C (2004) Pulmonary calcified micronodules. Ann Pathol 24:73–74

Boitsios G (2010) Diffuse pulmonary nodules. AJR Am J Roentgenol 194:W354–W366

Kim JS, Ryu CW, Lee SI, Sung DW, Park CK (1999) High-resolution CT findings of varicella-zoster pneumonia. AJR Am J Roentgenol 172:113–116

Kim EA, Lee KS, Primack SL, Yoon HK, Byun HS, Kim ST et al (2002) Viral pneumonias in adults: radiologic and pathologic findings. Radiographics 22:137–149

Marchiori E, Souza AS Jr, Franquet T, Müller NL (2005) Diffuse high-attenuation pulmonary abnormalities: a pattern-oriented diagnostic approach on high-resolution CT. AJR Am J Roentgenol 184:273–282

Mohsen AH, Peck RJ, Mason Z, Mattock L, McKendrick MW (2002) Risks factors for pneumonia in adults with chickenpox. J Infect Dis 186:1052–1053

Nishimura K, Itoh H, Kitaichi M et al (1993) Pulmonary sarcoidosis: correlation of CT and histopathologic findings. Radiology 189:105–109

Raider L (1991) Calcification in chickenpox pneumonia. Chest 60:504–507

Raoof S, Amchentsev A, Vlahos I et al (2006) Pictorial essay: multinodular disease. Chest 129:805–815

Rodríguez Borregan JC, Domínguez Artiga MJ, Miñambres E, Tejerina Álvarez E, Holanda Peña MS, Gónzalez Férnández C et al (2003) Neumonía varicelosa en adultos: 30 casos. An Med Interna (Madrid) 12:612–616

Ulbright TM, Katzenstein AL (1980) Solitary necrotizing granulomas of the lung: differentiating features and etiology. Am J Surg Pathol 4:13–28

Pulmonary Metastasis

Aquino SL (2005) Imaging of metastatic disease to the thorax. Radiol Clin North Am 43(3):481–495, vii

Cockshott WP, Hendrickse JP (1969) Pulmonary calcification at the site of trophoblastic metastases. Br J Radiol 42(493):17–20

de Santos LA, Lindell MM Jr, Goldman AM, Luna MA, Murray JA (1978) Calcification within metastatic pulmonary nodules from synovial sarcoma. Orthopedics 1(2):141–144

Jiménez JM, Casey SO, Citron M, Khan A (1995) Calcified pulmonary metastases from medullary carcinoma of the thyroid. Comput Med Imaging Graph 19(4):325–328

Murphey MD, Robbin MR, McRae GA, Flemming DJ, Temple HT, Kransdorf MJ (1997) The many faces of osteosarcoma. Radiographics 17(5):1205–1231

Seo JB, Im JG, Goo JM et al (2001) Atypical pulmonary metastases: spectrum of radiologic findings. Radiographics 21:403–417

Lymphangitic Carcinomatosis

Bhargava R, Winer-Muram HT, Kauffman WM et al (1994) Chest radiographic features of thoracic metastatic disease in adolescents with colon cancer. Pediatr Radiol 24(7):491–493

Davis SD (1991) CT evaluation for pulmonary metastases in patients with extrathoracic malignancy. Radiology 180(1):1–12

Hirakata K, Nakata H, Nakagawa T (1995) CT of pulmonary metastases with pathological correlation. Semin Ultrasound CT MR 16(5):379–394

Honda O, Johkoh T, Ichikado K et al (1999) Comparison of high resolution CT findings of sarcoidosis, lymphoma, and lymphangitic carcinoma: is there any difference of involved interstitium? J Comput Assist Tomogr 23(3):374–379

Johkoh T, Ikezoe J, Tomiyama N et al (1992) CT findings in lymphangitic carcinomatosis of the lung: correlation with histologic findings and pulmonary function tests. AJR Am J Roentgenol 158(6):1217–1222

Masson RG, Krikorian J, Lukl P et al (1989) Pulmonary microvascular cytology in the diagnosis of lymphangitic carcinomatosis. N Engl J Med 321(2):71–76

Munk PL, Muller NL, Miller RR et al (1988) Pulmonary lymphangitic carcinomatosis: CT and pathologic findings. Radiology 166(3):705–709

NEJM (1990) Pulmonary microvascular cytology in lymphangitic carcinomatosis. N Engl J Med. 322(1):59–60

Potente G, Bellelli A, Nardis P (1992) Specific diagnosis by CT and HRCT in six chronic lung diseases. Comput Med Imaging Graph 16(4):277–282

Rastogi R, Garg R, Thulkar S et al (2008) Unusual thoracic CT manifestations of osteosarcoma: review of 16 cases. Pediatr Radiol 38(5):551–558

Spillane RM, Shepard JA, DeLuca SA (1993) High-resolution CT of the lungs. Am Fam Physician 48(3):493–498

Pulmonary Leukemic Infiltrates

Barnes DJ, Melo J (2003) Management of chronic myeloid leukemia. Targets for molecular therapy. Semin Hematol 40:34–49

Cortés J, Kantarjian H (2004) Advanced phase chronic myeloid leukemia. Semin Hematol 40:79–86

Goldman J (2003) Chronic myeloid leukemia. Past, present and future. Semin Hematol 40:1–3

Goldman J, Melo J (2003) Chronic myeloid leukemia. Advances in biology and new approaches to treatment. N Engl J Med 349:1451–1464

Hernández P (2001) Nueva opción terapéutica en la leucemia mieloide crónica. Rev Cubana Hematol Inmunol Hemoter 40:205–210

Heyneman LE, Johkoh T, Ward S et al (2000) Pulmonary leukemic infiltrates: high-resolution CT findings in 10 patients. AJR Am J Roentgenol 174(2):517–521

Hochhaus A, Kreil S, Corbin AS, La Rosée P, Muller MC, Lahaye T et al (2002) Molecular and chromosomal resistance to Imatinib (STI571) therapy. Leukemia 16:2190–2196

Hudgues TP, Kaeda J, Brandford S, Rudzki P, Hochhaus A, Hensley ML et al (2003) Frequency of major molecular responses to Imatinib or interferon alfa plus cytarabine in newly diagnosed chronic myeloid leukemia. N Engl J Med 9:1423–1432

Melo JV, Hughues TP, Apperly JF (2003) Chronic myeloid leukemia. Hematology Am Soc Hematol Educ Program. 132–152

Remy-Jardin M, Remy J, Deffontaines C et al (1991) Assessment of diffuse infiltrative lung disease: comparison of conventional CT and high resolution CT. Radiology 181(1):157–162

Stone R (2004) Optimizing treatment of chronic myeloid leukemia: a rational approach. Oncologist 9:259–270

Tanaka N, Matsumoto T, Miura G et al (2002a) CT findings of leukemic pulmonary infiltration with pathologic correlation. Eur Radiol 12(1):166–174

Tanaka N, Matsumoto T, Miura G et al (2002b) HRCT findings of chest complications in patients with leukemia. Eur Radiol 12(6):1512–1522

Lung Cystic

Cloutier MM, Schaeffer DA, Hight D (1993) Congenital cystic adenomatoid malformation. Chest 103(3):761–764

Grant LA, Babar J, Griffin N (2009) Cysts, cavities, and honeycombing in multisystem disorders: differential diagnosis and findings on thin-section CT. Clin Radiol 64(4):439–448

Hansell DM, Bankier AA, MacMahon H, McLoud TC, Müller NL, Remy J (2008) Fleischner Society: glossary of terms for thoracic imaging. Radiology 246(3):697–722

Kim WS, Lee KS, Kim IO et al (1997) Congenital cystic adenomatoid malformation of the lung: CT-pathologic correlation. AJR Am J Roentgenol 168(1):47–53

Lee KH, Lee JS, Lynch DA, Song KS, Lim TH (2002) The radiologic differential diagnosis of diffuse lung diseases characterized by multiple cysts or cavities. J Comput Assist Tomogr 26(1):5–12

McGarry T, Giosa R, Rohman M, Huang CT (1987) Pneumatocele formation in adult pneumonia. Chest 92(4):717–720

Ryu JH, Swensen SJ (2003) Cystic and cavitary lung diseases: focal and diffuse. Mayo Clin Proc 78: 744–752

Seaman DM, Meyer CA, Gilman MD, McCormack FX (2011) Diffuse cystic lung disease at high-resolution CT. AJR Am J Roentgenol 196(6):1305–1311

Atelectasis

Ashizawa K, Hayashi K, Aso N, Minami K (2001) Lobar atelectasis: diagnostic pitfalls on chest radiography. Br J Radiol 74(877):89–97

Chinski A, Foltran F, Gregori D, Passali D, Bellussi L (2010) Foreign bodies causing asphyxiation in children: the experience of the Buenos Aires paediatric ORL clinic. J Int Med Res 38(2):655–660

Gurney JW (1996) Atypical manifestations of pulmonary atelectasis. J Thorac Imaging 11(3):165–175

Hansell DM, Bankier AA, MacMahon H, McLoud TC, Müller NL, Remy J (2008) Fleischner Society: glossary of terms for thoracic imaging. Radiology 246(3): 697–722

Herold CJ, Kuhlman JE, Zerhouni EA (1991) Pulmonary atelectasis: signal patterns with MR imaging. Radiology 178(3):715–720

Hopkinson NS (2007) Bronchoscopic lung volume reduction: indications, effects and prospects. Curr Opin Pulm Med 13(2):125–130

Kattan KR, Eyler WR, Felson B (1980) The juxtaphrenic peak in upper lobe collapse. Semin Roentgenol 15(2):187–193

Khoury MB, Godwin JD, Halvorsen RA Jr, Putman CE (1985) CT of obstructive lobar collapse. Invest Radiol 20(7):708–716

Lee KS, Logan PM, Primack SL, Müller NL (1994) Combined lobar atelectasis of the right lung: imaging findings. AJR Am J Roentgenol 163(1):43–47

McHugh K, Blaquiere RM (1989) CT features of rounded atelectasis. AJR Am J Roentgenol 153(2):257–260

Molina PL, Hiken JN, Glazer HS (1996) Imaging evaluation of obstructive atelectasis. J Thorac Imaging 11(3): 176–186

Naidich DP, McCauley DI, Khouri NF et al (1983) Computed tomography of lobar collapse: 1. Endobronchial obstruction. J Comput Assist Tomogr 7(5):745–757

Partap VA (1999) The comet tail sign. Radiology 213(2):553–554

Proto AV, Tocino I (1980) Radiographic manifestations of lobar collapse. Semin Roentgenol 15(2):117–173

Stark P, Leung A (1996) Effects of lobar atelectasis on the distribution of pleural effusion and pneumothorax. J Thorac Imaging 11(2):145–149

Woodring JH (1988) Determining the cause of pulmonary atelectasis: a comparison of plain radiography and CT. AJR Am J Roentgenol 150(4):757–763

Woodring JH, Reed JC (1996) Radiographic manifestations of lobar atelectasis. J Thorac Imaging 11(2): 109–144

Cavitary Lung

Abramson S (2001) The air crescent sign. Radiology 218:230–232

Fraser RG, Pare JAP (1978) Diagnosis of diseases of the chest, vol 2, 2nd edn. W.B. Saunders, Philadelphia, 1132pp

Godwin JD, Webb WR, Savoca CJ et al (1980) Multiple, thin-walled cystic lesions of the lung. AJR Am J Roentgenol 135:593–604

Hansell DM, Bankier AA, MacMahon H, McLoud TC, Müller NL, Remy J (2008) Fleischner Society: glossary of terms for thoracic imaging. Radiology 246(3): 697–722

Honda O, Tsubamoto M, Inoue A et al (2007) Pulmonary cavitary nodules on computed tomography: differentiation of malignancy and benignancy. J Comput Assist Tomogr 31:943–949

Jackson SA, Tung KT, Mead GM (1994) Multiple cavitating pulmonary lesions in non-Hodgkin's lymphoma. Clin Radiol 49:883–885

Liao WY, Liaw YS, Wang HC et al (2000) Bacteriology of infected cavitating lung tumor. Am J Respir Crit Care Med 161:1750–1753

Mondschein JF, Lazarus AA (1993) Multiple bilateral upper lobe cavitary lesions in a patient with inguinal diffuse large cell lymphoma. Chest 103:583–584

Ryu JH, Swensen SJ (2003) Cystic and cavitary lung diseases: focal and diffuse. Mayo Clin Proc 78:744–752

Seo JB, Im JG, Goo JM et al (2001) Atypical pulmonary metastasis: spectrum of radiologic findings. Radiographics 21:403–417

Shuji B, Jiro F, Yoko F et al (1999) Cavitary lung cancer with an aspergilloma-like shadow. Lung Cancer 26: 195–198

Souilamas R, Danel C, Chauffour X, Riquet M (2001) Lung cancer occurring with Mycobacterium xenopi and Aspergillus. Eur J Cardiothorac Surg 20:211–213

Torpoco JO, Yousuffuddin M, Pate JW (1976) Aspergilloma within a malignant pulmonary cavity. Chest 69: 561–563

Wang LF, Chu H, Chen YM, Perng RP (2007) Adenocarcinoma of the lung presenting as a mycetoma with an air crescent sign. Chest 131:1239–1242

Weisbrod GL, Towers MJ, Chamberlain DW et al (1992) Thin-walled cystic lesions in bronchioalveolar carcinoma. Radiology 185:401–405

Woodring JH, Fried AM (1983) Significance of wall thickness in solitary cavities of the lung: a follow-up study. AJR Am J Roentgenol 140:473–474

Woodring JH, Fried AM, Chuang VP (1980) Solitary cavities of the lung: diagnostic implications of cavity wall thickness. AJR Am J Roentgenol 135:1269–1271

Pneumonia P. jiroveci

Bessis L, Callard P, Gotheil C, Biaggi A, Grenier P (1992) High-resolution CT of parenchymal lung disease: precise correlation with histologic findings. Radiographics 12(1):45–58

Boiselle PM, Crans CA Jr, Kaplan MA (1999) The changing face of Pneumocystis carinii pneumonia in AIDS patients. AJR Am J Roentgenol 172(5):1301–1309

Bollée G, Sarfati C, Thiéry G et al (2007) Clinical picture of Pneumocystis jiroveci pneumonia in cancer patients. Chest 132(4):1305–1310

Crans CA Jr, Boiselle PM (1999) Imaging features of Pneumocystis carinii pneumonia. Crit Rev Diagn Imaging 40(4):251–284

Daly KR, Fichtenbaum CJ, Tanaka R, Linke MJ, O'Bert R, Thullen TD, Hui MS, Smulian AG, Walzer PD (2002) Serologic responses to epitopes of the major surface glycoprotein of Pneumocystis jiroveci differ in human immunodeficiency virus-infected and uninfected persons. J Infect Dis 186(5):644–651

Gruden JF, Huang L, Turner J et al (1997) High-resolution CT in the evaluation of clinically suspected Pneumocystis carinii pneumonia in AIDS patients with normal, equivocal, or nonspecific radiographic findings. AJR Am J Roentgenol 169(4):967–975

Richards PJ, Riddell L, Reznek RH et al (1996) High resolution computed tomography in HIV patients with suspected Pneumocystis carinii pneumonia and a normal chest radiograph. Clin Radiol 51(10):689–693

Stringer JR, Beard CB, Miller RF, Wakefield AE (2002) New name (Pneumocystis jiroveci) for Pneumocystis from humans. Emerg Infect Dis 8(9):891–896

Radiation Pneumonitis

Choi YW et al (2004) Effects of radiation therapy on the lung: radiologic appearances and differential diagnosis. Radiographics 24:985–998

Hirsch A, Van der Els N, Straus DJ, Gomez E, Leung D, Portlock CS, Yahalom J (1996) Effect of AVBD chemotherapy with and without mantle or mediastinal irradiation on pulmonary function and symptoms in early stage Hodgkin's disease. J Clin Oncol 14(4):1297–1305

Makimoto T, Tsuchiya S, Hayakawa K, Sayito R, Mori M (1997) Risk factors for severe radiation pneumonitis in lung cancer. Jpn J Clin Oncol 29(4):192–197

Marks LB, Yu X, Vujaskovic Z, Small W Jr, Folz R, Anscher MS (2003) Radiation induced lung injury. Semin Radiat Oncol 13(3):333–345

Morgan GW, Pharm B, Breit S (1995) Radiation and the lung: a reevaluation of the mechanisms mediating pulmonary injury. Int J Radiat Oncol Biol Phys 31(2):361–369

Intralobar Sequestration

Berrocal T, Madridi C et al (2004) Congenital anomalies of the tracheobronchial tree, lung, and mediastinum: embryology, radiology, and pathology. Radiographics 24:e17

Frazier AA et al (1997) Intralobar sequestration: radiologic-pathologic correlation. Radiographics 17:725–745

Ko SF et al (2000) Noninvasive imaging of bronchopulmonary sequestration. AJR Am J Roentgenol 175:1005–1012

Zylak CL, WilliEyler WR, Spizarny DL, Stone CH (2002) Developmental lung anomalies in the adult: radiologic-pathologic correlation. Radiographics 22:S25–S43

Lipoid Pneumonia

Baron SE, Haramati LB, Rivera VT (2003) Radiological and clinical findings in acute and chronic exogenous lipoid pneumonia. J Thorac Imaging 18:217–224

Betancourt SL, Martinez-Jimenez S, Rossi SE, Truong MT, Carrillo J, Erasmus JJ (2010) Lipoid pneumonia: spectrum of clinical and radiologic manifestations. AJR Am J Roentgenol 194:103–109

Kennedy JD, Costello P, Balikian JP, Herman PG (1981) Exogenous lipoid pneumonia. AJR Am J Roentgenol 136:1145–1149

Kitchen JM, O'Brien DE, McLaughlin AM (2008) Perils of fire eating: an acute form of lipoid pneumonia or fire eater's lung. Thorax 63:401–439

Air Space and Bronchi – II

5

John C. Pedrozo Pupo, Robin Rada Escobar, Eidelman Gonzalez Mejia, and Carlos de la Rosa Pérez

Contents

J.C. Pedrozo Pupo (ed.), *Learning Chest Imaging*, Learning Imaging,
DOI 10.1007/978-3-642-34147-2_5, © Springer-Verlag Berlin Heidelberg 2013

Case 1: Bacterial Pneumonia

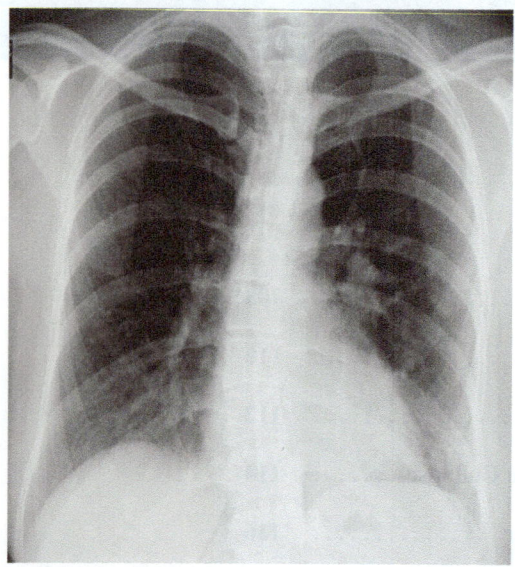

Fig. 5.1.1

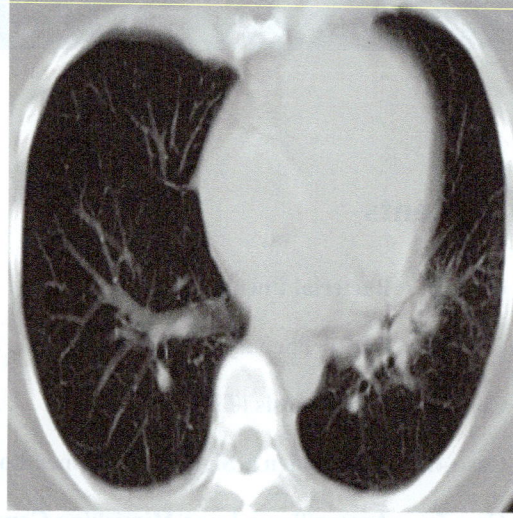

Fig. 5.1.2

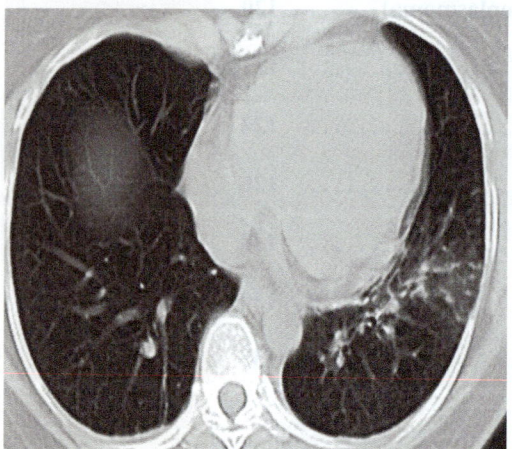

Fig. 5.1.3

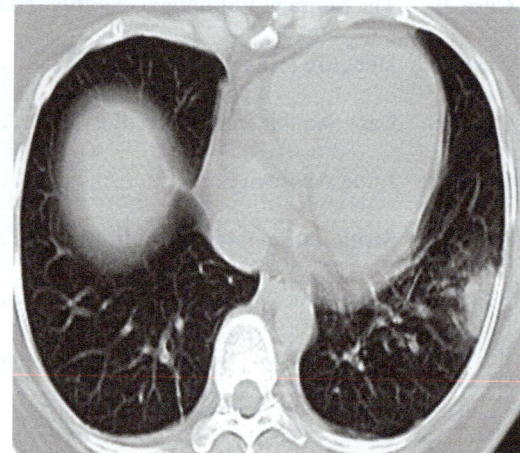

Fig. 5.1.4

A 38-year-old woman with symptoms of 10 days fever and dry cough. Blood cell count: no leukocytosis.

Computed tomography (CT) scanning is increasingly used in clinical practice, but various groups have questioned its usefulness in evaluating pneumonia. Their reports have suggested that its usefulness in the diagnosis of pneumonia is limited to the following settings:

- Evaluation of an indistinct, abnormal opacity depicted on a chest radiograph
- Assessment of patchy, ground-glass, or linear/reticular opacities on chest radiographs
- Confirmation of pleural effusion
- Examination of neutropenic patients with fever of unknown origin (with the use of ultrathin-section CT scanning)

The pneumonia is one of the most frequent causes of acute alveolar filling disorders. Radiologic and pathologic findings vary by types of pneumonia, namely, bacterial pneumonia and atypical pneumonia. Bacterial pneumonia, especially pneumonia induced by gram-positive organisms, creates an inflammatory response in the peripheral lung and produces an outpouring of edema fluid that rapidly spreads to the adjacent acini, lobules, segments, and a lobe. These rapidly progressing changes cause relatively large consolidative lesions (the same size or larger than acinar nodules) on CT. Smaller shadows, such as centrilobular nodules and branching linear structures (tree-in-bud), are significantly fewer, and ground-glass opacity, which indicates incomplete filling of alveoli, is seen only around air space consolidation.

The plain chest film is the imaging procedure of choice for detecting pneumonia and is the cornerstone of diagnosis. Examination with a stethoscope is less sensitive. The primary role of the chest radiograph is to differentiate pneumonia from other conditions that produce opacities (e.g., atelectasis, pleural effusion, pulmonary embolus, aspiration, pulmonary contusion, mass lesions). The chest radiograph is also helpful in following the progress of pneumonia, evaluating the response to therapy, and detecting complications (e.g., pleural effusion, empyema, congestive heart failure).

Follow-up X-rays showed complete clearance in 51 % of patients at 2 weeks, 85 % at 8 weeks, and 94 % at 24 weeks. Signs of consolidation cleared particularly rapidly; only 15 % of X-rays showed such signs at 4 weeks. The clearance rate was significantly faster among younger patients and those with single-lobe involvement.

CRX film shows alveolar infiltrate at the left hilar (Fig. 5.1.1). CT scan (lung window) shows alveolar infiltrate at the right lower lobe (Figs. 5.1.2, 5.1.3, and 5.1.4).

Comments

Radiological Findings

Case 2: COPD Phenotype Emphysema

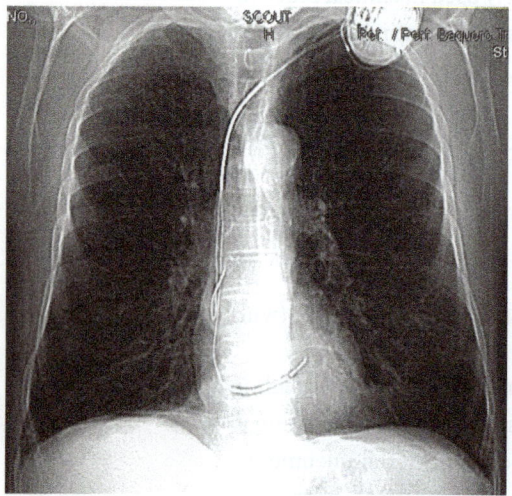

Fig. 5.2.1

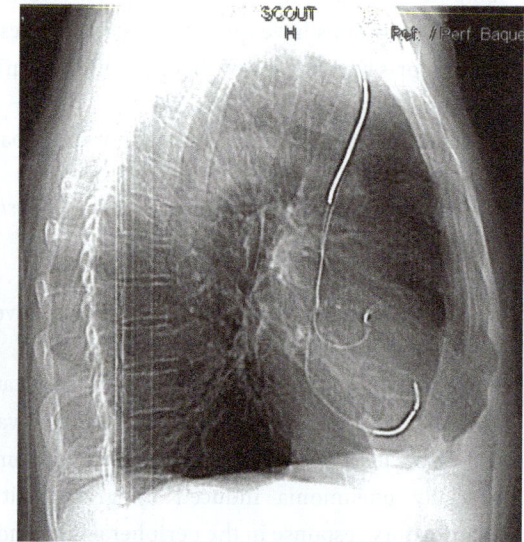

Fig. 5.2.2

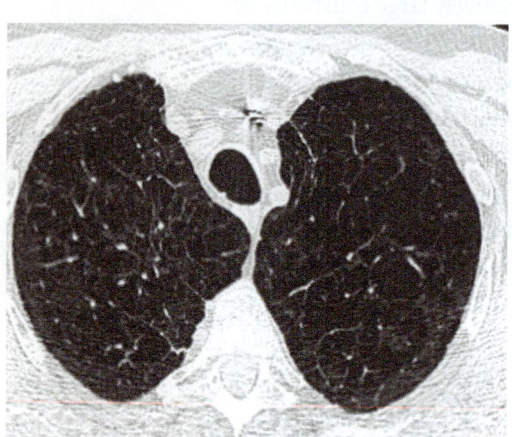

Fig. 5.2.3

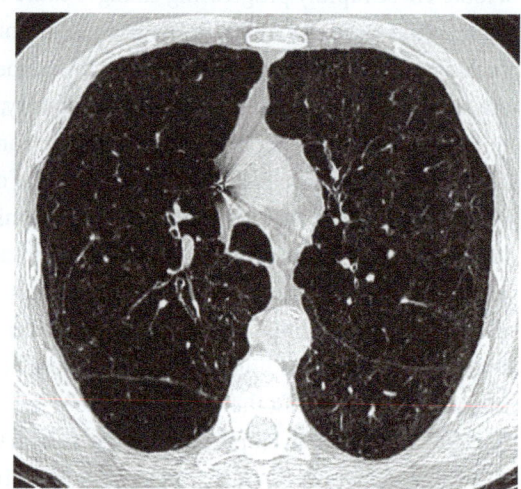

Fig. 5.2.4

A 68-year-old man with pacemaker, congestive heart failure, COPD pheno-type emphysema with a history of 9 years of evolution cough, dyspnea, and weight loss. A smoker of 35 pack years.

In computed tomography (CT), the following parameters are found in the HRCT:

Comments

1. Tracheal index: A ratio of transverse/anteroposterior diameter at a plane 1 cm above the aortic arch. Saber-sheath trachea is described as when the tracheal index was <2/3.
2. Thoracic cage ratio: A ratio of anteroposterior/transverse diameter. It was evaluated at two planes: tracheal carina and 5 cm below the carina.
3. Sterno-aortic distance: Distance from the posterior surface of the sternum to the anterior margin of the aorta at the carinal level.
4. Vascular attenuation: Vascular attenuation was considered when there was a thinning of pulmonary vessels and a reduction in their number.
5. Vascular distortion: An increased branching angle and/or excessive straightening of pulmonary vessels was described as vascular distortion.
6. Mosaic attenuation pattern: Mosaic attenuation meant nonhomogeneous lung density that later was described as areas that remain relatively lucent, interspersed with areas of normal higher lung density.
7. Directly visible small airways: The airways with an internal diameter of less than 2 mm.
8. Thoracic cross-sectional area: Thoracic cross-sectional area (TCSA) was measured on HRCT images made 1 cm below the top of the aortic arch. The ratio of TCSA over square of height (TCSA/height^2) was calculated for each patient.
9. Low attenuation areas of emphysema were assessed on HRCT.

These focal areas of decreased attenuation present differently in different types of emphysema:

(a) In centriacinar emphysema, focal areas of decreased attenuation with no discernable wall are found in association with respiratory bronchioles and usually have a focal arteriole at/or near the center of the lesion.
(b) Panacinar emphysema is characterized by large areas of decreased lung density with poorly defined margins, and these abnormally enlarged air spaces are evenly distributed within and across acinar units.
(c) Paraseptal emphysema where the enlarged air spaces are along the edge of the acinar unit but only where it abuts against a fixed structure, such as the pleura or a vessel.

CRX film shows oligemia and bilateral diaphragmatic flattening (Figs. 5.2.1 and 5.2.2). CT scan (lung window) shows decrease in lung density associated with panlobular and centrilobular emphysema (Figs. 5.2.3 and 5.2.4).

Radiological Findings

Case 3: Tuberculosis (TB)

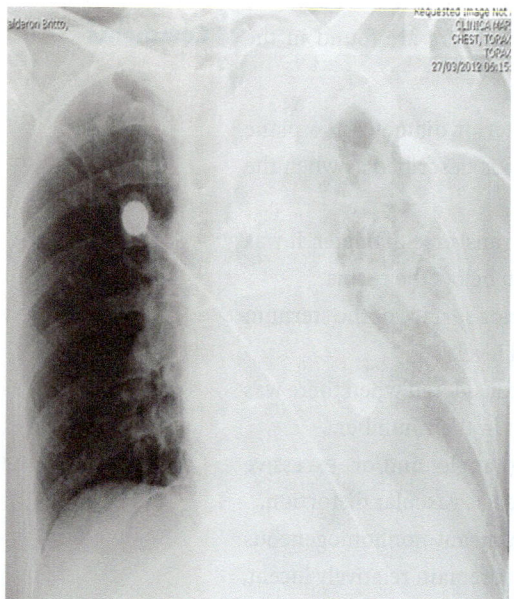

Fig. 5.3.1

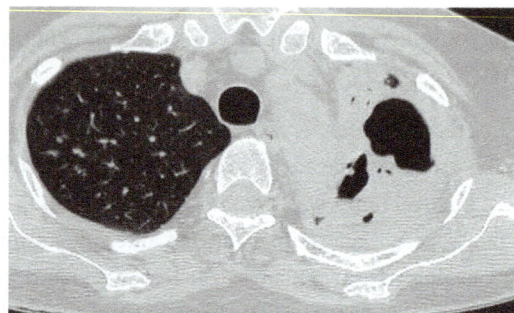

Fig. 5.3.2

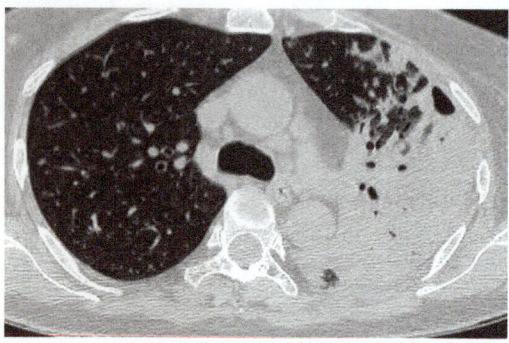

Fig. 5.3.3

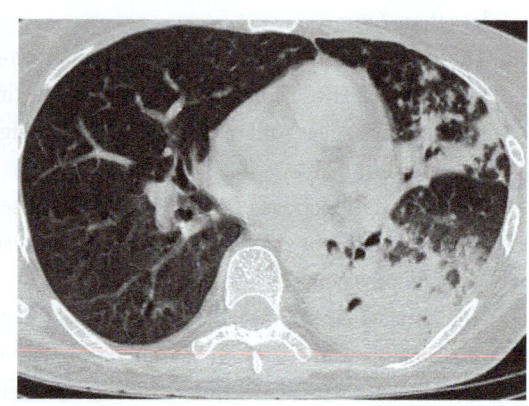

Fig. 5.3.4

A 53-year-old woman, with arthritis, type 2 diabetes, and hypertension with symptoms of 1 month of dry cough, intermittent fever, dyspnea, and weight loss. Ziehl-Neelsen staining is positive + +.

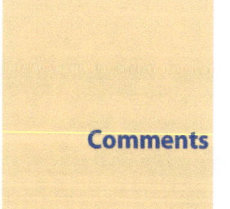

Comments

Primary infection typically presents as a segmental or lobar consolidation usually involving the lower lobes (although any lobe may be involved), and the appearance is often indistinguishable from bacterial pneumonia. Multifocal involvement is seen in 12–24 % of cases. Cavitation occurs in 10–60 % of cases. Unilateral adenopathy is seen in 60–80 % of cases and paratracheal adenopathy in 40 %. The prevalence of lymphadenopathy is greatest in the pediatric age group (about 90–96 % of affected children) and is seen in about 43 % of adults. Lymphadenopathy may be the only finding on chest radiograph, particularly in infants.

A normal chest radiograph has a high negative predictive value for the presence of active TB. The frequency of false-negative chest radiographs is about 1 % in the adult immunocompetent population and between 7 and 15 % in HIV patients. Computed tomography can detect the presence of adenopathy, parenchymal consolidations, or evidence of endobronchial spread not seen on plain film radiographs.

Disseminated (miliary) TB is a manifestation of primary infection that is seen in 1–7 % of patients (about 3 % of children and 6 % of adults). Typical miliary lesions may not be visible for 3–6 weeks after hematogenous dissemination. CRX reveals micronodular densities (1–2 mm) diffuse throughout both lungs. Associated mediastinal/hilar adenopathy is common, especially in children. HRCT demonstrates a combination of sharp and poorly defined 1- to 3-mm nodules distributed throughout the lungs and has no relationship to the airways in their distribution.

Progressive primary TB is widespread pulmonary infection due to impaired host immunity and develops in approximately 5 % of infected individuals.

Reactivation or postprimary TB: The infection usually appears as a patchy alveolar infiltrate involving the apical or posterior segments of the upper lobes, but it may cavitate in up to 50 % of patients. The cavities typically have thick, irregular walls which become smooth and thin with successful treatment. In about 5 % of patients, reactivation manifests as a sharply marginated round, oval, or irregular lesion (also called a tuberculoma). Satellite nodules around the tuberculoma may be present in up to 80 % of cases. Hilar or mediastinal adenopathy is unusual in reactivation TB (about 5–10 % of cases). Pleural effusion can be found in 15–20 % of cases of postprimary TB. Spread to other portions of the lung may occur via the bronchi – typically the lower lung zones (bronchogenic spread occurs in 20 % of cases of postprimary TB). On plain film, bronchogenic spread appears as multiple ill-defined nodules distant from the site of cavity formation.

Pleural effusion (about 18 % of patients) is found less commonly than with primary TB and is usually small. On CT, bronchogenic spread of tuberculosis commonly results in the presence of centrilobular opacities (70–95 % of cases) either as nodules or branching linear structures 2–4 mm in diameter. A tree-in-bud appearance correlates with filling of the bronchioles by caseous material and peribronchial extension of the inflammatory process.

Imaging Findings

CRX film shows cavitary lesion with alveolar infiltration and loss of volume in the left lung (Fig. 5.3.1). CT scan (lung window) shows cavitary lesion with alveolar infiltration and loss of volume in upper and lower left lobe (Figs. 5.3.2, 5.3.3, and 5.3.4).

Case 4: The Golden S Sign (Right Upper Lobe Collapse)

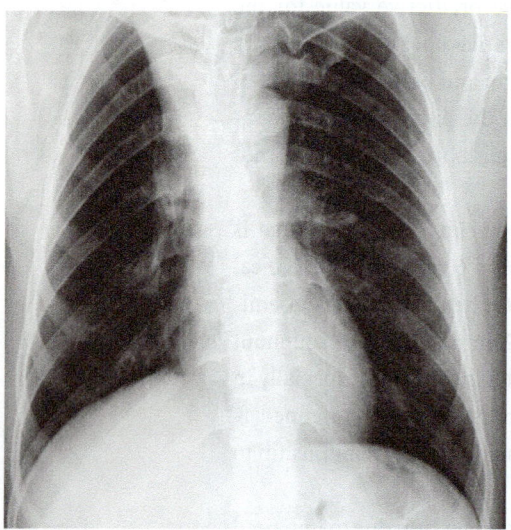

Fig. 5.4.1

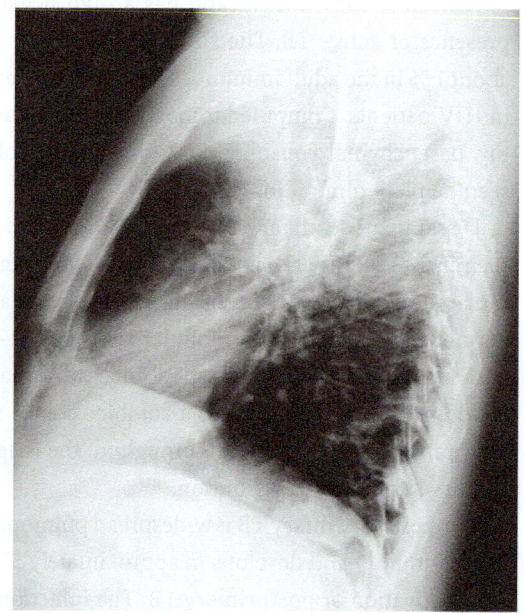

Fig. 5.4.2

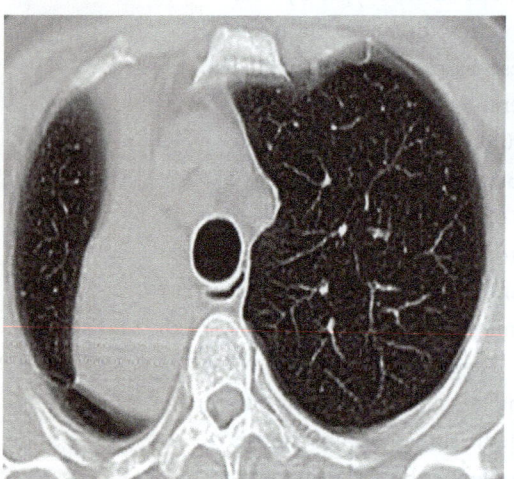

Fig. 5.4.3

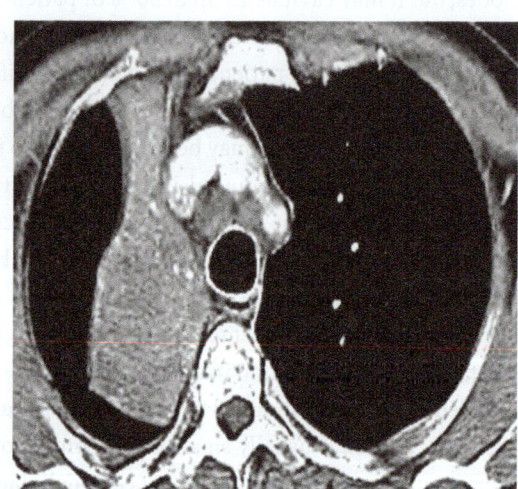

Fig. 5.4.4

A 59-year-old man, a smoker of 1 pack/day, went to the emergency due to an increase in the usual dyspnea, hemoptysis, chest pain, and weight loss. At bronchoscopy, there were neoplastic infiltration and obstruction of 100 % of the lumen of the bronchus of the RUL. Histopathological findings were consistent with adenocarcinoma.

Comments

Lung collapse, or atelectasis, is defined as reduced inflation of all or part of the lung. When collapse involves part of a lobe of a lung, it is called partial or linear atelectasis; when it involves a single lobe of the lung, it is called lobar collapse. Direct signs are related to the presence of the horizontal fissure and the middle lobe on the right side. The horizontal fissure is displaced superiorly on the frontal view, with its lateral margin being higher than its medial margin. The indirect signs of right upper lobe collapse are elevation of the right hilum, tracheal shift to the right, and compensatory hyperinflation of the right lower and middle lobes.

A specific sign which deserves mention is the "Golden S sign," first described by Ross Golden in 1925. The Golden S sign is created by a central mass and should raise suspicion of a central neoplasm, such as primary bronchial carcinoma. Golden S sign should alert the physician in charge and lead to further investigations to confirm the first suspected diagnosis, which is lung cancer. Differential diagnosis includes metastasis, primary mediastinal tumor, voluminous lymph nodes, and lymphoma. Eighty percent of lung cancers are non-small-cell lung carcinomas, which include adenocarcinoma, squamous cell carcinoma, and large cell carcinoma. Small cell lung carcinoma is the most aggressive and has the worst prognosis.

The computed tomography of the chest shows a mass that may also form a convex bulge at the fissural margin to produce an S shape.

The Golden S sign can be seen on posteroanterior chest radiographs of right upper lobe collapse when a large enough central mass is present to produce a downward convexity of the medial or proximal portion of the minor fissure. The proximal or medial portion of the minor fissure is convex inferiorly, and the distal or lateral portion of the fissure is concave inferiorly.

Imaging Findings

CRX film shows opacity associated with shift of the minor fissure due to loss of volume of right upper lobe (Figs. 5.4.1 and 5.4.2). CT scan (lung window) shows lung mass with displacement of the dome-shaped minor fissure producing a reverse S (the Golden S sign) (Fig. 5.4.3). CT scan (mediastinal window) arterial phase shows the Golden S sign (right upper lobe collapse) associated with lung mass (Fig. 5.4.4).

Case 5: Aspergilloma Lung Mimicking Cancer

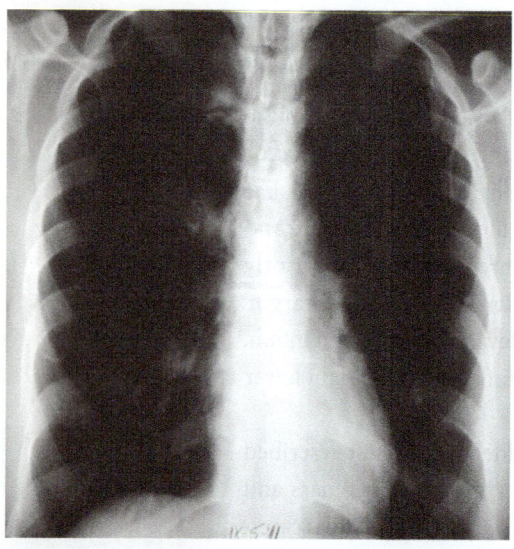

Fig. 5.5.1

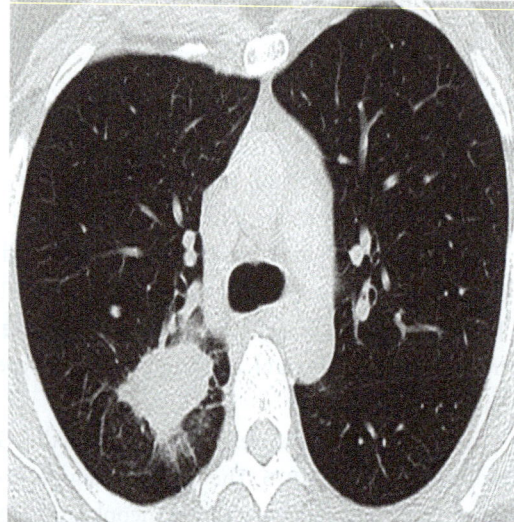

Fig. 5.5.2

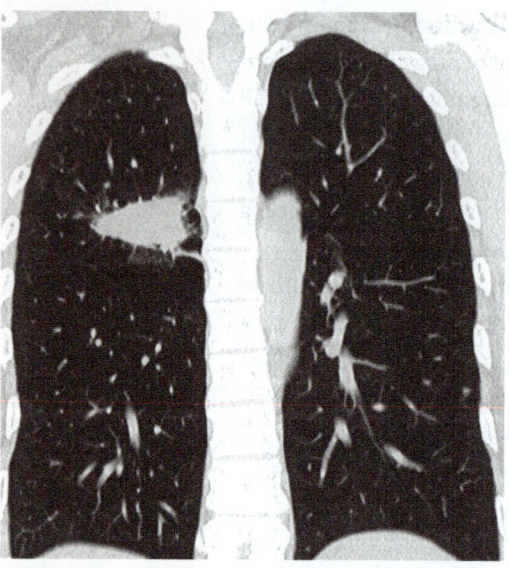

Fig. 5.5.3

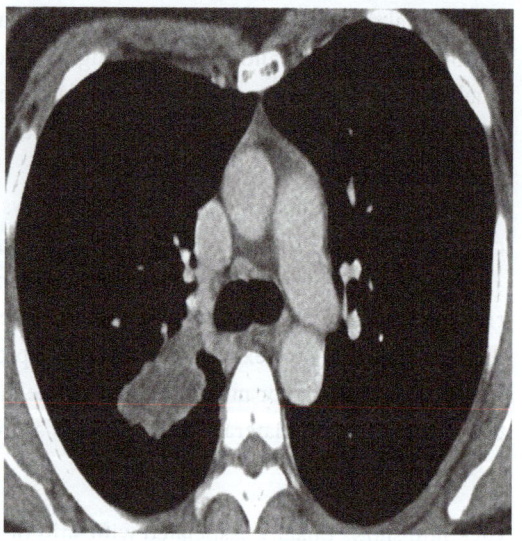

Fig. 5.5.4

A 43-year-old woman with a history of cough and dyspnea. Crepitus auscultation is scarce in the upper right chest. She does not smoke and her HIV serology was negative. Thoracoscopic lung biopsy findings are consistent with pneumonia cavitated septate hyphae of Aspergillus.

Pulmonary aspergillosis in immunocompetent hosts without a preexisting underlying lung lesion may manifest primarily as a single nodule or mass with or without an air crescent or as a localized consolidation on CT; these appearances differ from the well-known pattern of aspergilloma within preexisting structural lung disease and primary invasive aspergillosis in immunocompetent hosts.

The term aspergilloma was first used by Dave almost a century later to describe a discrete lesion that classically colonizes the cavities of healed pulmonary tuberculosis and other fibrotic lung diseases.

Aspergilloma, or secondary noninvasive aspergillosis, is the most common pattern of pulmonary aspergillosis in a healthy host. An aspergilloma is a mass of *Aspergillus* mycelia that accumulates in a preexisting cavity, bulla, or cyst. Preexisting diseases that are associated with aspergilloma include tuberculosis, bronchiectasis, pneumoconiosis, sarcoidosis, and pneumonia; in addition, preexisting bronchial cyst, bulla, or lung abscess and sites of prior surgery are associated with aspergilloma.

In this case, although not radiologically demonstrated some type of structural lesion of the lung parenchyma, if a cavity was demonstrated histopathologically.

With appropriate preoperative evaluation and judicious surgical technique, surgery is the preferred treatment for pulmonary aspergilloma, both for eradicating the tumor and for curing the underlying disease.

Computed tomography (CT) may be more accurate than conventional radiography in evaluating this condition. The classic appearance is seen on CT scans; mobility is easily demonstrated with the use of prone and supine positions. In other cases, the aspergilloma appears as an irregular spongework containing air spaces and filling the cavity, obliterating the air-crescent sign. The fungus ball is therefore fixed and immobile. Forming aspergillomas can also be identified by the fungal strands that fall into the cavity lumen, trapping air and initiating the spongework appearance. The CT appearance in patients with positive precipitins is characteristic and allows earlier diagnosis than does conventional tomography.

Aspergillomas typically appear as rounded or ovoid soft tissue attenuating masses located in a surrounding cavity and outlined by a crescent of air. Altering the position of the patient usually demonstrates that the mass is mobile, thus confirming the diagnosis. Other causes of the air-crescent sign include angioinvasive aspergillosis, echinococcal cyst, and, rarely, tuberculosis, Rasmussen aneurysm in a tuberculous cavity, lung abscess, bronchogenic carcinoma, hematoma, and *P. carinii* pneumonia.

CRX film shows pulmonary opacity in the right upper lobe (Fig. 5.5.1). CT scan (lung window) shows lung mass spiculated soft tissue in the right upper lobe (Figs. 5.5.2 and 5.5.3). CT scan (mediastinal window) shows pulmonary mass in the right upper lobe (Fig. 5.5.4).

Radiological Findings

Case 6: Bronchiectasis

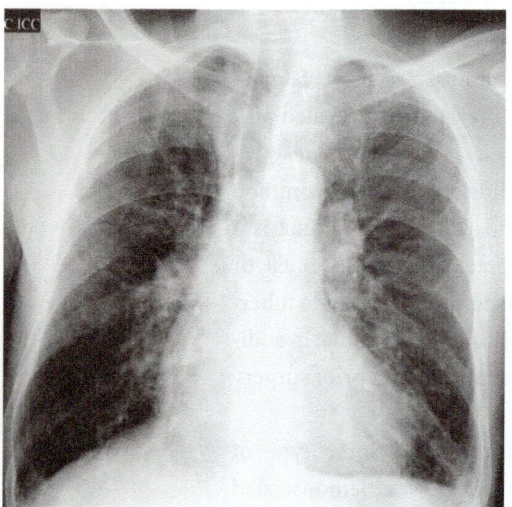

Fig. 5.6.1

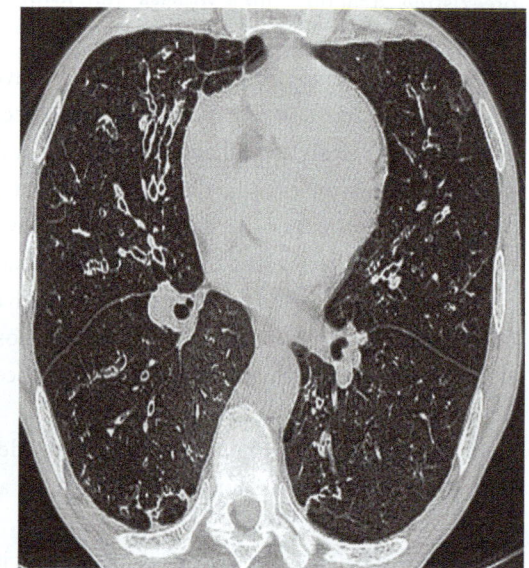

Fig. 5.6.2

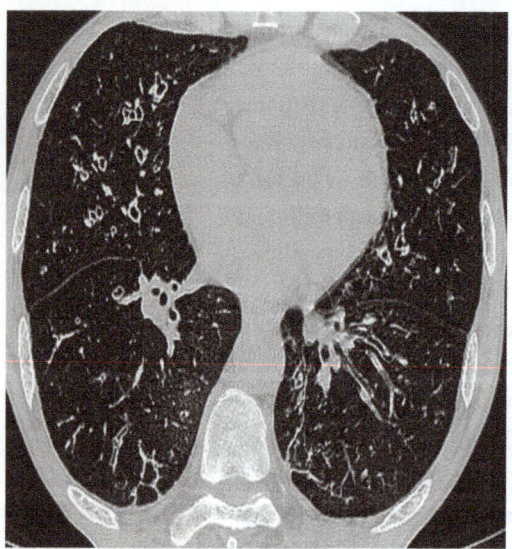

Fig. 5.6.3

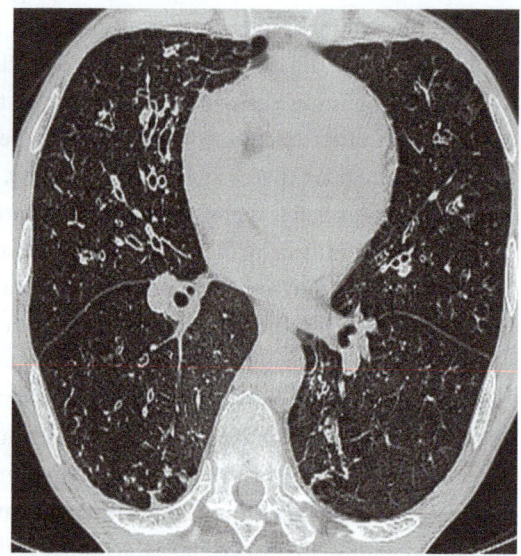

Fig. 5.6.4

A 59-year-old man with a history of 6 years of evolution bronchorrhea, dyspnea, fever, and malaise. He has been in the same clinical urgency several times; he is a smoker.

Bronchiectasis is defined as irreversible abnormal bronchial dilatation. Dilatation of the bronchi usually is most extensive in medium-sized bronchi. Bronchiectasis is commonly classified into three morphologic categories. Cylindrical bronchiectasis, the mildest form, is characterized by mildly and uniformly dilated bronchi. Varicose bronchiectasis is the term used to describe moderately dilated and irregularly beaded bronchi. Cystic bronchiectasis is the more severe: Marked cyst-like dilatations of the bronchi are found, and these dilatations contain variable amount of pooled secretions.

The high-resolution computed tomography (HRCT) is considered the test of choice for diagnosis of bronchiectasis. HRCT of the lung is a noninvasive test, which for many years has replaced bronchography. HRCT also serves to determine the morphology of the airway and the extent of disease. HRCT has a sensitivity of 87–97 % and specificity of 93–100 % for detection of bronchiectasis.

HRCT Findings

Direct Signs

1. Bronchial dilatation: Increased broncho-arterial ratio, contour abnormalities
2. Lack of airway tapering >2 cm distal to point of bifurcation
3. Airway visibility within 1 cm of the costal pleura of fissures

Indirect Signs

1. Bronchial wall thickening: Best assessed visually on images obtained at right angles through vertically oriented airways
2. Mucoid impaction/fluid-filled airways: Tubular or Y-shaped structures, branching or rounded opacities in cross section ± air-fluid levels
3. Bronchiolitis: Clustered ill-defined centrilobular nodules with a tree-in-bud configuration
4. Mosaic attenuation caused by air trapping: Best identified on expiratory HRCT images
5. Mosaic perfusion of the pulmonary identified on contrast-enhanced dual energy CT of the pulmonary parenchyma
6. Bronchial artery hyperplasia

The chest radiograph is very useful in the initial evaluation of many patients with suspected bronchiectasis. Findings related to the abnormal bronchi include tramline opacities and ring shadows, occasionally with air-fluid levels and a loss of definition of vessel markings due to peribronchial fibrosis. Retained mucus may be manifested as tubular opacities, which are sometimes branched, and there may be volume loss of a lobe or lung.

CRX film shows bronchial wall thickening (Fig. 5.6.1). CT scan (lung window) shows ill-defined centrilobular nodules, bronchial dilatation, and signet ring sign (Figs. 5.6.2, 5.6.3, and 5.6.4).

Case 7: The Solitary Pulmonary Nodule (Histoplasmoma)

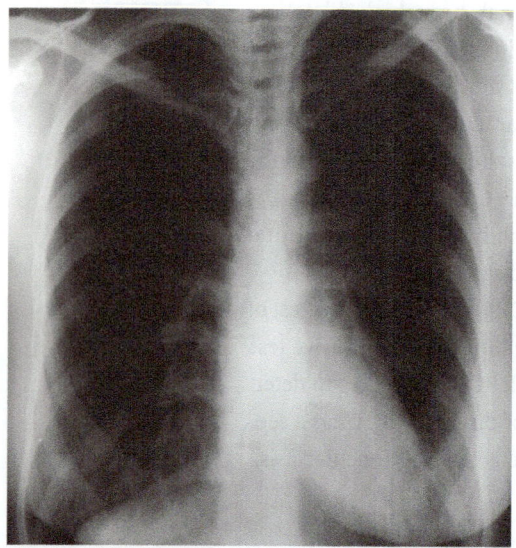

Fig. 5.7.1

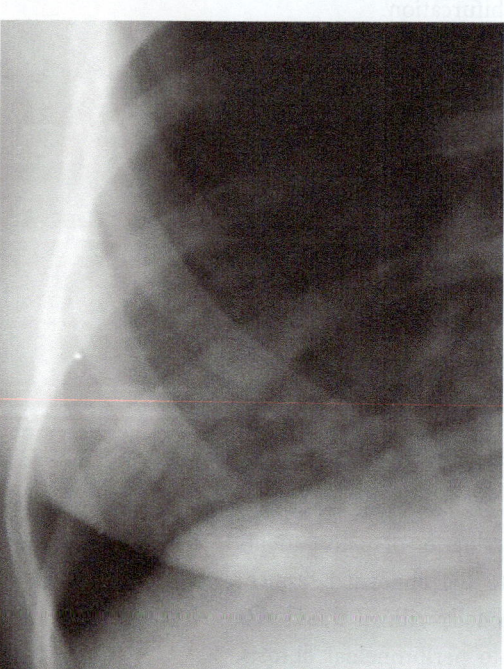

Fig. 5.7.2

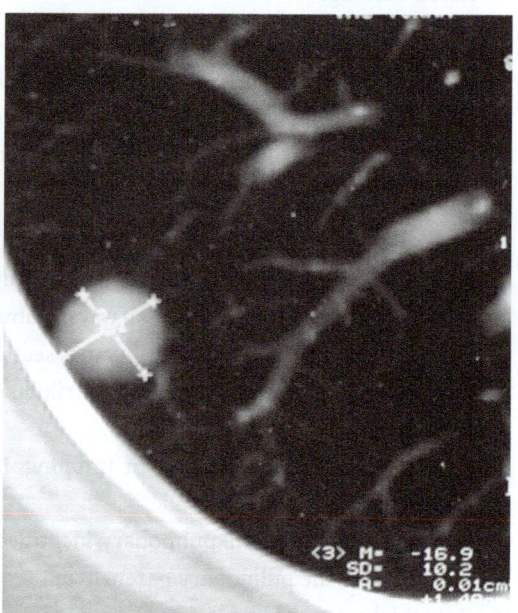

Fig. 5.7.3

Fig. 5.7.4

A 42-year-old woman, consulted for flu and solitary pulmonary nodule was demonstrated radiologically with smooth walls and calcification inside. Open thoracotomy was performed per medical decision. The histopathology is compatible with fungal origin node (*H. capsulatum*).

The solitary pulmonary nodule (SPN) is a round or oval opacity smaller than 3 cm in diameter that is completely surrounded by pulmonary parenchyma and is not associated with lymphadenopathy, atelectasis, or pneumonia.

The differential diagnosis for SPN is extensive; most SPNs are found to be granulomas, lung cancers, or hamartomas. Benign nodules can be confidently diagnosed if the lesion is smaller than 2 cm in diameter and exhibits one of the following patterns of calcification: central nidus, laminated, popcorn, or diffuse.

The probability of malignancy is high (90 % if the patient is older than 60 years) with positive fluoro-2-deoxy-D-glucose (FDG) PET findings and low (<5 %) with negative (FDG) PET findings. Nodules with low likelihood for malignancy that are at least 5 mm and smaller than 10 mm can be observed with CT for a 2-year period, while nodules with intermediate or high likelihood for malignancy can be sampled with FNAB or resected.

Histoplasmosis is a primarily pulmonary originated mycosis which is acquired by inhalation. In the majority of the cases, infection goes unnoticed or gets manifested by slight respiratory symptoms. Pulmonary histoplasmosis should be considered in patients with the following clinical presentations, particularly in the appropriate epidemiologic setting: pneumonia with mediastinal or hilar lymphadenopathy, mediastinal or hilar masses, pulmonary nodule, cavitary lung disease, pericarditis with mediastinal lymphadenopathy, pulmonary manifestations with arthritis or arthralgia plus erythema nodosum, dysphagia caused by esophageal narrowing, superior vena cava syndrome, or obstruction of other mediastinal structures.

Histoplasmoma is a relatively common form of acute lung histoplasmosis, in the form of nodules, which is generally accompanied by calcification that can increase in size and simulate a lung neoplasia.

CT scanning is helpful in detecting calcification in a lung nodule (histoplasmoma). The modality is more sensitive in detecting subtle calcification in a nodule and may identify other smaller nodules that are not seen on chest radiographs.

A solitary pulmonary nodule is a frequent finding on chest radiographs of the patient with asymptomatic primary infection. These nodules vary from a few millimeters to several centimeters. Most of these nodules have well-defined margins and central, laminar, or diffuse calcification patterns. Interestingly, some nodules slowly enlarge because of continued elaboration of collagen at the periphery of the lesion; in such cases, histoplasmosis may be difficult to distinguish from malignancy.

CRX film shows nodular lesion in the right lower lobe (Figs. 5.7.1 and 5.7.2). CT scan (lung window) shows soft tissue mass lesion with calcification located inside the right lower lobe (Figs. 5.7.3 and 5.7.4).

Comments

Imaging Findings

Case 8: Hodgkin's Lymphoma

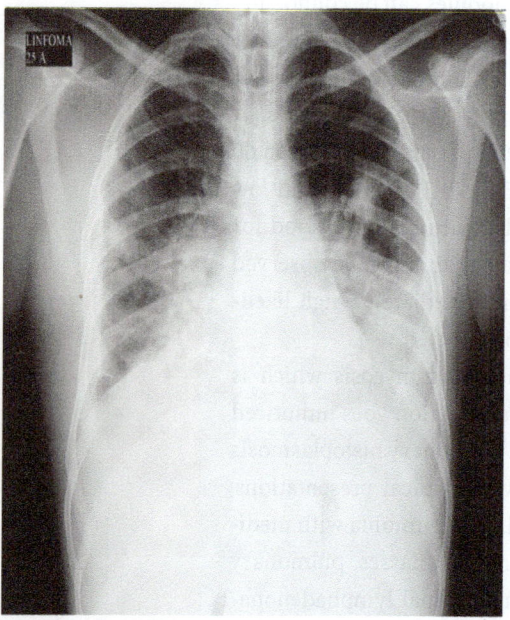

Fig. 5.8.1

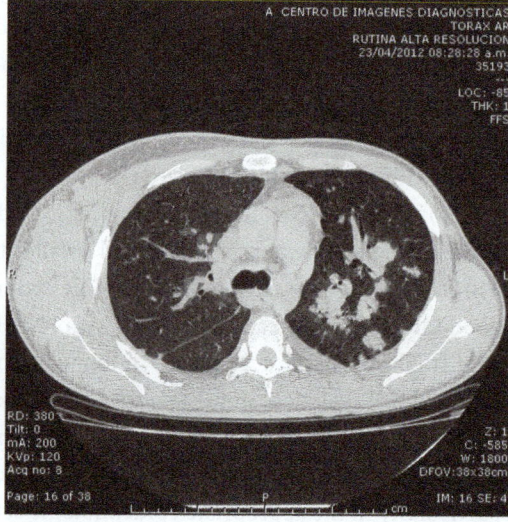

Fig. 5.8.2

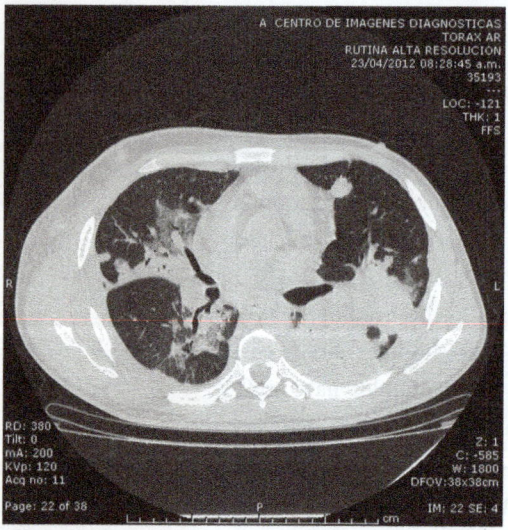

Fig. 5.8.3

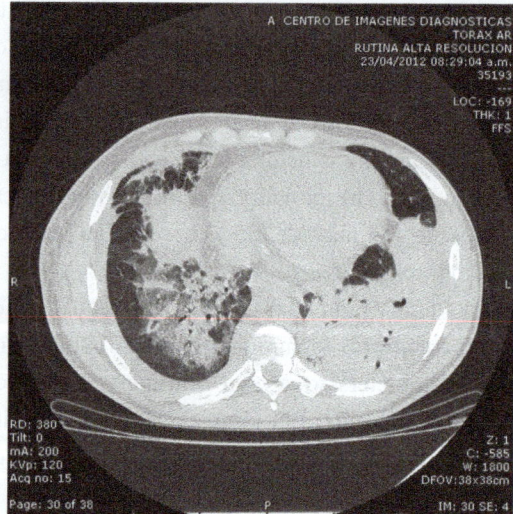

Fig. 5.8.4

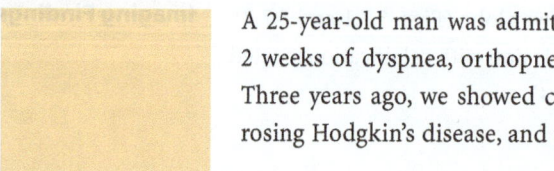

A 25-year-old man was admitted to the emergency room for symptoms of 2 weeks of dyspnea, orthopnea, dry cough, fatigue, weakness, and malaise. Three years ago, we showed cervical lymph node biopsy and nodular sclerosing Hodgkin's disease, and the patient received autologous hematopoietic transplantation, chemotherapy, and radiotherapy. It is currently considered advanced stage disease relapse.

Comments

In 80–90 % of patients with Hodgkin's disease, the first manifestation is lymphadenopathy, most frequently located supradiaphragmatically. Hodgkin's disease is usually almost entirely confined to the lymph nodes while extranodal involvement is much less common compared to non-Hodgkin's lymphoma. Extranodal invasion of adjacent tissue is seen in up to 15 % of cases and hematogenous spread in 5–10 %. Even when dissemination occurs beyond the lymphoreticular system, certain patterns of associated spread are frequently evident.

On chest radiographs of the left side, the normal aortopulmonary window is slightly concave, straight, or invisible. In the perivascular area, adenopathy is the most common cause for convexity of the aortopulmonary bay toward the left lung. On chest radiographs of the right side, the azygos node lies variably in relation to the azygos vein as the vein passes forward above the right bronchus to enter the superior vena cava (SVC). This node is the lowest member of the group of right paratracheal lymph nodes. Any convexity in this region that has a greater part of its curvature above the right main bronchus probably should be regarded as abnormal. Lower right perivascular nodal enlargement also can distort this region.

CT scanning has the additional advantage of depicting other areas of lymph node enlargement that are not obvious on chest radiographs. Some areas of lymph node enlargement that are difficult to detect by using radiography include paracardiac, supradiaphragmatic, and internal mammary chain lymph nodes; these can be detected easily via CT scanning. The modality also helps in formulating treatment plans and radiation fields. CT scans depicting characteristics of Hodgkin's disease are presented below. Involvement of the lungs and pericardium can occasionally be detected on CT scans; these exclude treatment by radiation therapy.

CT size criteria for lymph node involvement in the mediastinum are well defined. According to the criteria, subcarinal, paracardiac, and retrocrural lymph nodes are considered enlarged if they are larger than 12, 8, and 6 mm in their short-axis diameter, respectively. The remaining lymph nodes in the body are considered enlarged if they are larger than 10 cm in their short-axis diameter.

On CT scans, lymph node enlargement can be seen as multiple, rounded soft tissue masses or bulky soft tissue masses caused by nodal aggregation. Usually, a homogeneous soft tissue mass is noted; it may be heterogeneous when it is large, with areas of low attenuation representing necrosis, hemorrhage, or cyst formation.

Imaging Findings

CRX film shows bilateral alveolar infiltration (Fig. 5.8.1). CT scan (lung window) shows alveolar consolidation, with areas of patchy ground-glass with superimposed interlobular septal thickening (crazy paving) and soft tissue nodule with spiculated margins in both lungs (Figs. 5.8.2, 5.8.3, and 5.8.4).

Case 9: Late Sequelae in Tuberculosis

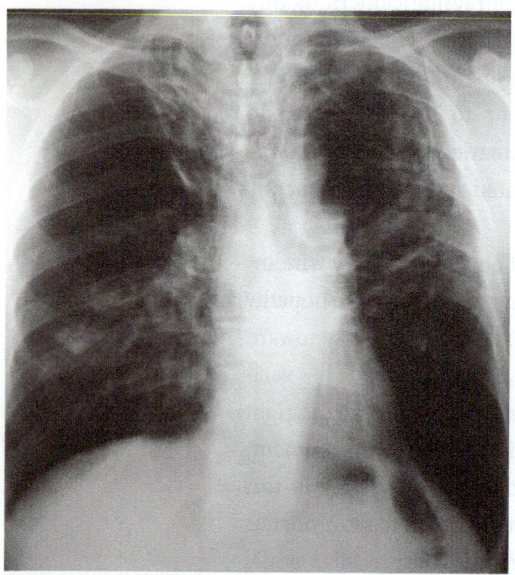

Fig. 5.9.1

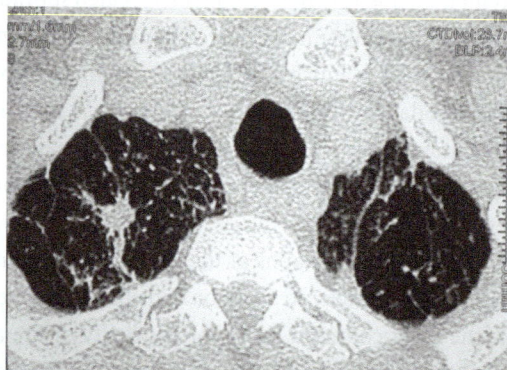

Fig. 5.9.2

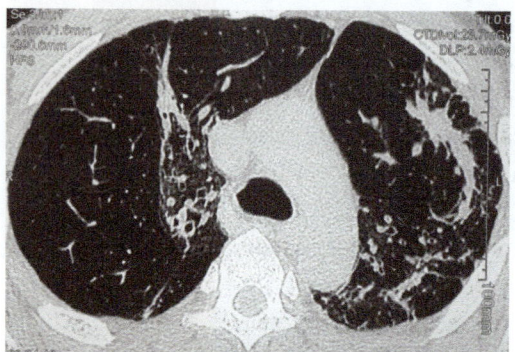

Fig. 5.9.3

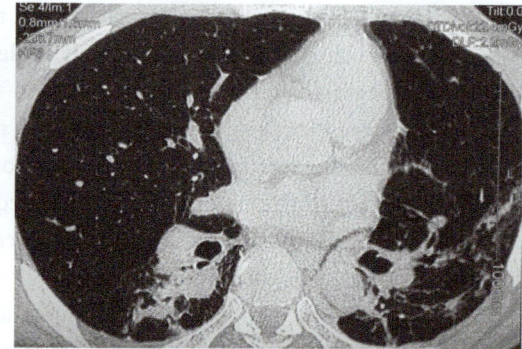

Fig. 5.9.4

A 52-year-old man had tuberculosis for 2 years, with symptoms of dry cough and dyspnea. Moderate restrictive defect on spirometry.

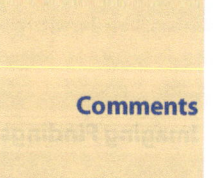

Comments   Pulmonary TB is a disease that usually when it does not heal any sequels, whose magnitude is related to the severity and extent of the previous process. Usually, they are grouped together according to the organ, and in Table 5.1, the most relevant are presented.

Table 5.1 Sequelae of tuberculosis

Parenchymal lesions
Scars
Destroyed lung
Airway lesions
Central and peripheral bronchiectasis
Tracheobronchial stenosis
Mediastinal lesions
Calcified adenopathies
Fibrosing mediastinitis
Pleural lesions
Fibrothorax
Loculated pneumothorax

Sequelae have also been reported in lung function. The obstructive pattern without bronchodilator reversibility is the most common spirometric alterations found in patients with sequelae of pulmonary tuberculosis.

A nonspecific radiologic pattern of fibrosis consisting of parenchymal bands, fibrotic nodules, and cavities or traction bronchiectasis is occasionally encountered. Apical pleural thickening associated with fibrosis may reveal proliferation of extrapleural fatty tissue and peripheral atelectasis at CT.

At radiography, a mobile, rounded mass surrounded by a crescentic air shadow is noted inside a lung cavity (air-crescent sign). CT demonstrates a mobile fungus ball, usually with air interspersed between the masses of mycelia. Calcification of the mycelial ball occurs in some cases.

Bronchiectasis is seen in 30–60 % of patients with active postprimary tuberculosis and in 71–86 % of patients with inactive disease at high-resolution CT. Although bronchiectasis in postprimary tuberculosis can be a result of cicatricial bronchostenosis after local infection, more commonly it occurs by destruction and fibrosis of the lung parenchyma with secondary bronchial dilatation (traction bronchiectasis).

On CT scans, irregular luminal narrowing with wall thickening, enhancement, and enlarged adjacent mediastinal nodes are common findings in the active stage of stenosis. The CT findings include concentric narrowing of the lumen, uniform thickening of the wall, and involvement of a long bronchial segment in the fibrotic stage.

Imaging Findings

CRX film shows bilateral parenchymal bands (Fig. 5.9.1). CT scan (lung window) shows bilateral parenchymal bands with traction bronchiectasis in the upper and middle lobes (Figs. 5.9.2, 5.9.3, and 5.9.4).

Case 10: Lung Abscess

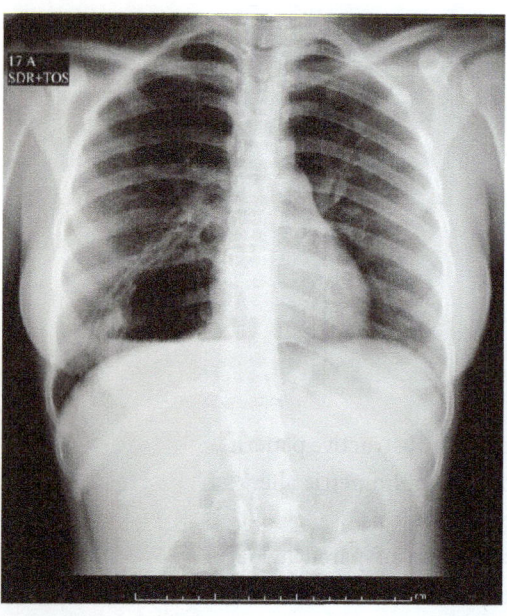

Fig. 5.10.1

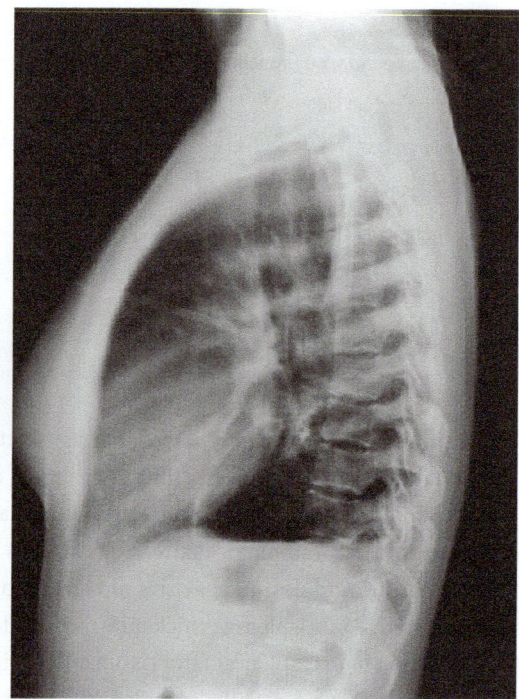

Fig. 5.10.2

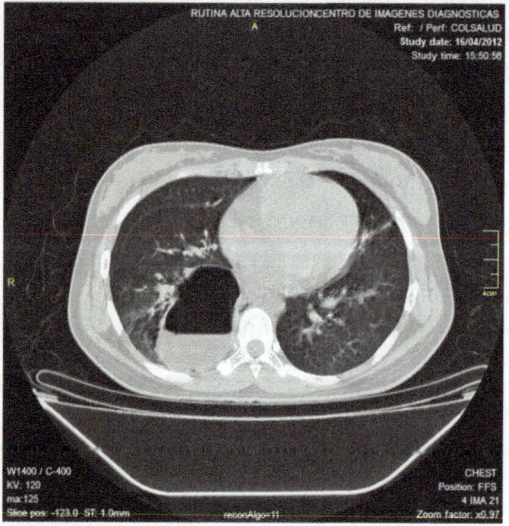

Fig. 5.10.3

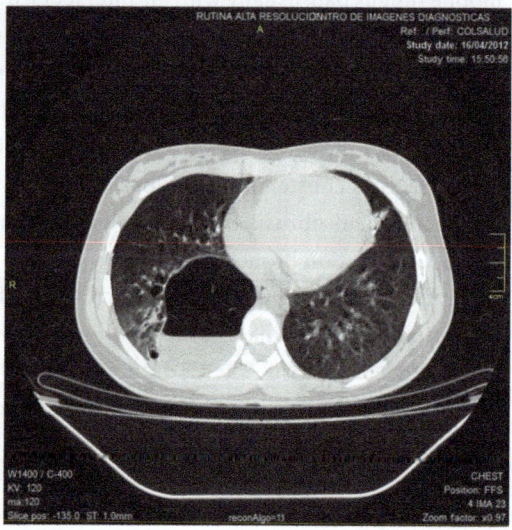

Fig. 5.10.4

A 17-year-old woman with a history of 1 week of evolution productive cough, fever, dyspnea, pleuritic pain, and malaise. She is a non-smoker.

Lung abscesses can be classified based on the duration and the likely etiology. Acute abscesses are less than 4–6 weeks old, whereas chronic abscesses are of longer duration. Primary abscess is infectious in origin caused by aspiration or pneumonia in the healthy host; secondary abscess is caused by a preexisting condition (e.g., obstruction), spread from an extrapulmonary site, bronchiectasis, and/or an immunocompromised state. Lung abscesses can be further characterized by the responsible pathogen, such as *Staphylococcus* lung abscess and anaerobic or *Aspergillus* lung abscess.

CT is the most sensitive and specific imaging modality to diagnose a lung abscess. Contrast should be administered, as this enables the identification of the abscess margins, which can otherwise blend with surrounding consolidated lung. It is helpful in differentiating between a lung abscess and an empyema. Cavity may be seen as rounded with a thick wall and an air-fluid level.

Abscesses vary in size and are generally rounded in shape. Lung abscesses, being intraparenchymal, form an acute angle where they meet the chest wall. Bronchial vessels and bronchi can be traced as far as the wall of the abscess, whereupon they are truncated. The differential diagnosis includes cavitary bronchogenic carcinoma, TB, pulmonary metastasis, pulmonary cavitating granulomatous disease (e.g., Wegener's granulomatosis), large pneumatocele, and hiatus hernia (especially for a retrocardiac abscess).

Usually, it is a single cavity. The classical appearance of a pulmonary abscess is its cavities typically have a thick wall (which may become thinner as the surrounding inflammation resolves), smooth inner margin, and air-fluid level, although adjacent consolidation may make assessment of this difficult.

It affects more frequently superior segments of lower lobes or posterior segments of lower lobes. Unlike pleural collections, lung abscesses frequently have a fluid level which is approximately the same length on both the frontal and lateral projection. About 1/3 may have an associated empyema.

CRX film shows level of lung injury with hydro-air with a diameter similar in both projections (Figs. 5.10.1 and 5.10.2). CT scan (lung window) shows cavitation level of hydro-air with thin walls located in the right lower lobe (Figs. 5.10.3 and 5.10.4).

Case 11: Septic Pulmonary Embolism

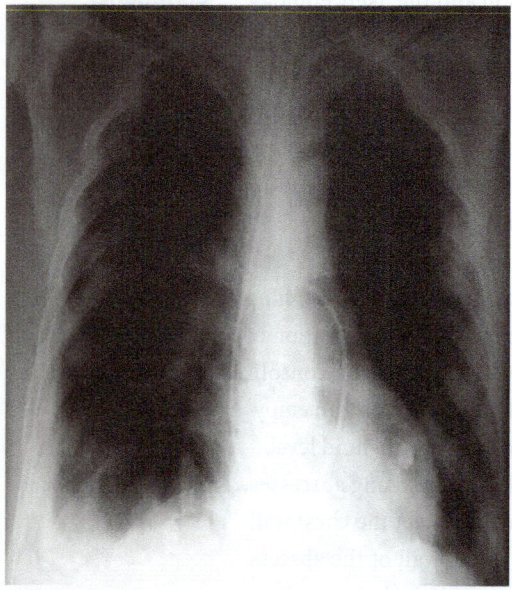

Fig. 5.11.1

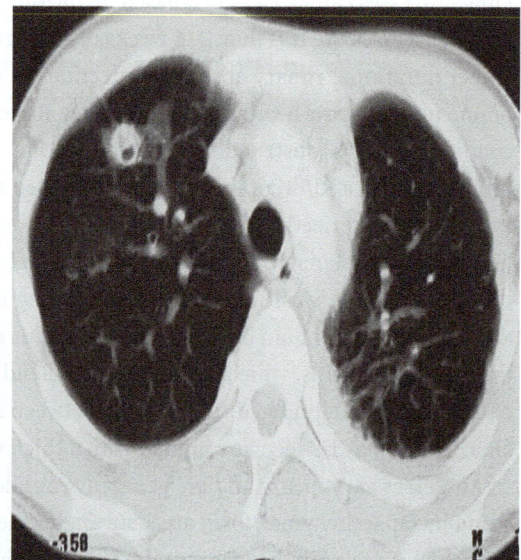

Fig. 5.11.2

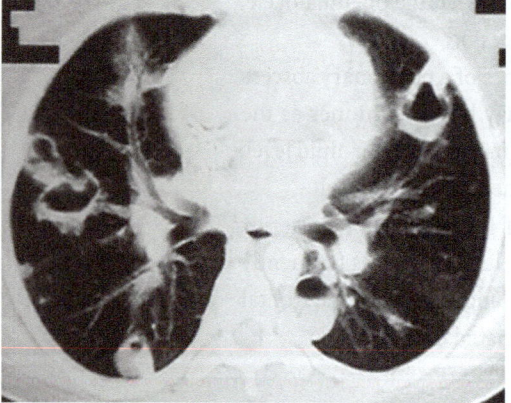

Fig. 5.11.3

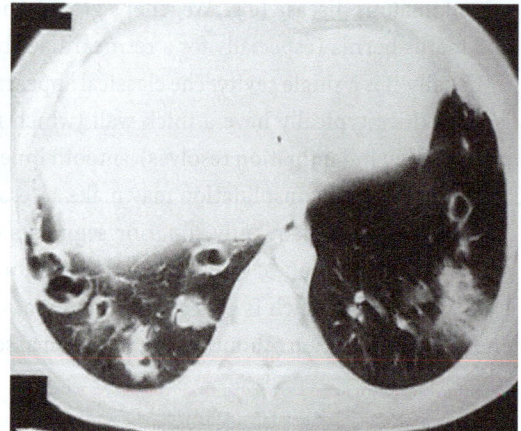

Fig. 5.11.4

A 51-year-old man was referred for dyspnea, cough, fever, fatigue, and weakness and soft tissue infection of scalp at right retroauricular region.

Septic pulmonary embolism (SPE) is an uncommon disorder that generally presents with an insidious onset of fever, respiratory symptoms, and lung infiltrates. Clinical and radiologic features at presentation are usually nonspecific, and the diagnosis of this disorder is frequently delayed.

Historically, SPE has been associated with risk factors such as IV drug use, pelvic thrombophlebitis, infective endocarditis, infected venous catheters or pacemaker leads, periodontal disease soft tissue infection, and suppurative processes in the head and neck. However, increasing use of indwelling catheters and devices as well as increasing numbers of immunocompromised patients has changed the epidemiology and clinical manifestations of SPE. In SPE, the embolic blood clot that leads to an infarction in the pulmonary vasculature also contains microorganisms that incite a focal abscess.

Imaging findings on CRX tend to be nonspecific, may reveal poorly marginated peripheral lung nodules. CT may yield helpful clues that may suggest the diagnosis of SPE.

CT scanning demonstrates bilateral nodules or multifocal infiltrates, commonly involving peripheral lung zones (subpleural), often associated with cavitation and the "feeding vessel" sign (a vessel leading to a peripheral lung lesion). The feeding vessel sign consists of a distinct vessel leading directly into the center of a nodule. This sign has been considered highly suggestive of septic embolism, the prevalence varying from 67 to 100 % in various series. The feeding vessel sign also occurs in pulmonary metastasis. In a careful stereomicroscopic CT–pathologic correlation of pulmonary vasculature to pulmonary metastasis found that only 18 % of nodules identified had a definitive pulmonary arterial branch entering the center of the nodule. In 58 % of nodules, stereomicroscopic examination showed that the vessel did not enter the nodule but coursed along its border, being displaced by the nodule.

CRX film shows multiple nodules of various sizes (Fig. 5.11.1). CT scan shows multiple and bilateral cavitated nodules (the feeding vessel sign) and subpleural distribution (Figs. 5.11.2, 5.11.3, and 5.11.4).

Case 12: Congenital Lobar Emphysema

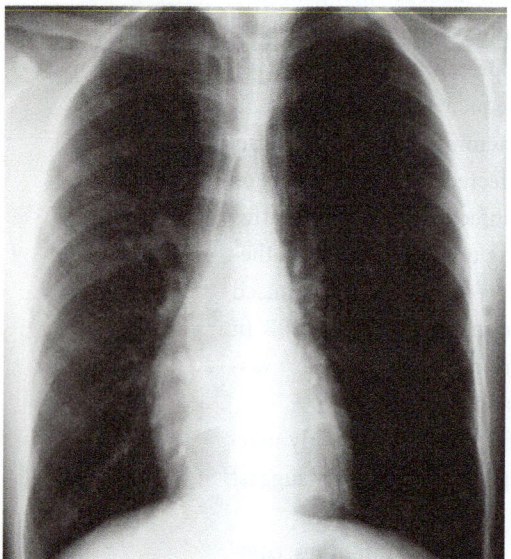

Fig. 5.12.1

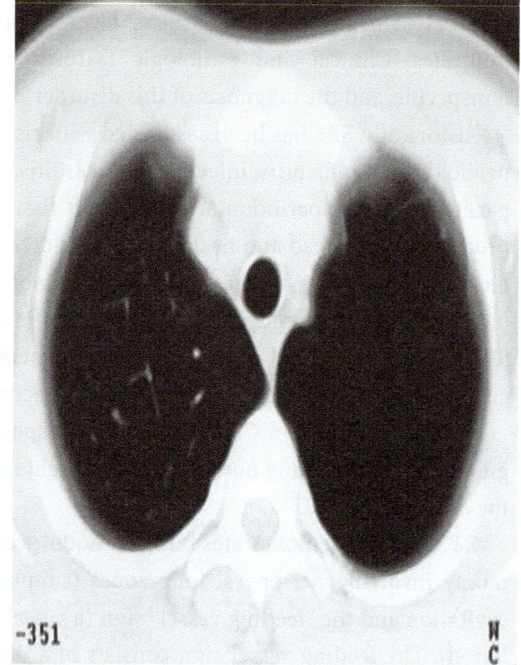

Fig. 5.12.2

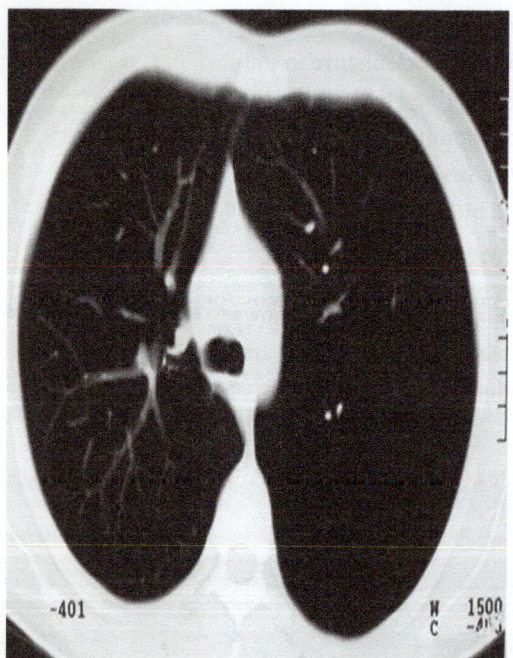

Fig. 5.12.3

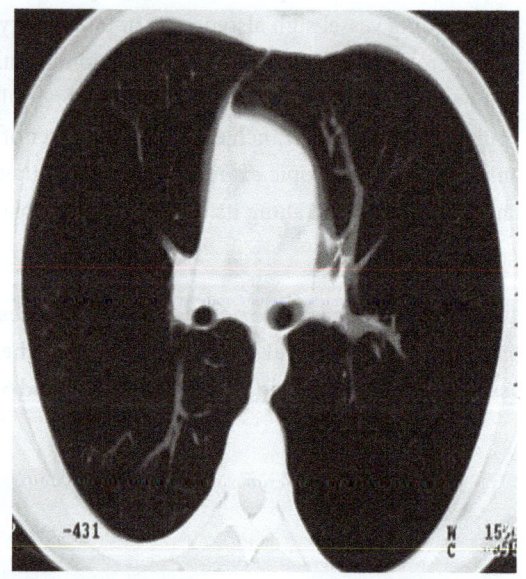

Fig. 5.12.4

A 25-year-old man refers dyspnea and dry cough. No evidence of a smoker.

Comments

Congenital lobar emphysema (CLE) is a developmental anomaly of the lower respiratory tract that is characterized by hyperinflation of one or more of the pulmonary lobes. Other terms for CLE include congenital lobar overinflation and infantile lobar emphysema. CLE is a rare congenital malformation, with a prevalence of 1 in 20,000 to 1 in 30,000. Depending upon the pattern of referrals, other tertiary medical centers may treat one or two cases per year. Males appear to be affected more than females, in a ratio of 3:1. The reason for the male predominance is unknown.

The most commonly affected lobe is the left upper lobe, followed by the middle lobe. The distribution of lobar involvement is 42.2 % in the left upper lobe, 35.3 % in the right middle lobe, 20.7 % in the right upper lobe, and 0.9 % in each lower lobe. There is no destruction of alveolar walls. In 50–55 % of cases, the cause of congenital lobar emphysema is unknown, although areas of malacia or stenosis of the bronchial cartilage were found in these patients, and these are considered the most likely explanations. Congenital lobar emphysema may be associated with other anomalies (cardiovascular system is involved in 12–14 %). It is more common among males than females; it is not familial and occurs predominantly in Caucasians. Most patients become symptomatic during the neonatal period, most before 6 months of age. Three clinical types are classified according to whether congenital lobar emphysema becomes symptomatic in infancy (type I), in older children (type II), or is an incidental finding in asymptomatic patients (type III). Types II and III are rare.

Findings of air trapping with lobar hyperinflation, mediastinal shift away from the involved lung, and compression of the ipsilateral and contralateral lung develop. CT shows an expanded lobe with attenuated vascular structures. CT is useful for diagnosis of multilobar involvement and mass effect on the remaining adjacent ipsilateral lung and mediastinal structures.

CRX film shows left unilateral hyperlucency (Fig. 5.12.1). CT scan (lung window) shows lobar hyperinflation in the left lung with air trapping (Figs. 5.12.2, 5.12.3, and 5.12.4).

Imaging Findings

Further Reading

Bacterial Pneumonia

Lee KS, Kim EA (2001) High-resolution CT of alveolar filling disorders. Radiol Clin North Am 39(6):1–14

Mittl RL Jr et al (1994) Radiographic resolution of community-acquired pneumonia. Am J Respir Crit Care Med 149:630–635

Reynold JH, McDonald G (2010) Pneumonia in the immunocompetent patient. Br J Radiol 83:998–1009

COPD Phenotype Emphysema

Gupta PP, Yadav R, Verma M, Gupta KB, Agarwal D (2009) High-resolution computed tomography features in patients with chronic obstructive pulmonary disease. Singapore Med J 50(2):193

Müller NL, Coxson H (2002) Imaging the lungs in patients with chronic obstructive pulmonary. Thorax 57:982–985

Orlandi I, Moroni C, Camiciottoli G et al (2005) Chronic obstructive pulmonary disease: thin-section CT measurement of airway wall thickness and lung attenuation. Radiology 234:604–610

Takasugi JE, Godwin JD (1998) Radiology of chronic pulmonary disease. Radiol Clin North Am 36(1):29–55

Webb WR (1997) Radiology of obstructive pulmonary disease. AJR Am J Roentgenol 169:637–647

Tuberculosis

Burrill J, Williams CJ et al (2007) Tuberculosis: a radiologic review. Radiographics 27:1255–1273

Choi YW, Jeon SC et al (2002) Tuberculous pleural effusion: new pulmonary lesions during treatment. Radiology 224:493–502

Curvo-Semedo L, Teixeira L et al (2005) Tuberculosis of the chest. Eur J Radiol 55:158–172

Domínguez Del Valle FJ, Fernández M et al (2007) Clinical manifestations and radiology of thoracic tuberculosis. An Sist Sanit Navar 30(Suppl 2):33–48

Hatipoglu N, Osma E et al (1996) High resolution computed tomographic findings in pulmonary tuberculosis. Thorax 51:397–402

Jeong YJ, Lee KS (2008) Pulmonary tuberculosis: up-to-date imaging and management. AJR Am J Roentgenol 191:834–844

Kim HY, Song K-S et al (2001) Thoracic sequelae and complications of tuberculosis. Radiographics 21:839–860

Lee KS, Im J-G (1995) CT in adults with tuberculosis of the chest: characteristic findings and role in management. AJR Am J Roentgenol 164:1361–1367

Lee KS et al (1993) Adult-onset pulmonary tuberculosis: findings on chest radiographs and CT scans. AJR Am J Roentgenol 160:753–758

Lee KS, Hwang JW et al (1996) Utility of CT in the evaluation of pulmonary tuberculosis in patients without AIDS. Chest 110:977–984

Leung AN (1999) Pulmonary tuberculosis: the essentials. Radiology 210:307–322

Marciniuk DD, McNab BD et al (1999) Detection of pulmonary tuberculosis in patients with a normal chest radiograph. Chest 115:445–452

Morris BS, Maheshwari M et al (2004) Chest wall tuberculosis: a review of CT appearances. Br J Radiol 77:449–457

Poey C, Verhaegen F et al (1997) High resolution chest CT in tuberculosis: evolutive patterns and signs of activity. J Comput Assist Tomogr 21(4):601–607

Rossi SE, Tomas FT et al (2005) Tree-in-bud pattern at thin-section CT of the lungs: radiologic-pathologic overview. Radiographics 25:789–801

Woodring JH, Vandiviere HM et al (1986) Update: the radiographic features of pulmonary tuberculosis. AJR Am J Roentgenol 146:497–506

The Golden S Sign (Right Upper Lobe Collapse)

Geoffrey MB, Brenda FA et al (2006) Signs in thoracic imaging. J Thorac Imaging 21(1):76–90

Golden R (1925) The effect of bronchostenosis upon the roentgen-ray shadows in carcinoma of the bronchus. AJR Am J Roentgenol 13:21–30

Gupta P (2004) The golden S sign. Radiology 233:790–791

Lemyze M, Van Grunderbeeck N, Gasan G et al (2011) Golden S sign. Am J Respir Crit Care Med 183:131

Mullett R, Jain A, Kotugodella S et al (2012) Lobar collapse demystified: the chest radiograph with CT correlation. Postgrad Med J. doi:10.1136/postgradmedj-2011-130213

Aspergilloma Lung Mimicking Cancer

Chen JC, Chang YL et al (1997) Surgical treatment for pulmonary aspergilloma: a 28 year experience. Thorax 52:810–813

Franquet T, Muller NL et al (2001) Spectrum of pulmonary aspergillosis: histologic, clinical, and radiologic findings. Radiographics 21:825–837

Roberts CM, Citron KM, Strickland B (1987) Intrathoracic aspergilloma: role of CT in diagnosis and treatment. Radiology 165:123–128

Sakarya ME, Özbay B et al (1998) Aspergillomas in the lung cavities. East J Med 3(1):7–9

Bronchiectasis

Bonavita J, Naidich DP (2012) Imaging of bronchiectasis. Clin Chest Med 33:233–248

Grenier P, Maurice F et al (1986) Bronchiectasis: assessment by thin – section CT. Radiology 161:95–99

Ooi GC, Khong PL, Chan-Yeung M et al (2002) High-resolution CT quantification of bronchiectasis: clinical and functional correlation. Radiology 225:663–672

Ouellette H (1999) The signet ring sign. Radiology 212:67–68

Smith IE, Flower CDR (1996) Imaging in bronchiectasis. Br J Radiol 69:589 593

The Solitary Pulmonary Nodule (Histoplasmoma)

Erasmus JJ (2000a) Solitary pulmonary nodules: part I. Morphologic evaluation for differentiation of benign and malignant lesions. Radiographics 20:43–58

Erasmus JJ (2000b) Solitary pulmonary nodules: part II. Evaluation of the indeterminate nodule. Radiographics 20:59–66

Li F et al (2004) Radiologists' performance for differentiating benign from malignant lung nodules on high-resolution CT using computer-estimated likelihood of malignancy. AJR Am J Roentgenol 183:1209–1215

Massaro M et al (2005) Histoplasmosis pulmonar Infección pulmonar primaria: histoplasmoma. Rev Col Radiol 16(3):1788–1790

McGuinness G, Naidich DP, Jagirdar J et al (1992) High resolution CT findings in miliary lung disease. J Comput Assist Tomogr 16(3):384–390

Midthun DE, Swensen SJ, Jett JR (1993) Approach to the solitary pulmonary nodule. Mayo Clin Proc 68:378–385

Winer-Muram HT (2006) The solitary pulmonary nodule. Radiology 239:34–49

Yi CA et al (2006) Tissue characterization of solitary pulmonary nodule: comparative study between helical dynamic CT and integrated PET/CT. J Nucl Med 47:443–450

Hodgkin's Lymphoma

Guermazi A, Brice P, de Kerviler EE, Ferme C, Hennequin C, Meignin V, Frija J (2001) Extranodal Hodgkin disease: spectrum of disease. Radiographics 21:161–179

Thoracic Sequelae in Tuberculosis

Castaner E, Gallardo X, Mata JM (1998) Common and uncommon complications of reactivation tuberculosis in immunocompetent patients. Eur J Radiol 27:43–52

Choi J-A et al (2001) CT manifestations of late sequelae in patients with tuberculous pleuritis. AJR Am J Roentgenol 176:441–445

Kim HY et al (2001) Thoracic sequelae and complications of tuberculosis. Radiographics 21:839–860

Leung AN (1999) State of the art. Pulmonary tuberculosis: the essentials. Radiology 210:307–322

Llanos-Tejada F (2010) Spirometrics alterations in patients with pulmonary tuberculosis sequelae. Rev Med Hered 21:77–78

Lung Abscess

César Pedrosa Rafael S (2000) Diagnóstico por Imagen – Compendio de Radiología Clínica. McGraw – Hill Interamericana, Madrid, pp 1–185

Fraser RS, Paré JAM, Fraser RG, Paré PD (1994) Synopsis of diseases of the chest, 2nd edn. W.B. Saunders Company, Philadelphia

Groskin SA (1993) Heiztman's the lung radiology-pathologic correlations, 3rd edn. Mosby Years Book, St. Louis

Katz D, Math KR, Groskin SA (1998) Radiology secrets. Hanley & Belfus Inc., Philadelphia, pp 1–11, 9–21, 41–100

Millar WT (1982) Introduction to clinical radiology. Editorial Manual Moderno S.A. Mcmillan, pp 11–107. ISBN:0023811706, 9780023811708

Santin G (2001) Vademecum Radiologico: Lo que Importa en la Clínica General. McGraw – Hill Interamericana, México, pp 83–91, 93 – 100

Stark DD, Federle MP, Goodman PC, Podrasky AE, Webb WR (1983) Differentiating lung abscess and empyema: radiography and computed tomography. AJR Am J Roentgenol 141(1):163–167

Stern E, White C (2000) Radiología del Tórax, 1st edn. McGraw-Hill, México

Takayanagi N, Kagiyama N, Ishiguro T et al (2010) Etiology and outcome of community-acquired lung abscess. Respiration 80:98–105

Taveras JM, Ferruchi JT (2000) Radiology: diagnosis, imaging, intervention. Lippincott William and Wilkins, Philadelphia

Williford ME, Godwin JD (1983) Computed tomography of lung abscess and empyema. Radiol Clin North Am 21(3):575–583

Septic Pulmonary Embolism

Cook RJ, Ashton RW, Aughenbaugh GL, Ryu JH (2005) Septic pulmonary embolism. Chest 128:162–166

Dodd JD, Souza CA, Müller NL (2006) High-resolution MDCT of pulmonary septic embolism: evaluation of the feeding vessel sign. AJR Am J Roentgenol 187:623–629

Jorens PG, Van Marck E, Snoeckx A, Parizel PM (2009) Nonthrombotic pulmonary embolism. Eur Respir J 34:452–474

Khashper A, Discepola F, Kosiuk J, Qanadli SD, Mesurolle B (2012) Nonthrombotic pulmonary embolism. AJR Am J Roentgenol 198:W152–W159

Lin MY, Rezal K, Schwartz DN (2008) Septic pulmonary emboli and bacteremia associated with deep tissue infections caused by community-acquired methicillin-resistant *Staphylococcus aureus*. J Clin Microbiol 46(4):1553

Congenital Lobar Emphysema

Zylak CJ, Eyler WR, Spizarny DL, Stone CH (2002) Developmental lung anomalies in the adult: radiologic-pathologic correlation. Radiographics 22:S25–S43

Daltro P, Fricke BL, Kuroki I, Domingues R, Donnelly LF (2004) CT of congenital lung lesions in pediatric patients. AJR Am J Roentgenol 183:1497–1506

Biyyam DR et al (2010) Congenital lung abnormalities: embryologic features, prenatal diagnosis, and postnatal radiologic-pathologic correlation. Radiographics 30:1721–1738

Berrocal T et al (2004) Congenital anomalies of the tracheobronchial tree, lung, and mediastinum: embryology, radiology, and pathology. Radiographics 24:e17

Lee EY et al (2008) Multidetector CT evaluation of congenital lung anomalies. Radiology 247:632–648

Trachea and Airway

6

John C. Pedrozo Pupo, Diego Pardo Pinzón, Manuel Pacheco, Paulina Ojeda León, Pedro Chaparro Mutis, and Manuel Garay Fernandez

Contents

J.C. Pedrozo Pupo (ed.), *Learning Chest Imaging*, Learning Imaging,
DOI 10.1007/978-3-642-34147-2_6, © Springer-Verlag Berlin Heidelberg 2013

Case 1: Tracheobronchopathia Osteochondroplastica

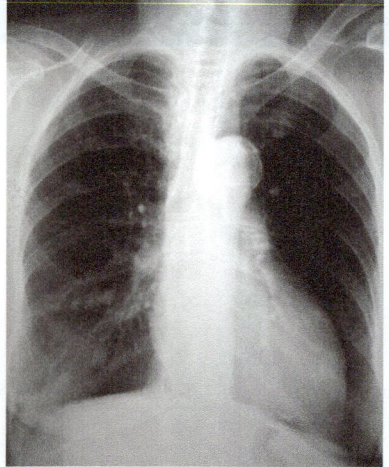

Fig. 6.1.1

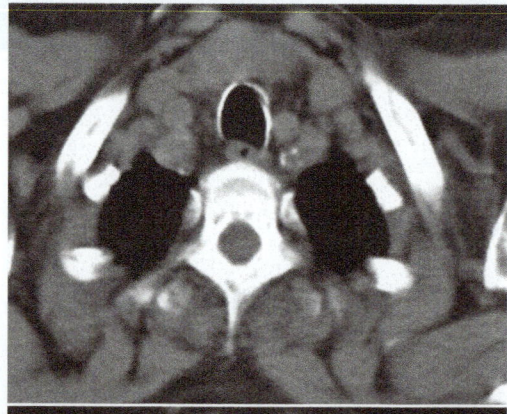

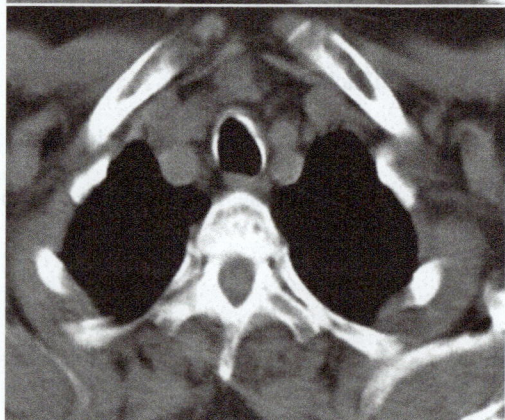

Fig. 6.1.2

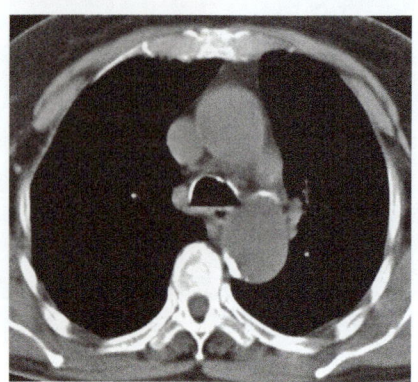

Fig. 6.1.3

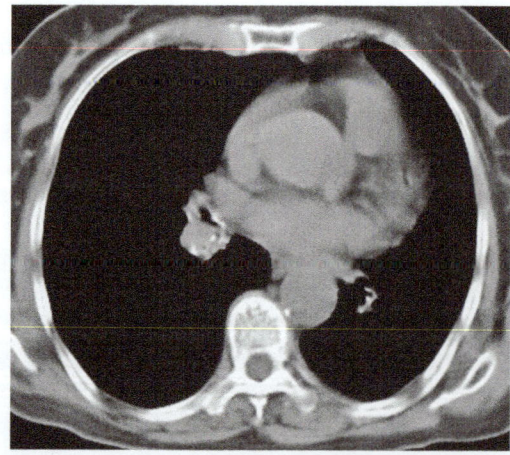

Fig. 6.1.4

A 65-year-old woman consulted for recurrent pneumonia.

The tracheobronchopathia osteochondroplastica (TBOC) is a rare benign disease of unknown etiology, characterized by multiple cartilaginous or bony submucosal nodules in the trachea, bronchi, and, less frequently, subglottic larynx. The clinical presentation of the disease varies from asymptomatic to severe disease with airway obstruction. The gold standard for diagnosis is bronchoscopy, which typically displays the presence of multiple submucosal nodules that project into the lumen of the airway. Biopsy is not required for diagnosis. The treatment of the disease is usually directed at symptom management. In patients with severe airway obstruction, bronchoscopic therapies have been performed such as laser ablation, cryotherapy, or divulsion mechanical injuries. Surgical resolution has also been attempted, being generally ineffective.

The TBOC usually involves the walls of the trachea, bronchi, and, less frequently, subglottic larynx. The incidence is low, with a reported figure of 0.11 % in patients undergoing bronchoscopy. The larynx and subglottic commitment is described in 40 % of patients with TBOC.

TBOC association with other pathologies such as amyloidosis, silicosis, and mycobacterial infection is uncertain. Its complications include recurrent respiratory infections, bronchiectasis, and atelectasis, there being sufficient evidence that associated with progression to malignancy.

The differential diagnosis of TBOC include tracheobronchial amyloidosis, calcified lesions secondary to tuberculosis, carcinoma, papilloma, fibroma, endobronchial sarcoidosis, polychondritis, and Wegener's granulomatosis of the proximal airways.

The chest X-ray is usually normal. Chest computed tomography discloses dense submucosal nodules protruding into the lumen of the trachea and main bronchi. They are calcified in half cases. The typical sparing of the posterior is usually visible.

Comments

CRX film shows thickening and calcification of the tracheal lumen associated with right perihilar alveolar infiltration (Fig. 6.1.1). CT scan (mediastinal window) shows calcification of the tracheal and bronchial lumen associated with marked narrowing of the intermediate bronchus (Figs. 6.1.2, 6.1.3, and 6.1.4).

Imaging Findings

Case 2: Tracheal Stenosis

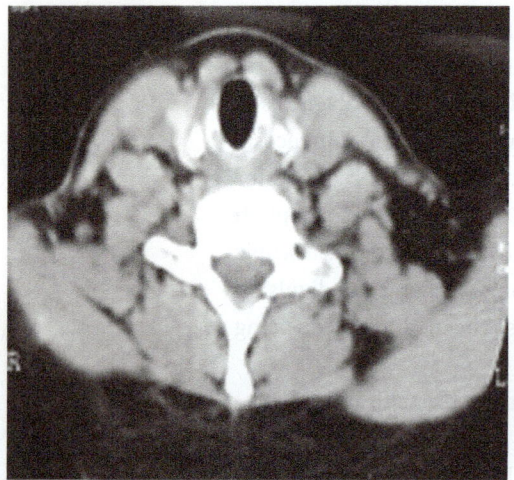

Fig. 6.2.1

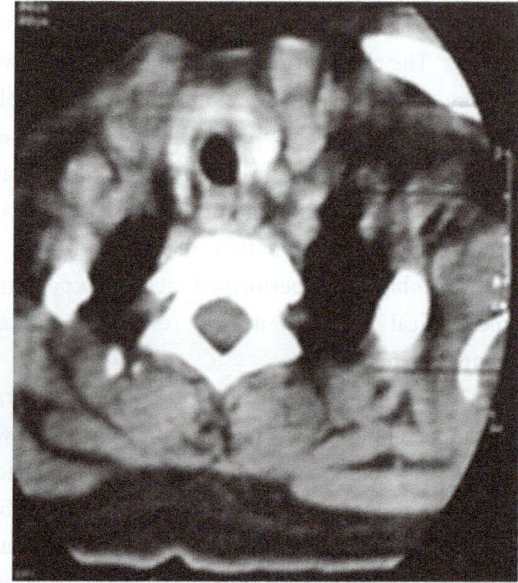

Fig. 6.2.2

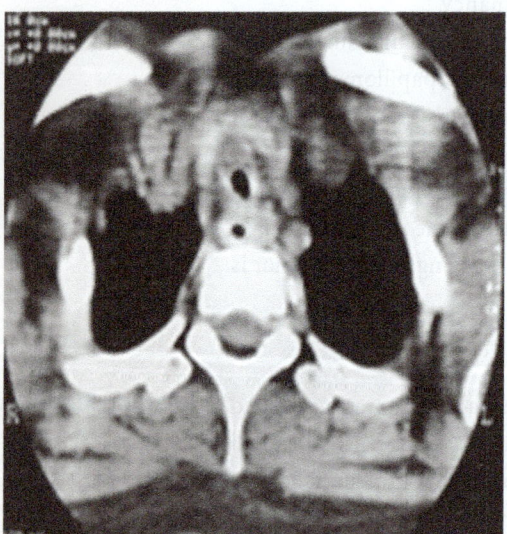

Fig. 6.2.3

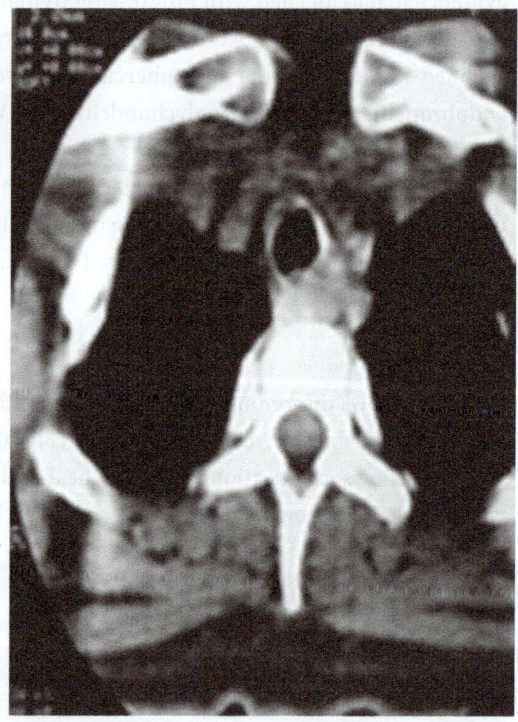

Fig. 6.2.4

A 43-year-old man has consultation for 2-month symptoms of dyspnea, stridor with expiration, and history of endotracheal intubation 8 months ago.

The causes of adult laryngeal and upper tracheal stenosis are trauma, chronic inflammatory diseases (e.g., amyloidosis, sarcoidosis, relapsing polychondritis), benign neoplasm (e.g., respiratory papillomatosis), malignant neoplasm (e.g., primary tracheal, secondary invasion, metastatic), and collagen vascular diseases (e.g., tracheopathia osteoplastica, Wegener granulomatosis).

The sequence of events that leads to laryngeal and upper tracheal stenosis in adults involves ulceration of the mucosa and cartilage, inflammatory reactions with associated granulation tissue, fibrous tissue formation, and contraction of fibrous scar tissue. Capillary perfusion pressure is a crucial consideration in mucosal injury, and mucosal ischemia is produced by direct contact with an endotracheal tube segment or by an increase in the pressure in the tube cuff. The radiographs can demonstrate soft tissue swelling, alterations of the cartilaginous framework (if it is sufficiently calcified), and the position of the air column.

On CT scan, this condition may be seen as eccentric or concentric soft tissue thickening internal to normal-appearing tracheal cartilage. The outer tracheal wall has a normal appearance without evidence of deformity or narrowing. Expiratory CT shows little change in tracheal diameter. In patients with chronic stricture, thickening of the mucosa and submucosa may be absent or of mild degree, with tracheal narrowing resulting from deformity of the tracheal cartilage or posterior membrane. This technique enables satisfactory analysis of the vertical extent of the tracheal stenosis or stricture, but conventional coronal CT scanning is only used occasionally because of its limited grayscale ability to differentiate soft tissue. Axial CT scan images can sufficiently evaluate the majority of airway abnormalities, but there are some limitations, including the following: (a) limited ability to detect subtle airway stenosis, (b) underestimation of the craniocaudal extent of disease, (c) difficulty displaying the relationships of the airway to the adjacent mediastinal structures, (d) inadequate representation of the airways that are oriented obliquely to the axial plane, (e) difficulty assessing the interfaces and surfaces of airways that lie parallel to the axial plane, and (f) generation of a large number of images for review.

The best compromise among the combined factors of CT scan airway measurement precision, patient breath-holding time, and total X-ray dose is the use of a 3-mm section thickness, a reconstruction interval of 1.5 mm, and a maximal pitch of 1.3–1.5, as well as the application of the edge-enhancing modus. CT scanning, sectional image data acquisition, and 3-dimensional (3D) airway image reconstruction have become increasingly useful in head and neck surgery. The sensitivity of CT scan-based virtual bronchoscopy (CTVB) in detecting central tumors is 93.3 %, with an accuracy of 93.5 %.

CT scan (mediastinal window) shows narrowing of tracheal lumen semicircular shape by 60–70 % (Figs. 6.2.1, 6.2.2, 6.2.3, and 6.2.4).

Case 3: Foreign Body Aspiration

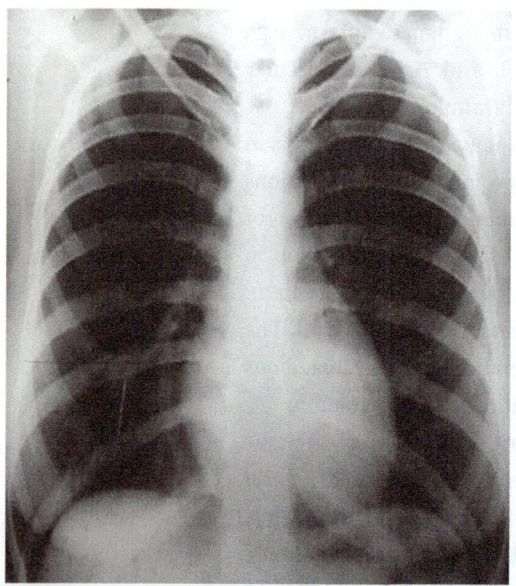

Fig. 6.3.1

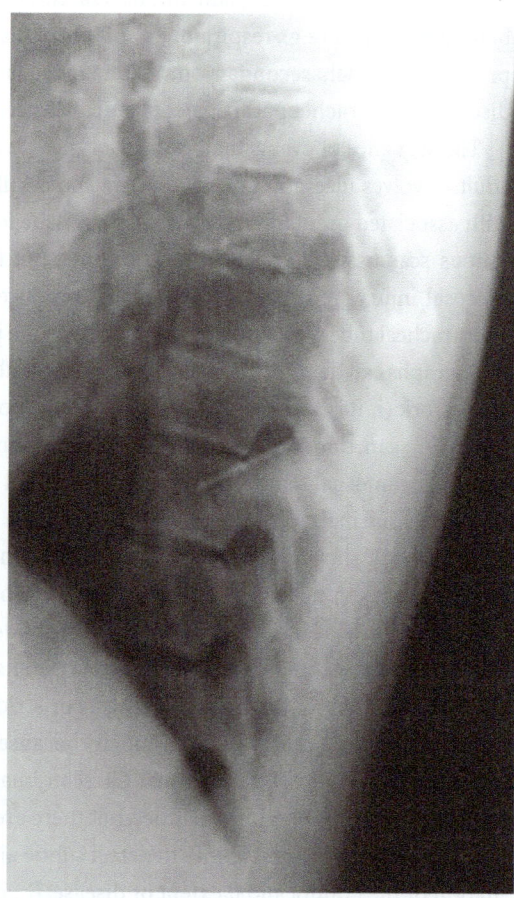

Fig. 6.3.2

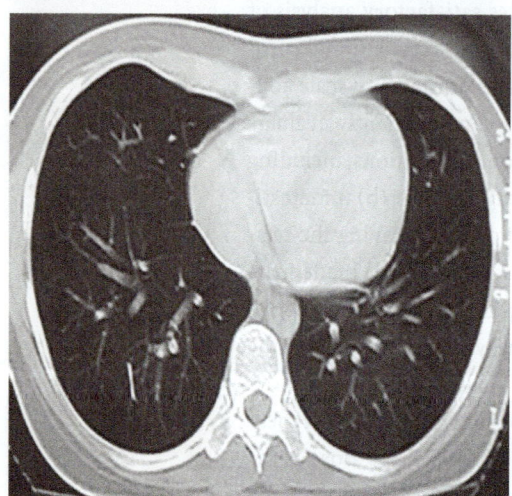

Fig. 6.3.3

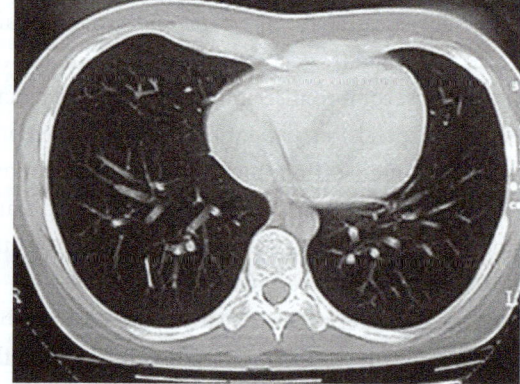

Fig. 6.3.4

A 25-year-old woman has consultation for cough after needle aspiration.

The death rate from asphyxia due to foreign body aspiration is 1.3 in 100,000. **Comments**
Death from foreign body aspiration has a bimodal pattern, with peaks at ages under 1 year (1.9 per 100,000) and over 75 years (10.7 per 100,000). Foreign body aspiration occurs commonly in childhood and to a lesser extent in adults. In adults, it happens more frequently in older people due to insufficient airway protective mechanism. The acute complications of non-asphyxiating foreign body aspiration are pneumothorax, pneumomediastinum, and obstructive emphysema, and in delayed cases may cause recurrent pneumonia and hemoptysis, bronchiectasis, infection, and abscess. A delay in diagnosis of over 24 h increases the incidence of complications.

In adults, the right lower lobe bronchus is more frequently affected because it is wider than the left bronchus and makes a wider angle with the trachea. It has been reported that 40–70 % of foreign body aspirations occur in the right bronchial system, 30–40 % in the left bronchial system, and 10–20 % in the laryngotracheal region.

Bronchoscopy is the standard procedure in the diagnosis and extraction of an airway FB. The development of the flexible bronchoscope has reduced the need for rigid bronchoscopy. Although most of the airway FBs in adult patients can be extracted with flexible bronchoscopy, rare cases with an airway FB may need to undergo rigid bronchoscopic extraction. Some patients will have retained foreign bodies after bronchoscopy, with the reported incidence ranging from 1 to 18 %.

If foreign body aspiration is suspected in a patient, screening radiographic studies employed include anteroposterior (AP) and lateral imaging of the soft tissues of the neck, inspiratory and expiratory posteroanterior (PA) chest radiographs (CRXs), and lateral CRXs. Radiologic diagnosis of foreign body aspiration is challenging for several reasons. Although radiopaque foreign bodies are obvious on radiographic studies, only 10 % of foreign bodies are radiopaque. The findings of chest radiography are normal in up to 30 % of children who aspirate a foreign body. The presence of pulmonary infiltrates may misdirect the management away from foreign body aspiration. Unilateral radiolucent lung is the most important radiographic finding in the diagnosis of bronchial foreign body. The sensitivity and specificity of chest radiography for foreign body detection were only 68 and 67 %, respectively, in a series of 83 patients.

CT is the most sensitive diagnostic imaging technique but is reserved for the diagnosis of elusive cases of a foreign body aspiration because of its radiation hazard and cost. CT not only shows both opaque and nonopaque foreign bodies in the bronchial tree in many cases but also sensitively detects subtle air trapping.

CRX film shows the presence of metallic density linear object in the right **Imaging Findings**
lower lobe (Figs. 6.3.1 and 6.3.2). CT scan (lung window) shows metal needle in the posterior segment of right lower lobe (Figs. 6.3.3 and 6.3.4).

Case 4: Tracheal Sarcoidosis

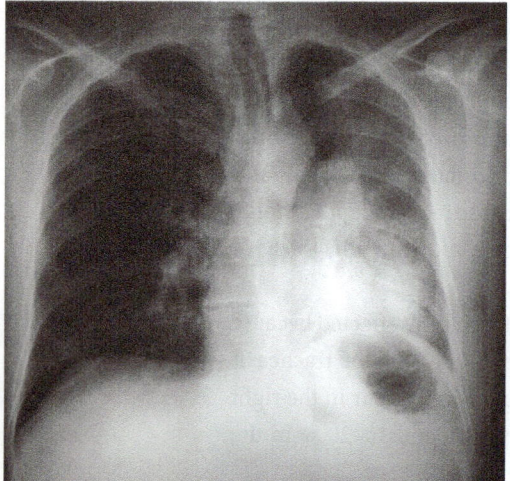

Fig. 6.4.1

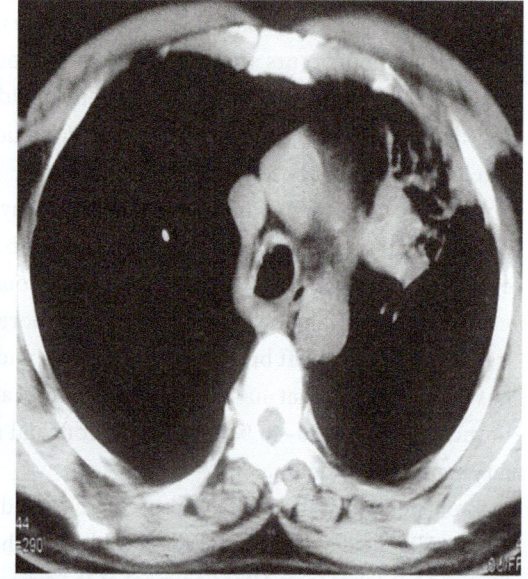

Fig. 6.4.2

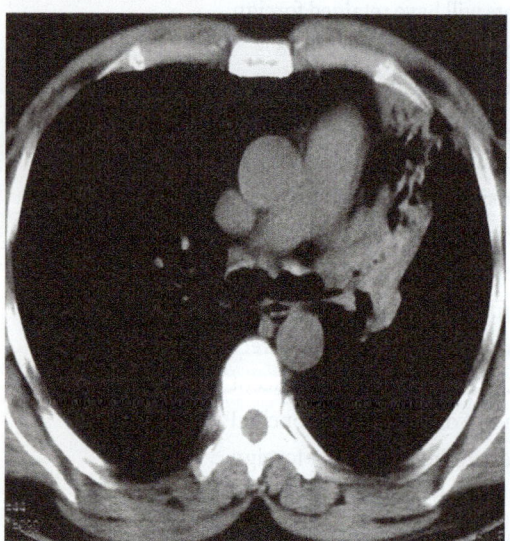

Fig. 6.4.3

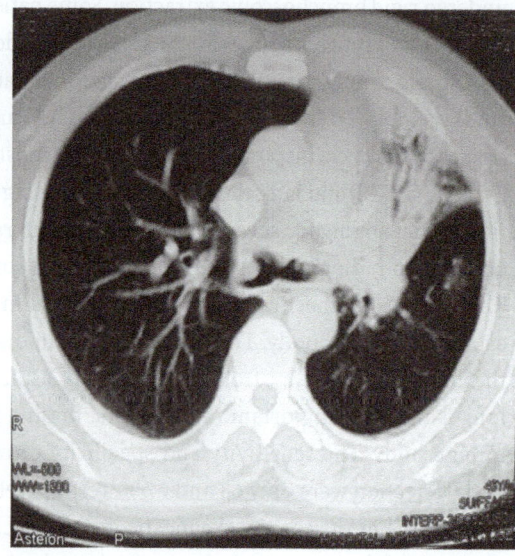

Fig. 6.1.1

A 50-year-old man with clinical symptoms of approximately 8 months of evolution characterized by symptoms of cough initially dry, then productive with whitish sputum, intermittent episodes of grade 2 dyspnea, weight loss, fever, and dysphonia

Sarcoidosis is a multisystemic granulomatous disease of unknown cause that is characterized by the formation of noncaseous epithelioid cell granulomas. Sarcoidosis primarily affects the lung and lymphatic systems. It is a relatively common disorder in most of parts of the world and usually affects those persons in the 25- to 50-year-old age group. Sarcoidosis involves the respiratory system in >90 % of cases, usually the hilar and mediastinal nodes and, less frequently, the lung tissue. Airway involvement, as judged by clinical features, physiologic testing, imaging techniques, bronchoscopy, and airway mucosal biopsy, has been observed in nearly two-thirds of patients with sarcoidosis.

Chest roentgenographic abnormalities are frequently the first indication of sarcoidosis, even in asymptomatic patients. Subtle airway involvement is not visible on plain chest films. Secondary traction bronchiectasis may be suggested by the prominent air bronchograms.

High-resolution CT scans may demonstrate bronchial distortion, angulation, and displacement. Decreased airway luminal diameter caused by endobronchial granulomas and evidence of bronchial mural thickening may be seen. Extrinsic compression of the airways by the enlarged lymph nodes may be depicted. Large airway involvement, on the other hand, is very uncommon. Airway abnormalities may result from extrinsic compression by adjacent diseased lymph nodes or from primary infiltration of the airway walls with noncaseating granulomas. Upper tracheal and laryngeal involvement is more common than distal central airway involvement.

CRX film shows opacity and signs of loss of volume in the left lower lobe (Fig. 6.4.1). CT scan (mediastinal window) shows nodular mucosa at the trachea and carina associated with left upper lobe collapse (Figs. 6.4.2 and 6.4.3). CT scan (lung window) shows nodular mucosa at the trachea and carina, decreasing the caliber of the left main bronchus and left upper lobe collapse (Fig. 6.4.4). Bronchoscopy shows alteration of the mucosa with presence of nodular lesions in size from 3 to 5 mm compromising the light in 30 % and diffuse localization to the carina (Fig. 6.4.5). HE staining 10× and 40× shows nonnecrotizing granulomatous reaction with ZN staining and Grocott negative for AFB and fungi. PCR was also performed for mycobacteria in paraffin block which was negative (Fig. 6.4.6).

Fig. 6.4.5

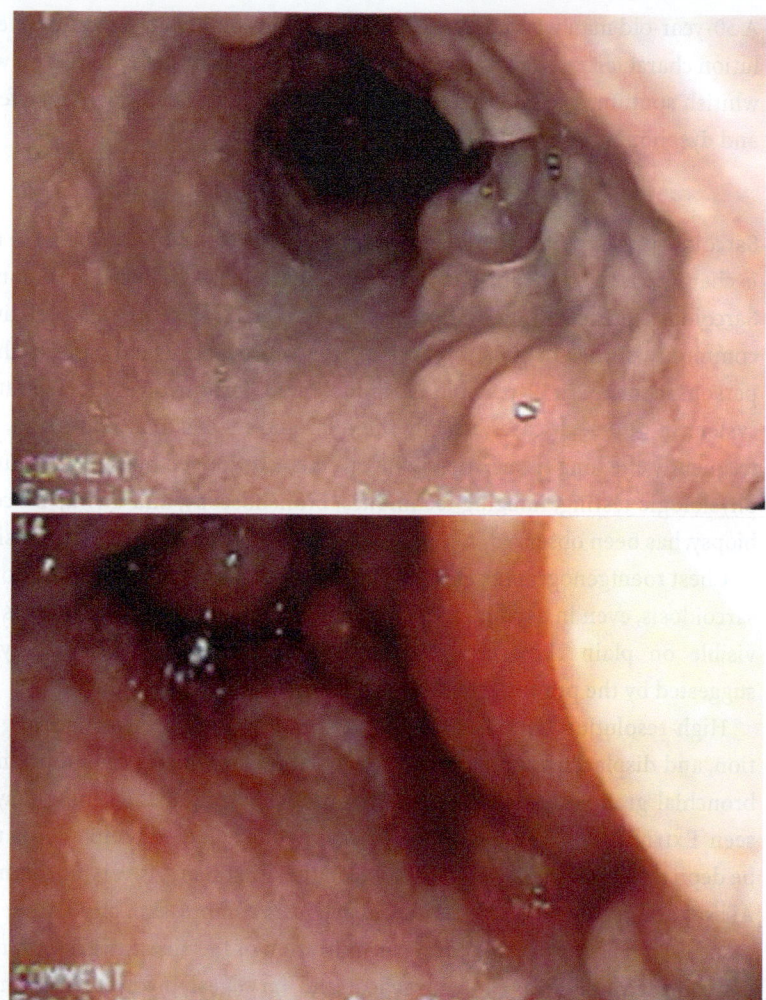

Fig. 6.4.6

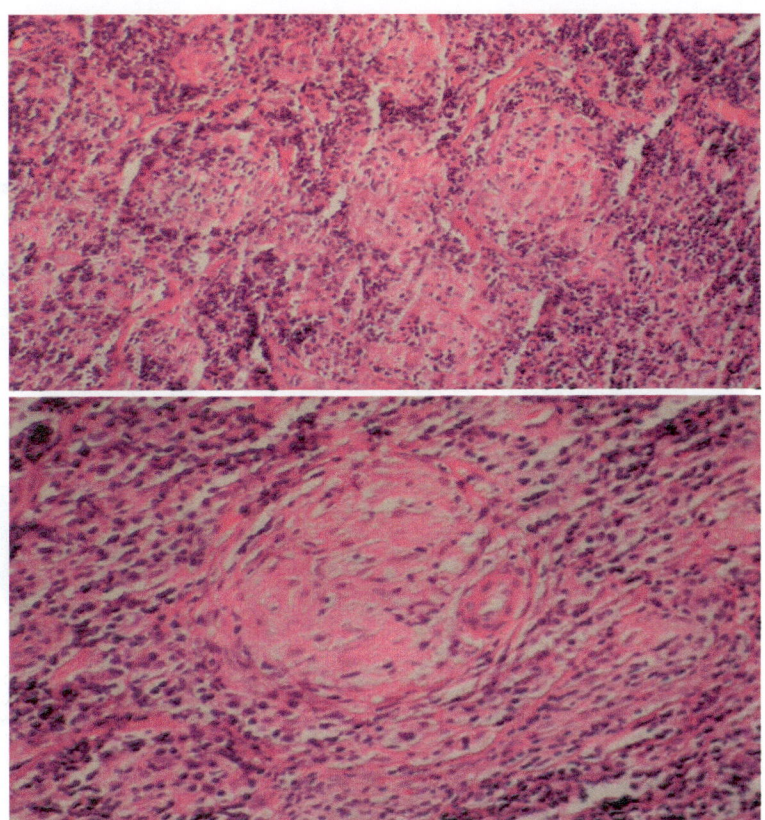

Case 5: Localized Tracheal Amyloidosis

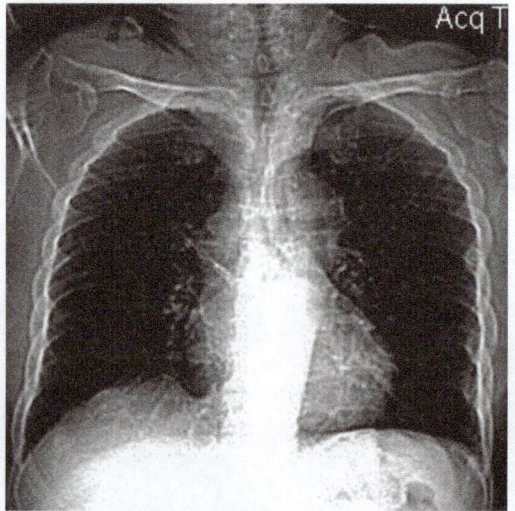

Fig. 6.5.1

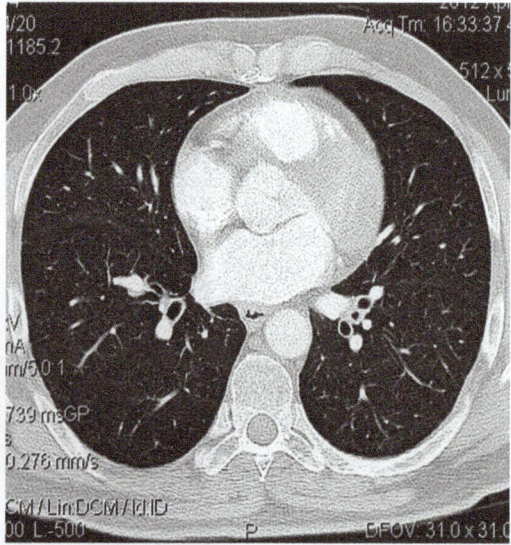

Fig. 6.5.2

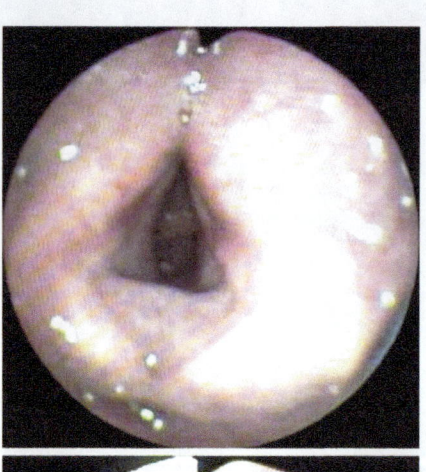

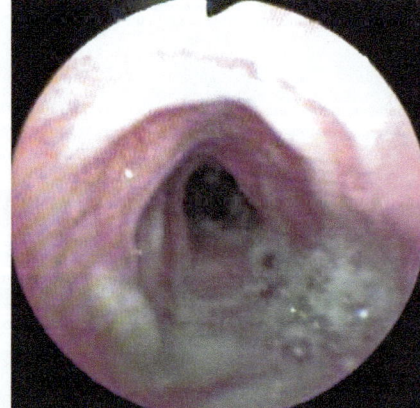

Fig. 6.5.3

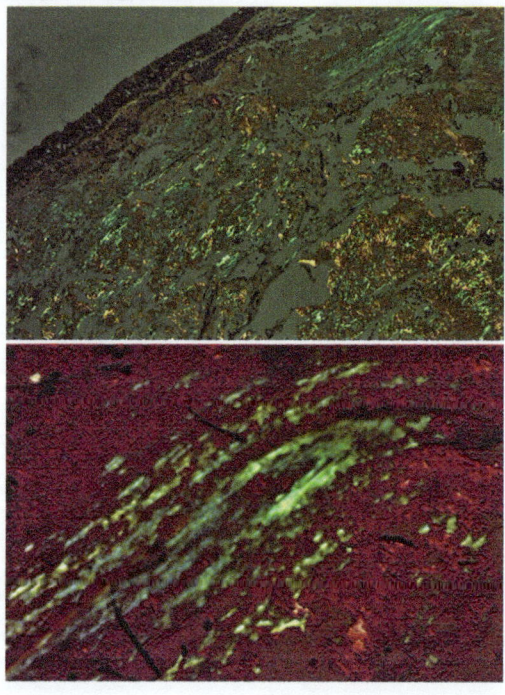

Fig. 6.5.4

A 61-year-old man with clinical symptoms of approximately 2 months of evolution characterized by intermittent episodes of dry cough without hemoptysis and persistent and progressive dysphonia.

Amyloidosis is a rare condition characterized by deposition of insoluble protein in the extracellular tissues. It may involve any portion of the respiratory tract. Within the lung parenchyma, abnormal amyloid deposition can appear as single or multiple nodules or diffuse interstitial opacities.

Tracheobronchial amyloidosis is a rare condition. Primary tracheobronchial amyloidosis is generally not associated with parenchymal abnormalities. Deposits are submucosal and most commonly involve the entire trachea. Infrequently, a solitary submucosal nodule is present.

The clinical profile is typically a male patient in the sixth decade of life, presenting cough, dyspnea, and occasional hemoptysis. Depending on the size and location of the lesion, pulmonary atelectasis can occur, as can obstructive pneumonia. If the obstruction is located in the trachea, the physical examination will reveal bilateral wheezing.

Radiological and endoscopic examinations are useful for locating the lesion and evaluating the architecture of the affected area, although the definitive diagnosis usually requires histopathological confirmation.

CT shows diffuse nodular thickening of the trachea and main bronchi, often involving the subglottic trachea. Bronchial stenosis or occlusion may result in lobar or segmental atelectasis [8]. Nodular calcified regions within the trachea are common, as in tracheobronchopathia osteochondroplastica. Amyloidosis typically involves the airway concentrically, whereas tracheobronchopathia osteochondroplastica and RPC characteristically spare the posterior tracheal and bronchial walls. In addition, amyloidosis may affect the larynx, pharynx, and superior trachea in contrast to tracheobronchopathia osteochondroplastica.

CRX film shows narrowing of the lumen of the trachea (Fig. 6.5.1). CT scan (lung window) shows no pulmonary involvement (Fig. 6.5.2). Bronchoscopy shows nodular lesions and white on the tracheal mucosa (Fig. 6.5.3). Congo red stain 10× and 40× shows amorphous material in the submucosa with amyloid deposits. In polarized light, apple-green shows Congo red positive (Fig. 6.5.4).

Case 6: Direct Tracheal Involvement of Lung Cancer

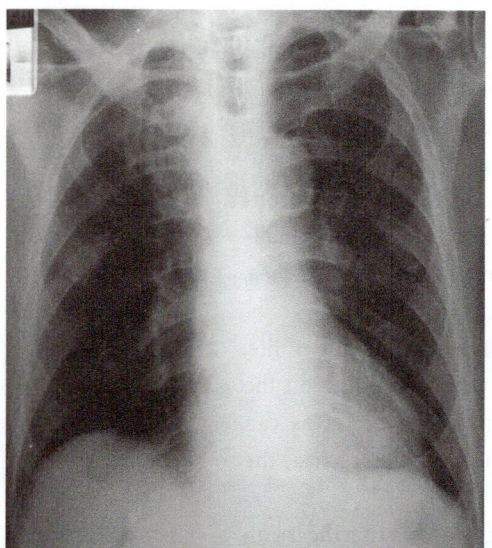

Fig. 6.6.1

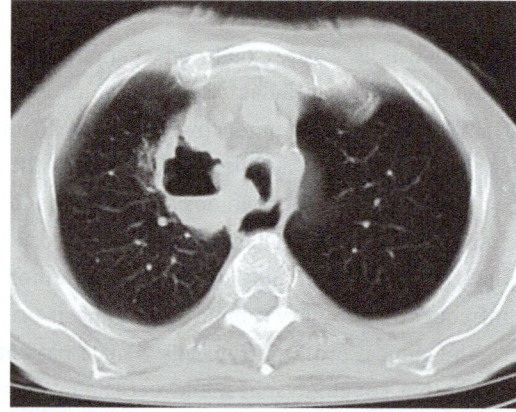

Fig. 6.6.2

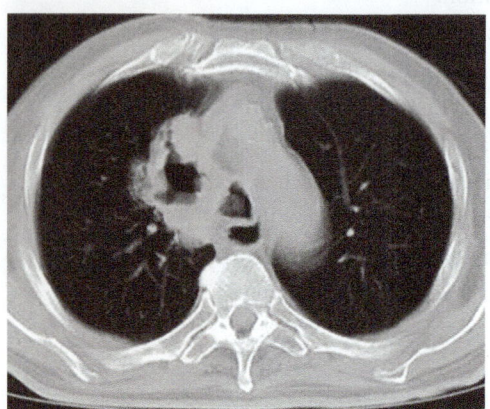

Fig. 6.6.3

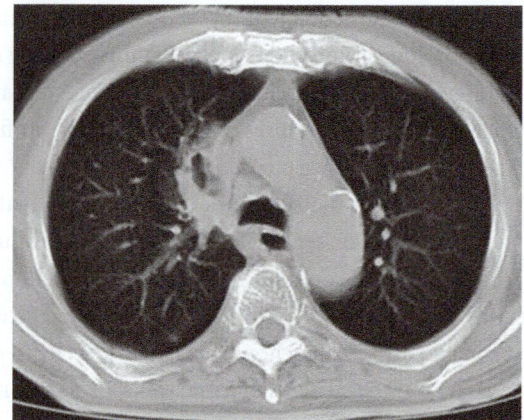

Fig. 6.6.4

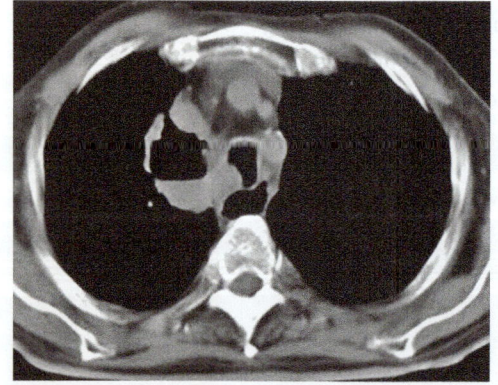

Fig. 6.6.5

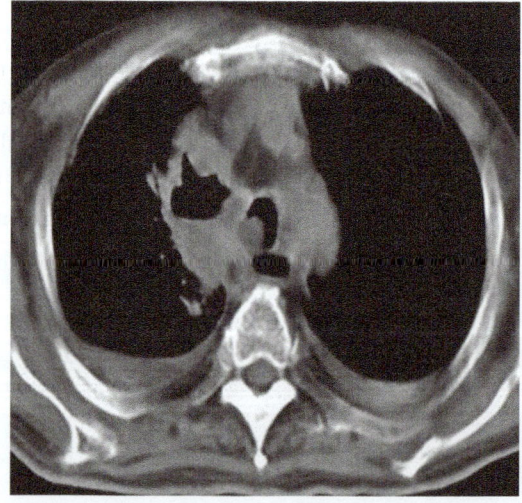

Fig. 6.6.6

A 76-year-old man is referred for inspiratory stridor, dyspnea, cough with bloody sputum, fatigue, weakness, and weight loss. Bronchoscopy showed tumor lesion which reduces the tracheal lumen by 70 %. Smoked for 30 years.

Comments

Tracheal metastasis of primary lung cancer is extremely rare, although direct tracheal involvement by primary lung cancer is often seen and classified as T4 lung cancer. Tracheal metastases from nonpulmonary malignancies such as breast cancer, colorectal carcinoma, renal carcinoma, and melanoma have been reported.

The incidence of endotracheal or endobronchial metastasis of primary lung cancer has not been reported in the literature. However, the incidence of endotracheal or endobronchial metastasis of nonpulmonary malignancies is known to vary, ranging from approximately 2–50 %, according to how they are defined.

The symptoms associated with endotracheal and endobronchial metastases regardless of its primary site are similar to those associated with primary endotracheal and endobronchial tumors. Hemoptysis with coughing is the most common symptom, with an incidence of 41–62 %.

In the endotracheal and endobronchial metastases is proposed four types of developmental modes of endotracheal and endobronchial metastases in a morphologic way: type 1, direct metastasis to the bronchus; type 2, bronchial invasion by a parenchymal lesion; type 3, bronchial invasion by mediastinal or hilar lymph node metastasis; and type 4, a peripheral lesion extending along the proximal bronchus.

The metastatic lesions may be asymptomatic or may present with cough, hemoptysis, dyspnea, and stridor. Bronchoscopy has 100 % diagnostic accuracy for identifying endoluminal lesions.

Squamous cell carcinoma (SCC) is the most common primary tracheobronchial malignancy and develops mainly in the sixth and seventh decades of life. This tumor is strongly associated with habitual cigarette smoking, affecting men two to four times more frequently than women. SCC can be exophytic or infiltrative and tends to involve the posterior wall of the lower two-thirds of the trachea. About one-third of patients have either mediastinal or pulmonary metastases at diagnosis. Furthermore, approximately 40 % of tracheobronchial SCCs have been reported to occur before, concurrently with, or after carcinoma of the oropharynx, larynx, or lung.

At CT, the tumor may appear as a polypoid lesion, a focal sessile lesion, eccentric narrowing of the airway lumen, or circumferential wall thickening. The majority of SCCs of the tracheobronchial tree show high uptake at FDG PET, apparently due to their increased metabolic activity.

Imaging Findings

CRX film shows ill-defined lesion in the right upper lobe that contacts the line right paratracheal (Fig. 6.6.1). CT scan (mediastinal and lung window) shows cavitary lung mass infiltrating the side wall of the trachea and occupies the lumen by 70 % lower third level (Figs. 6.6.2, 6.6.3, 6.6.4, 6.6.5, and 6.6.6).

Further Reading

Tracheobronchopathia Osteochondroplastica

Abu-Hijleh M, Lee D, Braman SS (2008) Tracheobronchopathia osteochondroplastica: a rare large airway disorder. Lung 186:353–359

Alroy GG, Lichtig C, Kaftori JK (1972) Tracheobronchopathia osteoplastica: end stage of primary lung amyloidosis? Chest 61(5):465–468

Harma RA, Suurkari S (1977) Tracheopathia chondroosteoplastica. A clinical study of thirty cases. Acta Otolaryngol 84(1–2):118–123

Hussain K, Gilbert S (2003) Tracheopathia osteochondroplastica. Clin Med Res 1(3):239–242

Jabbardarjani HR, Radpey B, Kharabian S, Masjedi MR (2008) Tracheobronchopathia osteochondroplastica: presentation of ten cases and review of the literature. Lung 186(5):293–297

Karlikaya C, Yüksel M, Kilicli S, Candan L (2000) Tracheobronchopathia osteochondroplastica. Respirology 5(4):377–380

Montufar FE, Echeverri JA, Baena J, Ojeda P (1994) Traqueobroncopatia osteocondroplástica. Aspectos clínicos y diagnóstico broncoscópico-radiográfico. Rev Colomb Neumol 6(1) Marzo

Nienhuis DM, Prakash UB, Edell ES (1990) Tracheobronchopathia osteochondroplastica. Ann Otol Rhinol Laryngol 99(9 Pt 1):689–694

Prakash UB (2002) Tracheobronchopathia osteochondroplastica. Semin Respir Crit Care Med 23:167–175

Vilkman S, Keistinen T (1995) Tracheobronchopathia osteochondroplastica. Report of a young man with severe disease and retrospective review of 18 cases. Respiration 62(3):151–154

Tracheal Stenosis

Gluecker T, Lang F, Bessler S et al (2001) 2D and 3D CT imaging correlated to rigid endoscopy in complex laryngo-tracheal stenoses. Eur Radiol 11(1):50–54

Grenier PA, Beigelman-Aubry C, Brillet PY (2009) Nonneoplastic tracheal and bronchial stenoses. Radiol Clin North Am 47(2):243–260

Rahman NA, Fruchter O, Shitrit D, Fox BD, Kramer MR (2010) Flexible bronchoscopic management of benign. tracheal stenosis: long term follow-up of 115 patients. J Cardiothorac Surg 5:2

Webb EM, Elicker BM, Webb WR (2000) Using CT to diagnose nonneoplastic tracheal abnormalities: appearance of the tracheal wall. AJR Am J Roentgenol 174:1315–1321

Foreign Body Aspiration

Applegate KE, Dardinger JT, Lieber ML et al (2001) Spiral CT scanning technique in the detection of aspiration of LEGO foreign bodies. Pediatr Radiol 31:836–840

Kosucu P, Ahmetoglu A, Koramaz I et al (2004) Low-dose MDCT and virtual bronchoscopy in pediatric patients with foreign body aspiration. AJR Am J Roentgenol 183:1771–1777

Limper AH, Prakash UB (1990) Tracheobronchial foreign bodies in adults. Ann Intern Med 15:604–609

Rafanan AL, Mehta AC (2004) Bronchoscopy in foreign body removal. In: Wang K, Mehta AC, Turner JF (eds) Flexible bronchoscopy, 2nd edn. Blackwell Publishing, Malden, MA, pp 197–208

Shin SM et al (2009) CT in children with suspected residual foreign body in airway after bronchoscopy. AJR Am J Roentgenol 192:1744–1751

Zissin R, Shapiro-Feinberg M, Rozenman J, Apter S, Smorjik J, Hertz M (2001) CT findings of the chest in adults with aspirated foreign bodies. Eur Radiol 11:606–611

Tracheal Sarcoidosis

Chung JH, Kanne JP, Gilman MD (2011) CT of diffuse tracheal diseases. AJR Am J Roentgenol 196:W240–W246

Marchiori E, Pozes AS, Souza Junior AS, Escuissato DL, Irion KL, Araujo Neto C, Barillo JL, Souza CA, Zanetti G (2008) Diffuse abnormalities of the trachea: computed tomography findings. J Bras Pneumol 34(1): 47–54

Marom EM, Goodman PC, McAdams HP (2001) Diffuse abnormalities of the trachea and main bronchi. AJR Am J Roentgenol 176(3):713–717

Polychronopoulos VS, Prakash UBS (2009) Airway involvement in sarcoidosis. Chest 136(5):1371–1380

Prince JS, Duhamel DR (2002) Nonneoplastic lesions of the tracheobronchial wall: radiologic findings with bronchoscopic correlation. Radiographics 22:S215–S230

Localized Tracheal Amyloidosis

Chung JH, Kanne JP, Gilman MD (2011b) CT of diffuse tracheal diseases. AJR Am J Roentgenol 196:W240–W246

Georgiades CS, Neyman EG, Barish MA, Fishman EK (2004) Amyloidosis: review and CT manifestations. Radiographics 24(2):405–416

Gilad R, Milillo P, Som P (2007) Severe diffuse systemic amyloidosis with involvement of the pharynx, larynx, and trachea: CT and MR findings. AJNR Am J Neuroradiol 28:1557–1558

Prince J, Duhamel D, Levin D, Harrell J, Friedman P (2002) Nonneoplastic lesions of the tracheobronchial wall: radiologic findings with bronchoscopic correlation. Radiographics 22(Spec No):S215–S230

Webb EM, Elicker BM, Webb WR (2000) Using CT to diagnose nonneoplastic tracheal abnormalities: appearance of the tracheal wall. AJR Am J Roentgenol 174:1315–1321

Direct Tracheal Involvement of Lung Cancer

Chong S, Kim TS, Han J (2006) Tracheal metastasis of lung cancer: CT findings in six patients. AJR Am J Roentgenol 186:220–224

De S (2009) Tracheal metastasis of small cell lung cancer. Lung India 26(4):162–164

Kiryu T, Hi HH, Matsui E et al (2001) Endotracheal/endobronchial metastases. Chest 119:768–775

Park CM, Goo JM et al (2009) Tumors in the tracheobronchial tree: CT and FDG PET features. Radiographics 29:55–71

Heart and Great Vessels

7

John C. Pedrozo Pupo and Alvaro Coral Martinez

Contents

J.C. Pedrozo Pupo (ed.), *Learning Chest Imaging*, Learning Imaging,
DOI 10.1007/978-3-642-34147-2_7, © Springer-Verlag Berlin Heidelberg 2013

Case 1: Cardiomegaly

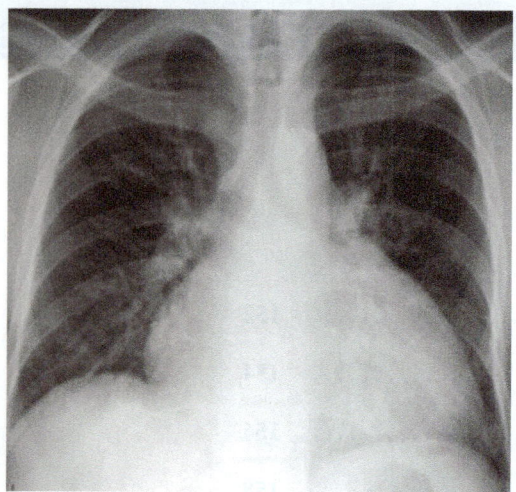

Fig. 7.1.1

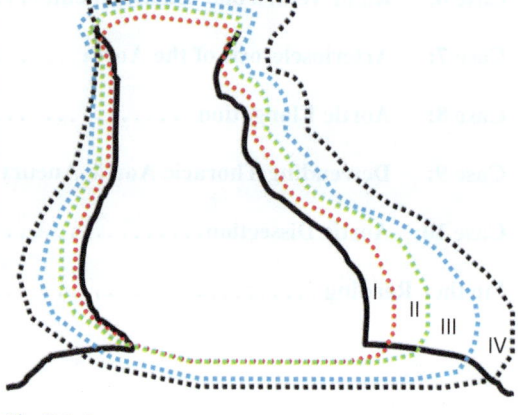

Fig. 7.1.2

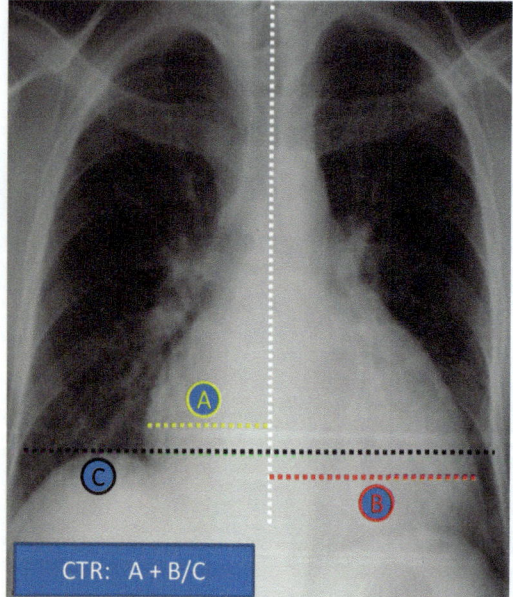

CTR: A + B/C

Fig. 7.1.3

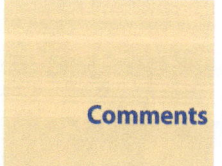

Fig. 7.1.4

Comments

A 65-year-old man with coronary artery disease and hypothyroidism is referred for 5 months of dyspnea functional class I/IV.

To make a proper systematic evaluation of the heart, we must consider the following: size, position, contour, density, pulmonary vascularization, and other chest abnormalities. Radiography contributes to the management in three ways, namely, (1) it can help exclude lung disease as the cause of symptoms. It can exclude gross pulmonary pathology and is valuable in pointing away from the lungs and toward the heart as the cause of symptoms. (2) It can make a positive diagnosis of heart disease. The demonstration of gross cardiac enlargement, abnormal shape, a grossly abnormal pulmonary vasculature, or possibly even pulmonary edema will all point to heart disease as the cause of symptoms. (3) A specific cardiac diagnosis may occasionally be possible on the radiograph.

Looking at the heart in an axial view, it would be easy to identify all cavities; in the frontal (AP, PA) view, this does not occur because the right edge of the heart corresponds to the right atrium (the first curve to the right) and the left edge corresponds to the left ventricle. The left atrium or right ventricle can be seen in this projection.

On the lateral view, the heart touches the sternum in less than 1/3 of the AP diameter and occupies less than half. The contour edge presents a higher heart, which is constituted by the right ventricle and posterior contour with a lower heart edge which constitutes the left ventricle. The left atrium cannot be observed in any forward conventional.

The size of the heart is established through two radiographic methods: the first is an objective method, which is performed by measuring the cardiothoracic ratio, and the second is a subjective method, which is established by direct visualization of the degree of cardiomegaly.

In adults, a CTR greater than 0.5 is considered to represent cardiomegaly. In aortic regurgitation, the left ventricle is often enlarged downward rather than horizontally. A high diaphragm position, as seen with obesity or shallow inspiration, will produce an erroneous CTR greater than 0.5. Pectus excavatum and the absence of pericardium displace the heart posteriorly and rotate the apex laterally, resulting in a CTR greater than 0.5 in the presence of a normal-sized heart. Large pericardial fat pads may give a falsely increased CTR. Because of these factors, one can be misled if relying on the CTR alone to diagnose cardiomegaly; however, it does serve as a baseline for future comparisons. A CTR > 0.5 with a normal heart size occurs with absent pericardium, pectus excavatum, obesity, and poor inspiration.

Imaging Findings

CRX film shows increased volume of cardiac chambers (Fig. 7.1.1). The formula used is ICT: $A + B / C$, the letter A represents the distance between the midline of the thorax and the more prominent right heart border, the letter B represents the distance between the midline of the chest with the most prominent left heart border, and the letter C represents the distance between the left and right costal arches with the reference the most prominent point of the diaphragm (Figs. 7.1.2 and 7.1.3). Schematic shows the subjective evaluation of cardiomegaly (Fig. 7.1.4).

Case 2: Dilated Cardiomyopathy

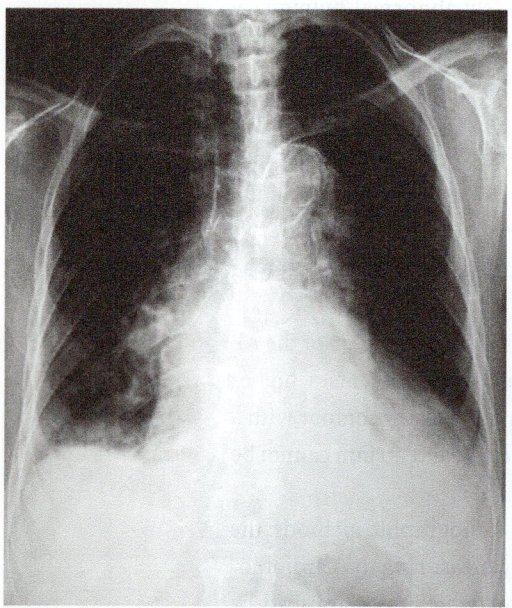

Fig. 7.2.1

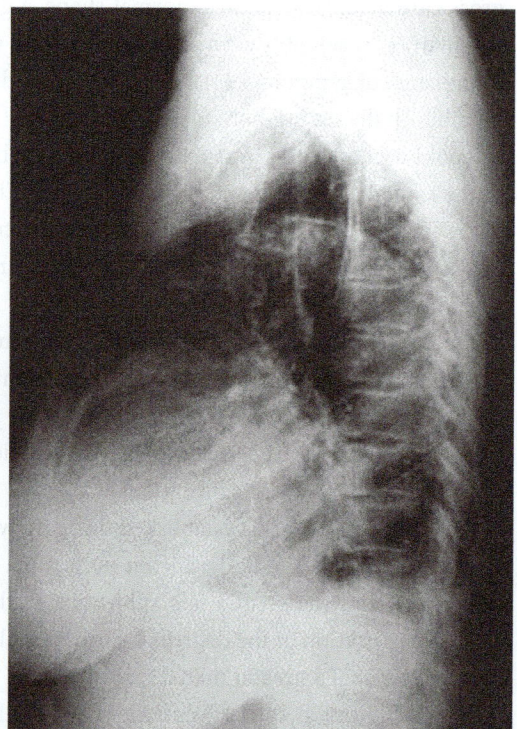

Fig. 7.2.2

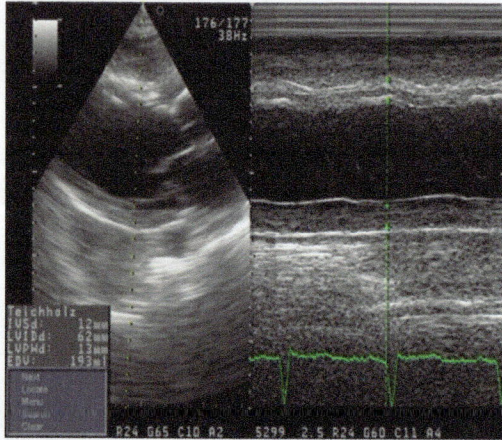

Fig. 7.2.3

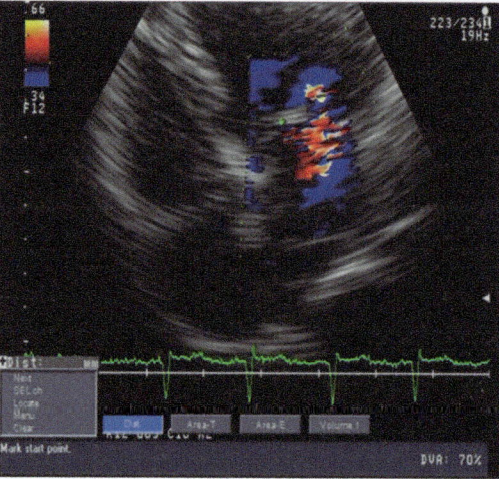

Fig. 7.2.4

A 78-year-old woman with hypertension and convulsion has had 6 days of dyspnea, orthopnea, abdominal distension, lower limb edema, and headache.

Dilated cardiomyopathy is characterized by left ventricular dilation that is associated with systolic dysfunction (a low < 40 % ejection fraction). Diastolic dysfunction and impaired right ventricular function can develop. Affected individuals are at risk of left or right ventricular failure, or both. Heart failure symptoms can be exercise-induced or persistent at rest. Many patients are asymptomatic. Chronically treated patients sometimes present acutely with decompensated heart failure. Other life-threatening risks are ventricular arrhythmias and atrioventricular block, syncope, and sudden death. Genetic inheritance arises in 30–48 % of patients, and inflammatory disorders such as myocarditis or toxic effects from medications, alcohol, or illicit drugs also result in dilated cardiomyopathy. Genes that cause dilated cardiomyopathy generally encode cytoskeletal and sarcomeric (contractile apparatus) proteins, although disturbance of calcium homeostasis also seems to be important.

The prevalence of heart failure is approximately 1–1.5 % in the adult population of Western countries. Dilated cardiomyopathy is associated with a large number of systemic or cardiac diseases, including specific heart muscle diseases (e.g., ischemic cardiomyopathy, diabetic cardiomyopathy, alcoholic cardiomyopathy).

Radiography is inexpensive and poses low risk to the patient. If the presenting symptom is dyspnea, radiographic findings may differentiate cardiac etiologies (e.g., alcoholic cardiomyopathy from pulmonary ones). Cardiomegaly (cardiac shadow >50 % of thorax width on the posteroanterior view), Kerley B lines prominent lines in the peripheral parts of the lungs, secondary to interstitial edema, pleural effusions, and cephalization of the pulmonary vasculature (as in the fifth image below) are consistent with a cardiac origin of dyspnea.

CT scanners (electron beam) and multidetector-row CT scanners can be used with ECG gating to assess ventricular function; little reason exists to employ this equipment.

MRI and MRA offer excellent noninvasive means of displaying cardiac and coronary anatomy. They provide high spatial and contrast resolution, which can be used to evaluate congenital and acquired abnormalities and assess results of therapy. Pulse sequences (e.g., cine MRA sequences) that provide high temporal resolution can be used to identify and quantify functional abnormalities.

Echocardiography is the next and, usually, most useful investigation after chest radiography. Two-dimensional echocardiography, with its superior spatial coverage, is used to guide the positioning of the M-mode sample for direct measurements of ventricular wall thickness, left ventricular volumes, and ejection fraction. An advantage of 2-dimensional echocardiography (compared with M-mode imaging) is that the myocardial mass, chamber volumes, and ejection fraction of an abnormally shaped ventricle can be measured.

Comments

CRX film shows enlargement of heart chambers associated with alveolar infiltration and small bilateral pleural effusion (Figs. 7.2.1 and 7.2.2). Echocardiogram shows ejection fraction (EF) of 23 %, dilated cardiomyopathy, and moderate mitral regurgitation (Figs. 7.2.3 and 7.2.4).

Imaging Findings

Case 3: Left Atrial Enlargement

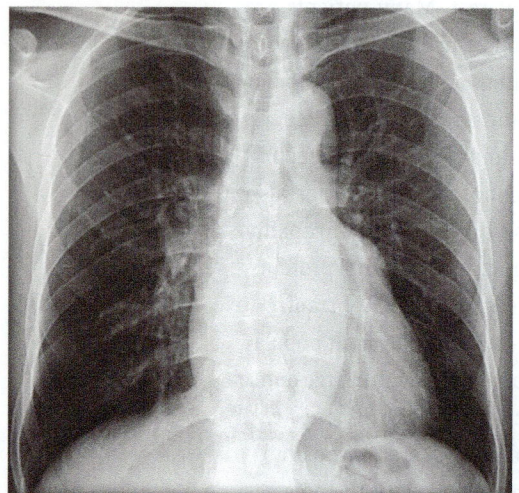

Fig. 7.3.1

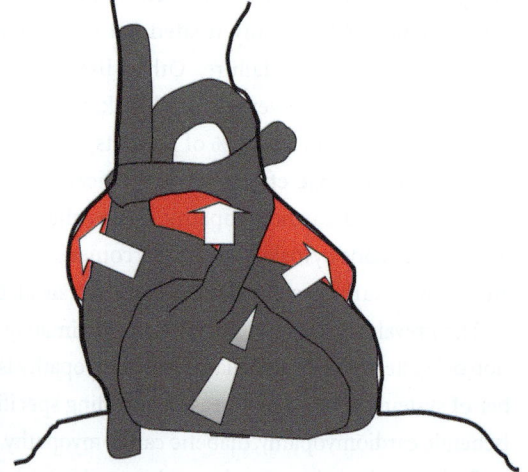

Fig. 7.3.3

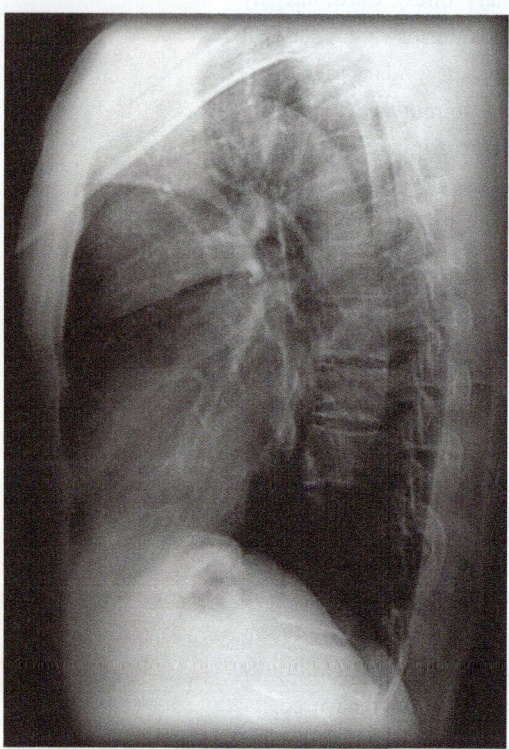

Fig. 7.3.2

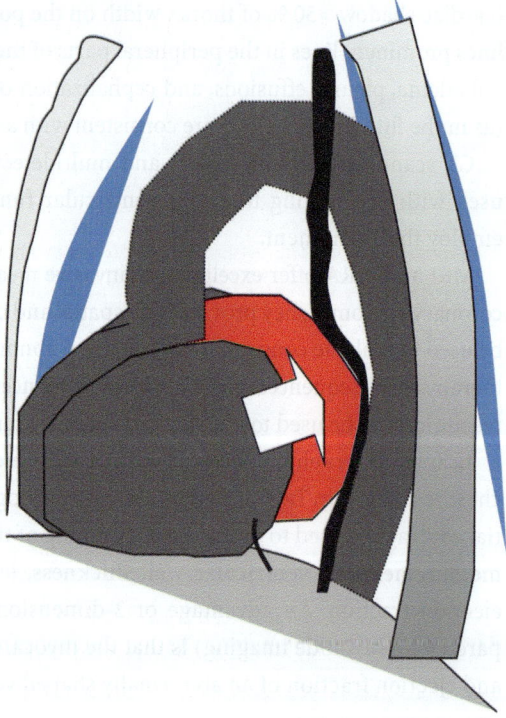

Fig. 7.3.4

A 49-year-old man with patent ductus arteriosus and pulmonary hypertension is referred for dyspnea, fatigue, weakness, and edema of the legs.

Left atrial enlargement can be the result of a number of conditions, including acquired (mitral stenosis, mitral regurgitation, left ventricular failure, left atrial myxoma) and congenital (ventricular septal defect – VSD, patent ductus arteriosus – PDA) heart diseases.

LA enlargement is best confirmed by measuring the distance from the mid-inferior border of the left main stem bronchus to the right lateral border of the left atrial density. This distance is less than 7 cm in 90 % of patients with LA enlargement, and this has been proven by echocardiography. Less sensitive signs of LA enlargement include splaying of the carinal angle, uplifting of the left main stem bronchus, and prominence of the LA appendage. The normal carinal angle is said to be 50–100°, a more obtuse angle reflecting left atrial enlargement. On occasion, the enlarged LA displaces the descending thoracic aorta to the left. Massive LA enlargement may result in the LA becoming border-forming on the right side, so-called atrial escape. On lateral views, an enlarged LA displaces the left bronchus posteriorly, with the bronchi creating right and left legs for the "walking man" sign. An enlarged LA may also indent the esophagus.

CRX film shows prominence of the auricle (Figs. 7.3.1 and 7.3.2; growth of the left atrium). AP view shows double right temple piece, prominent appendage, carinal increased angle, and aorta laterally offset (Fig. 7.3.3; growth of the left atrium). Lateral view shows increasing size of the silhouette and lateroposterior esophageal displacement (Fig. 7.3.4).

Case 4: Left Ventricular Enlargement

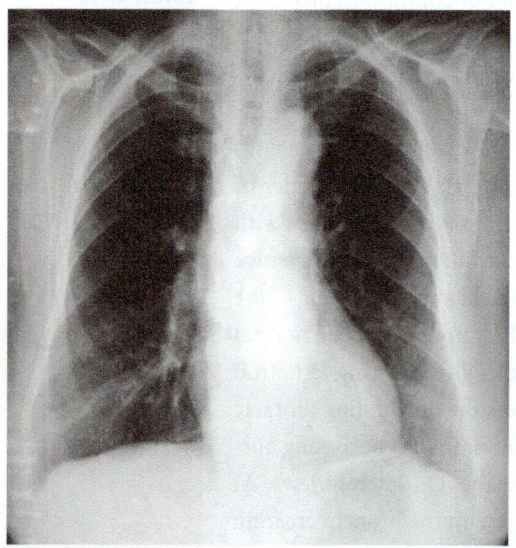

Fig. 7.4.1

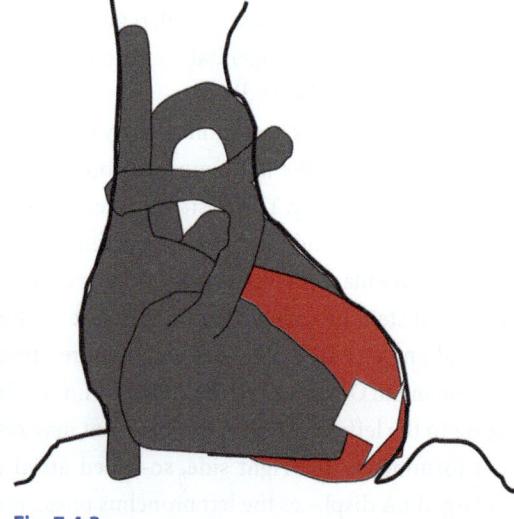

Fig. 7.4.3

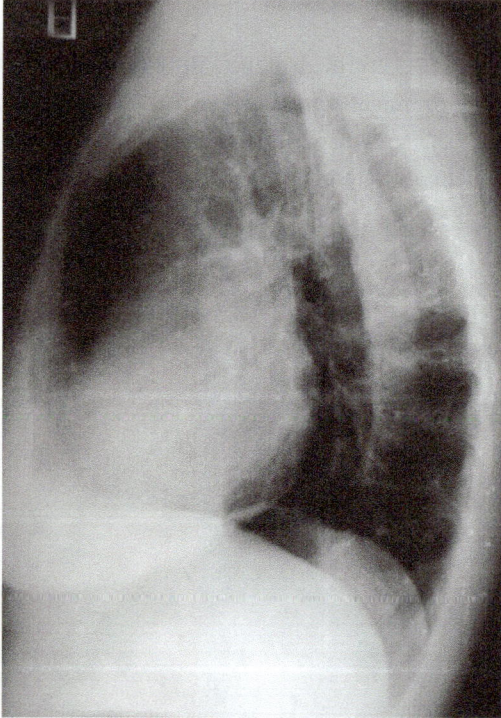

Fig. 7.4.2

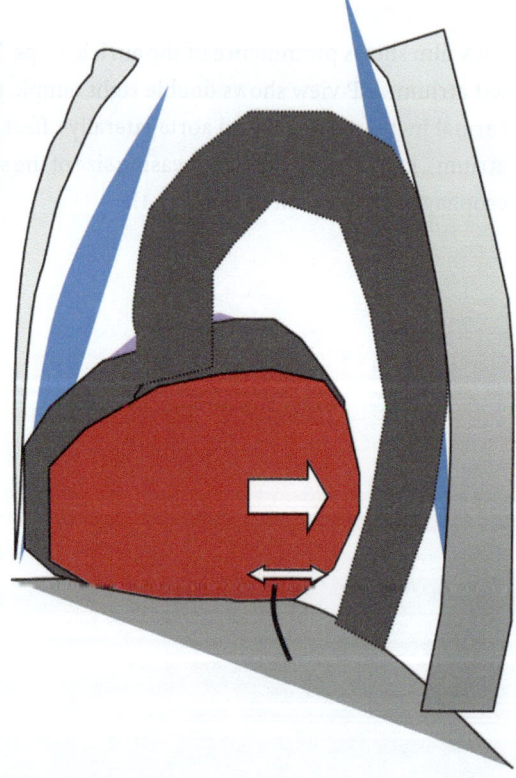

Fig. 7.4.4

A 68-year-old woman with hypertension is referred for 6 years of dyspnea functional class I/IV.

Comments

Left ventricular enlargement can be the result of a number of conditions, including pressure overload (hypertension, aortic stenosis), volume overload (aortic regurgitation, mitral regurgitation), and wall abnormalities (left ventricular aneurysm, hypertrophic cardiomyopathy).

Elongation of the LV outflow tract produces an increase in length of the LV segment making up the left lateral cardiac contour. The second sign of enlargement of this tract is rounding of the contour of the LV. As a result of this downward and leftward enlargement, the cardiac apex may extend below the dome of the diaphragm and be projected over the air-filled gastric fundus.

With counterclockwise rotation of the heart as viewed from the diaphragmatic side, the aortic knob and ascending aorta become prominent, the cardiac waist becomes concave, and the contour of the LV becomes round, producing the specific features of "aortic configuration." Enlargement of the LV inflow tract, which follows that of the outflow tract, produces posterior enlargement. In addition to the enlargement downward, to the left, as well as posteriorly, disease causing increased left ventricular work may result in concentric hypertrophy of this chamber. The lateral view shows an enlarged LV extending behind the esophagus.

At X-ray, there is a sign for determining left ventricle enlargement on a lateral view. The *Hoffman-Rigler sign* is a sign of left ventricular enlargement where an approximation of the distance between the inferior vena cava and left ventricle are used:

- Draw a 2-cm vertical line upward along the inferior vena cava from the point where the posterior wall of the left ventricle and inferior vena cava cross in the lateral projection.
- From this point, a second line is drawn parallel to the vertebral bodies.
- If the distance between the left ventricular border and the vertical line exceeds 1.8 cm, left ventricular enlargement is suggested.

Later investigators suggest this should be increased to 19 mm to decrease the number of false positives.

Prior to their publication in 1951, LV enlargement was suggested where the posterior border of LV was more than 1.5 cm behind IVC.

Imaging Findings

CRX film in the PA projection of the radiograph shows normal cardiac silhouette (cardiothoracic ratio normal) (Fig. 7.4.1). The lateral view shows an enlarged left ventricle (Fig. 7.4.2; left ventricular growth). AP view shows increased left edge, decrease of the cardiac apex (Fig. 7.4.3; growth of the left ventricle). Lateral view shows cardiac growth and lower back and increasing the distance between the inferior vena cava and the posterior edge of the left ventricle >1.5 cm (Fig. 7.4.4).

Case 5: Right Atrial Enlargement

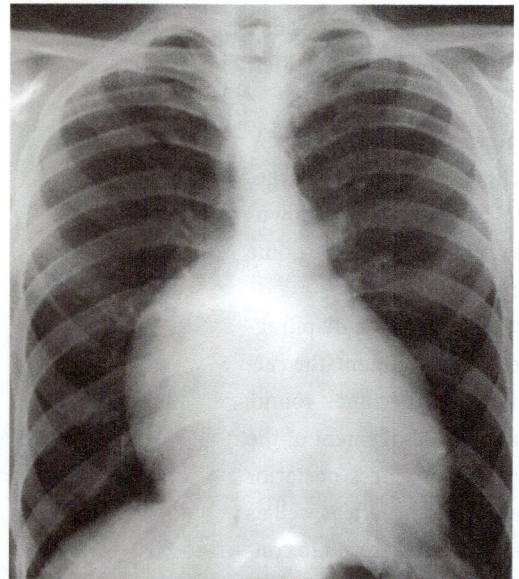

Fig. 7.5.1

Fig. 7.5.2

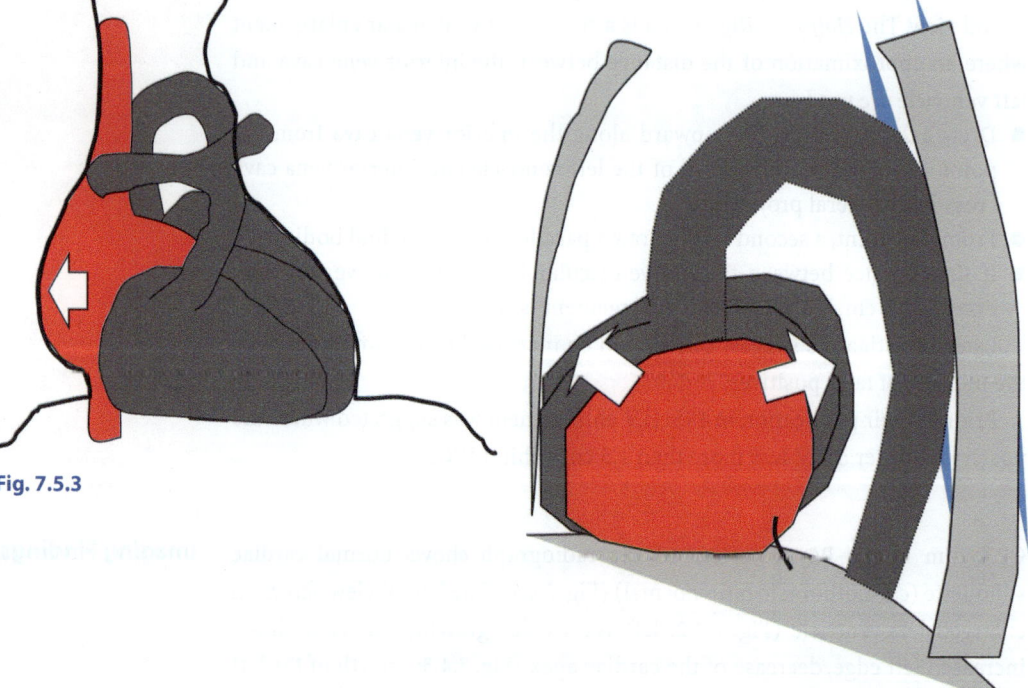

Fig. 7.5.3

Fig. 7.5.4

A 62-year-old man with septal defect atrial is referred for history of dyspnea of 1 year of evolution.

Comments

Isolated right atrial enlargement is uncommon and usually is due to tricuspid stenosis or right atrial tumor. Right atrial dilatation associated with other chamber enlargement, primarily right ventricular enlargement, can be seen in several conditions, such as tricuspid regurgitation, pulmonary arterial hypertension, shunts to the right atrium, and cardiomyopathies. Marked isolated right atrial enlargement resulting in a "box-shaped" heart is seen in Ebstein's malformation of the tricuspid valve. This configuration of the heart is the result of marked angulation at the superior vena caval right atrial junction as the right atrium enlarges. Ebstein's anomaly causes a "box-shaped" heart.

Isolated right atrial enlargement is detected best on a frontal film. Enlargement is to the right and causes increased fullness and convexity of the right cardiac contour and angulation of the junction of the superior vena cava and right atrium. There may be associated dilatation of the superior and inferior venae cavae that causes widening of the right superior mediastinum and an additional border in the right cardiophrenic angle.

On the lateral projection, right atrial dilatation is often difficult to appreciate. It causes a "filling-in" of the retrosternal clear space anteriorly and superiorly, with the cardiac silhouette extending behind the sternum more than one-third the way above the cardiophrenic angle, similar to that seen with right ventricular enlargement. There may be a double density that merges with the inferior vena caval shadow, which may be a slightly convex structure. Left atrial enlargement can be simulated by marked right atrial dilatation.

Clues include a prominent atrial bulge too far to the right of the spine, measuring more than 5.5 cm from the midline on a well-positioned posteroanterior radiograph. Another sign is elongation of the RA convexity to exceed 50 % of the mediastinal or cardiovascular shadow. RA enlargement usually accompanies RV enlargement.

CRX film shows growth of the right atrium (Figs. 7.5.1 and 7.5.2; growth of the right atrium). AP view shows increased cardiothoracic ratio at the expense of the right edge (Fig. 7.5.3; growth of the right atrium). Lateral view shows increased heart shadow anterior and posterior (Fig. 7.5.4).

Imaging Findings

Case 6: Right Ventricular Enlargement

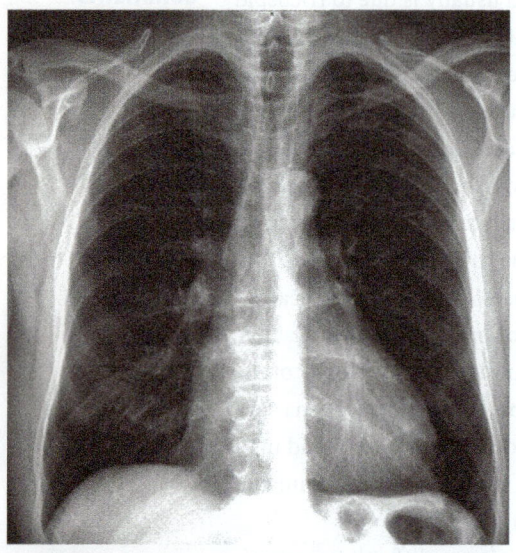

Fig. 7.6.1

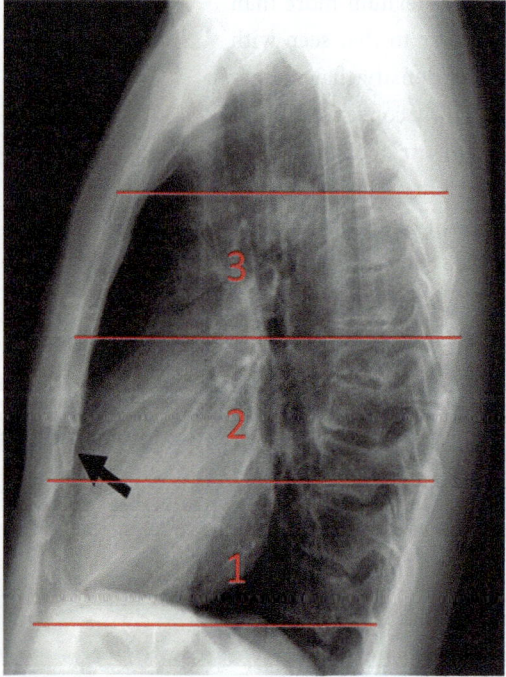

Fig. 7.6.2

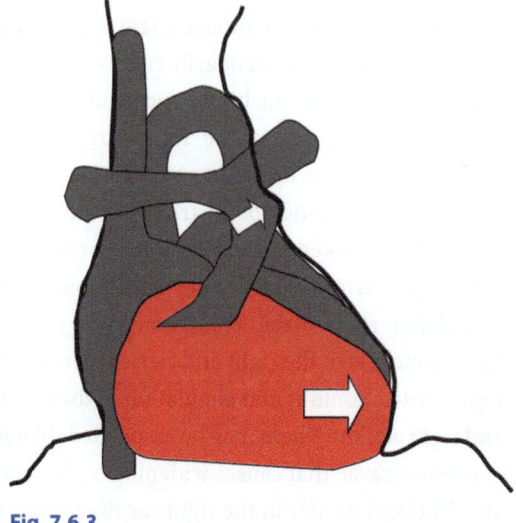

Fig. 7.6.3

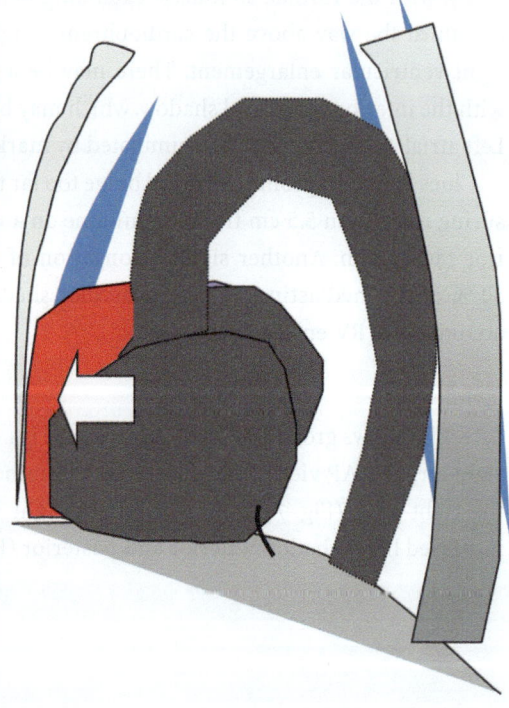

Fig. 7.6.4

A 49-year-old man, with hypertension and dilated cardiomyopathy, is referred for fatigue.

Comments

Right ventricular enlargement can be the result of a number of conditions, including pulmonary valve stenosis, pulmonary artery hypertension, atrial septal defect, tricuspid regurgitation, and dilated cardiomyopathy.

Enlargement of the RV outflow tract results in lengthening of the anterior ventricular wall, which is manifested radiographically by the prominence of the distal RV or pulmonary conus. The result is an anterior bulge in the upper anterior cardiac contour just below the PA. There often is associated enlargement of the PA, which adds to the anterior prominence of the upper border of the heart in this projection. When this occurs, there is more prominence and convexity of the PA segment in the frontal projection than in a normal subject. This results in straightening or convexity of the left upper cardiac contour below the aortic knob.

When the RV enlargement becomes greater, the heart tends to be rotated to the left, so that the conus of the RV may become border-forming. In the lateral projection, the anterolateral bulge in the region of the RV outflow tract reduces the size of the retrosternal space between the upper cardiac border and the sternum. The PA also contributes to this narrowing. When the RV inflow tract enlarges, the diaphragmatic portion of this ventricle is increased in length, resulting in an anterior rounding or bulging in the right ventricular area. This enlargement may displace the LV posteriorly and elevate the cardiac apex, as seen in the frontal projection.

Imaging Findings

CRX film shows elevated cardiac apex and increased retrosternal shadow over 1/3 lower sternum (Figs. 7.6.1 and 7.6.2; growth of the right ventricle). AP view shows increased heart shadow at the expense of the left border, elevation of the cardiac apex, pulmonary hypertension with prominence of the pulmonary artery cone (Fig. 7.6.3; growth of the right ventricle). Lateral view shows increased retrosternal shadow over 1/3 lower sternum (Fig. 7.6.4).

Case 7: Arteriosclerosis of the Aorta

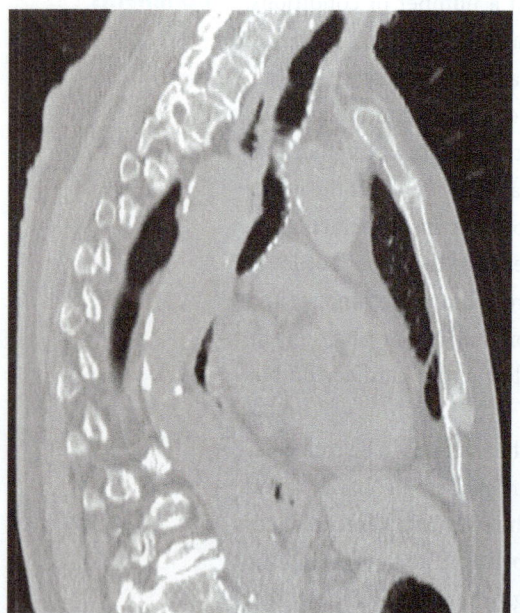

Fig. 7.7.1

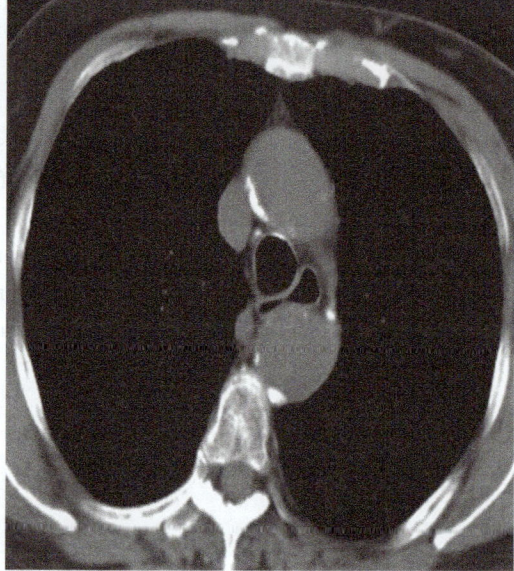

Fig. 7.7.2

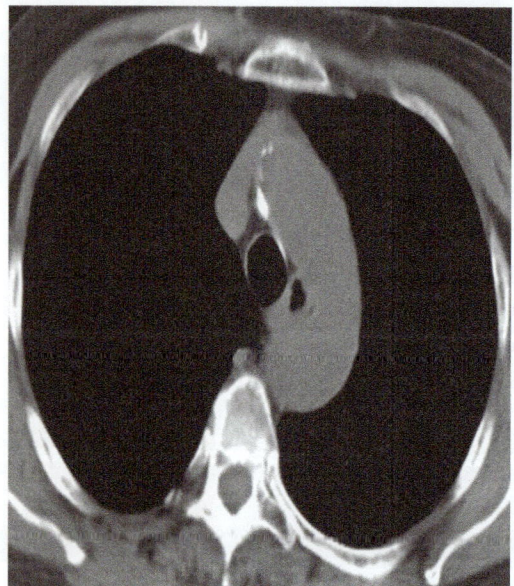

Fig. 7.7.3

Fig. 7.7.4

A 70-year-old woman is diagnosed with coronary disease.

Atherosclerosis is an inflammatory disease that causes most myocardial infarctions, strokes, and acute coronary syndromes. Despite the identification of multiple risk factors and widespread use of drug therapies, it still remains a global health concern with associated costs. It is well known that the risks of atherosclerotic plaque rupture are not well correlated with stenosis severity.

Aortic plaque is an expression of generalized atherosclerosis. As such, it is most often seen in the elderly. It also is more common in patients with hypertension and hypercholesterolemia and in those who smoke. The thoracic aorta has been implicated as a source of cryptogenic strokes and peripheral organ damage because imaging techniques, including transesophageal echocardiography, CT, MR imaging, and MR angiography, have allowed the visualization, characterization, and quantification of atherosclerotic lesions in the thoracic aorta.

Thoracic aortic atherosclerosis is an important cause of severe morbidity and mortality. Its presence in patients undergoing surgery requiring cardiopulmonary bypass dramatically increases the risk of complications such as stroke.

Routine posteroanterior chest films constitute a useful and easily applicable procedure in the detection of aortic atherosclerosis.

Transthoracic echocardiography (*TTE*): frequently visualizes the aortic root and proximal ascending aorta. In some patients, the aortic arch can be seen from the suprasternal notch and the descending aorta from that window and on apical views. Aortic plaque may be visualized with TTE B-mode imaging.

Transesophageal echocardiography (*TEE*): is the procedure of choice for the detection, measurement, and characterization of thoracic aortic atheromas. It is a noninvasive procedure with a low risk of complications. Not only the thickness of an intimal plaque is detected but also ulcerations, calcifications, and superimposed mobile thrombi. The identification of aortic plaques in the aorta could be a very useful noninvasive marker for coronary artery disease and their absence could be used to identify patients over 70 with a very low probability of CAD.

Computerized tomography scanning: is yet another modality frequently used to evaluate the aorta and its branches. Unenhanced dual-helical CT with thin sections has been reported to be successful in detecting protruding aortic plaque, especially in areas not visualized by TEE (94 % of plaques detected by TEE were seen with CT).

CT scan (mediastinal and lung window) shows elongation and atheromatous plaques in the ascending aorta, aortic arch, and descending aorta (Figs. 7.7.1, 7.7.2, 7.7.3, and 7.7.4).

Case 8: Aortic Elongation

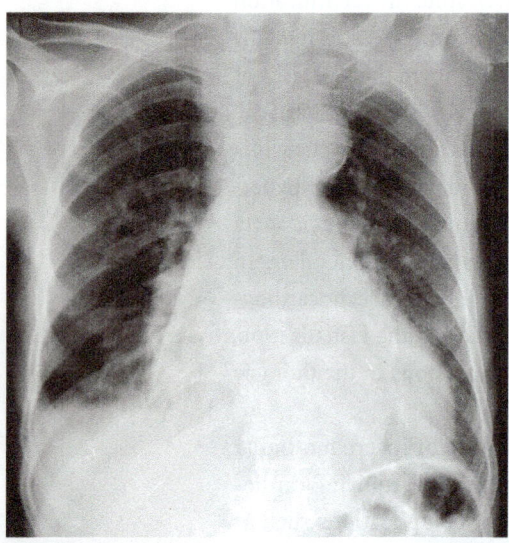

Fig. 7.8.1

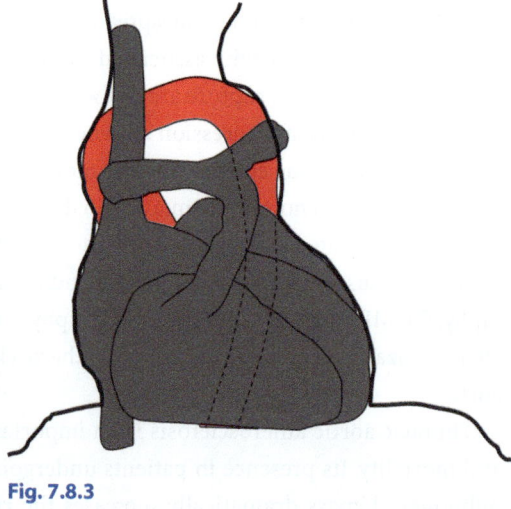

Fig. 7.8.3

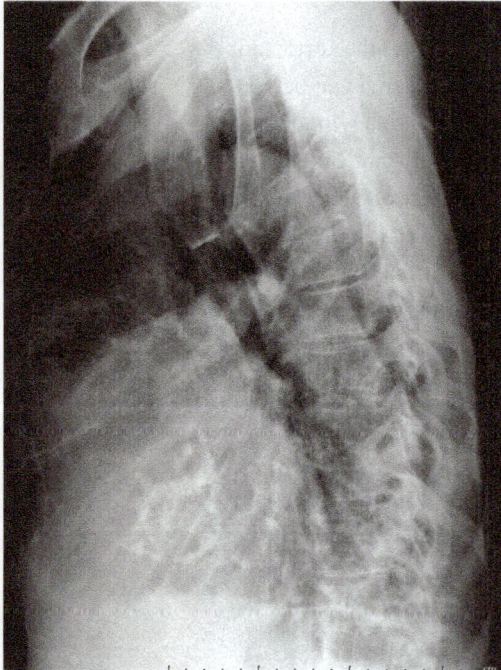

Fig. 7.8.2

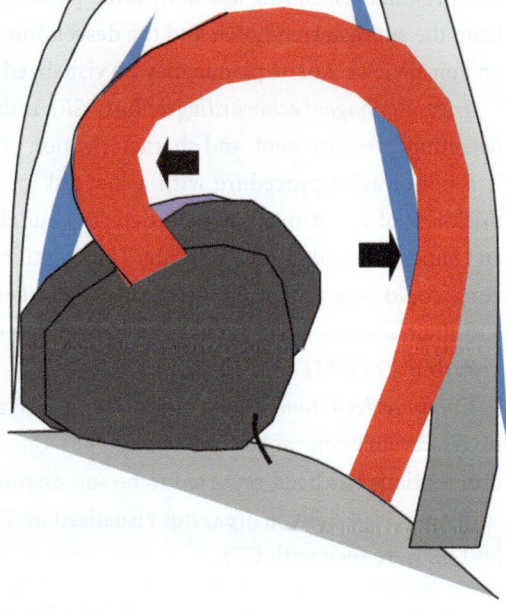

Fig. 7.8.4

A 79-year-old man with chronic bronchitis and hypertension and who is a smoker attends for 1 week symptom of cough, dyspnea, orthopnea, fatigue, and weakness, without paroxysmal nocturnal dyspnea.

The thoracic aorta is divided into 4 parts: the aortic root (which includes the aortic valve annulus, the aortic valve cusps, and the sinuses of Valsalva), the ascending aorta (which includes the tubular portion of the ascending aorta beginning at the sinotubular junction and extending to the brachiocephalic artery origin), the aortic arch (which begins at the origin of the brachiocephalic artery and is the origin of the head and neck arteries, coursing in front of the trachea and to the left of the esophagus and the trachea), and the descending aorta (which begins at the isthmus between the origin of the left subclavian artery and the ligamentum arteriosum and courses anterior to the vertebral column, and then through the diaphragm into the abdomen).

Age, arteriosclerosis, and hypertension all appear to produce aortic elongation and are additive in this respect. Visceral fat obesity is a novel contributor to tortuosity of the thoracic aorta, which may be as a shortening of the distance between aortic tethering points due to elevation of the diaphragm by excessive intra-abdominal fat and as a consequence of aortic elongation due to arteriosclerosis caused by obesity-related metabolic disorders.

It has also been reported cases of acquired forms subvalvular aortic stenosis through the impaction of the mitral valve due to the elongation of the ascending aorta.

The radiographic findings of aortic elongation in the chest radiograph are:

PA projection: aorta distortion, the ascending and descending aorta displacement exceeding the heart boundary, intruding the lung field; the demarcation between the ascending aorta and right atrium descend; aortic knob is high, above the clavicula sometimes. Lateral projection: Ascending and descending aorta bend forward and backward, respectively.

CRX film shows elongation with aortic atherosclerosis (Figs. 7.8.1 and 7.8.2; aortic elongation). AP view shows prominence on the right edge, prominence of the aortic arch and curvature of the descending aorta (Fig. 7.8.3; aortic elongation). Lateral view shows former prominence with straight edge and overlap with the column (Fig. 7.8.4).

Case 9: Descending Thoracic Aortic Aneurysm

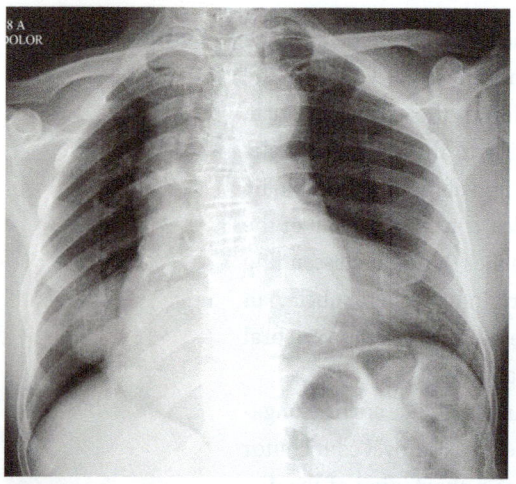

Fig. 7.9.1

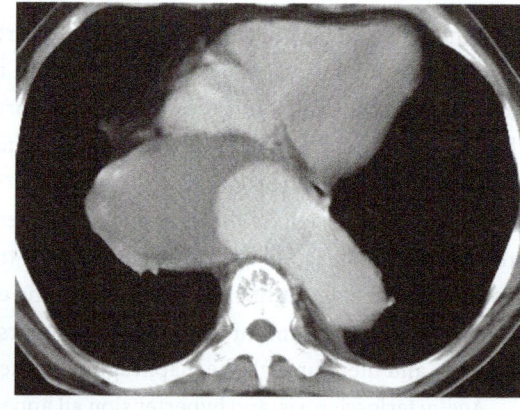

Fig. 7.9.2

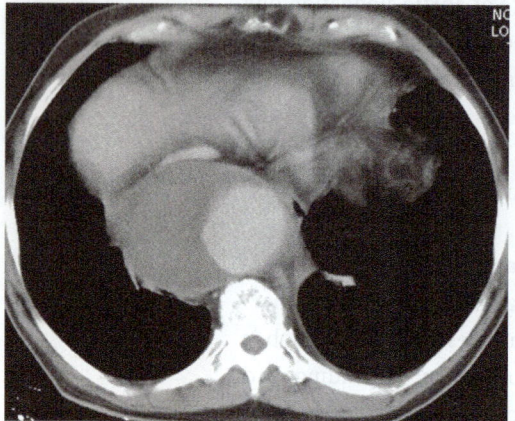

Fig. 7.9.3

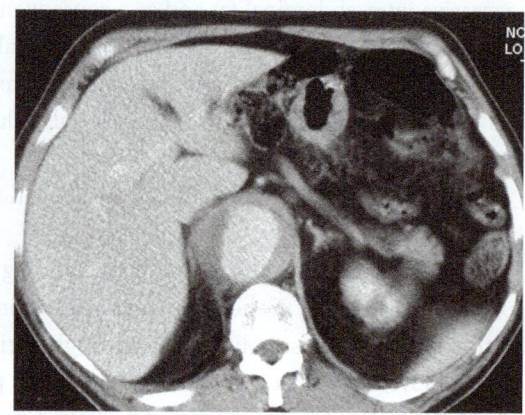

Fig. 7.9.4

A 78-year-old man with hypertension and stroke 5 years ago is referred for chest pain of 4 days and systolic blood pressure of 170 and diastolic pressure of 100.

Comments   Aneurysm of the aorta is defined as a permanent localized dilatation of the aorta, at least 50 % greater than normal and involving all three wall layers. The lesser degree of dilatation generally is referred to as "ectasia." Most aneurysms of the thoracic aorta are atherosclerotic in origin. Other causes are infection (mycotic aneurysms) and cystic medial necrosis (annuloaortic ectasia). Frequent comorbidities include hypertension, coronary artery disease, obstructive pulmonary disease, and congestive heart failure.

Imaging characteristics important in aortic aneurysms are the maximum diameter, length, and the condition of major branches. The aneurysmal thoracic aorta grows at an average speed of 1 mm per year, with a high risk of complications (tear or dissection) when it reaches 6 cm for the ascending aorta and 7 cm for the descending aorta. The annual risk that rupture, dissection, or death of a patient by a thoracic aneurysm >6 cm in diameter is more than 14 %.

Aneurysms of the descending aorta are most common, followed by aneurysms of the ascending aorta; aneurysms of the arch occur less often. In addition, descending aortic thoracic aneurysms may extend distally to involve the abdominal aorta and create a thoracoabdominal aortic aneurysm.

At radiography, the characteristic findings are (1) widening of the mediastinal silhouette, (2) enlargement of the aortic knob, or (3) displacement of the trachea from the midline (see the first image below). Chest radiographs display abnormalities in 80–90 % of patients, but the abnormalities are nonspecific.

On CT scans, thoracic aortic aneurysms are characterized by an increase in aortic diameter and outward displacement of calcium of the aortic wall (see the images below). CT scanning is an effective method for defining the maximum diameter of the aneurysm and monitoring the diameter over time. A diameter exceeding 4 cm is considered aneurysmal. A diameter exceeding 6 cm is usually an indication for surgery of thoracic aortic aneurysm. Multidetector computed tomographic (CT) angiography is routinely performed for the diagnosis and evaluation of thoracic aortic aneurysms (TAAs), having essentially replaced diagnostic angiography.

MRI and CT scanning are now the modalities most frequently used for diagnosing and monitoring thoracic aortic diseases.

Transesophageal echocardiography (TEE) provides an assessment of cardiac structure and function and is highly sensitive in the diagnosis of aortic pathologies. Intraoperatively, TEE may be used to monitor cardiac function; detect atherosclerosis in the thoracic aorta; establish the competency of the aortic valve before surgery; and lower the incidence of stroke, by enabling surgeons to better navigate the placement of clamps and to avoid loosening any atherosclerotic plaques, which could otherwise cause brain embolism.

The findings of aortic dissection seen at angiography include the following: (1) filling of a false channel with or without an intervening intimal flap, (2) distortion of the true lumen by either a patent or a thrombosed false lumen, (3) thickening of the aortic wall by more than 0.5 cm from a thrombosed false lumen, and (4) displaced intimal calcification.

Imaging Findings

CRX film shows marked dilatation of the descending aorta aneurysmal producing double contour on the right edge of the heart (Fig. 7.9.1). CT scan (arterial phase) shows aneurysmal dilatation with intimal flap secondary to thrombus in the wall of the descending aorta (Figs. 7.9.2, 7.9.3, and 7.9.4).

Case 10: Aortic Dissection

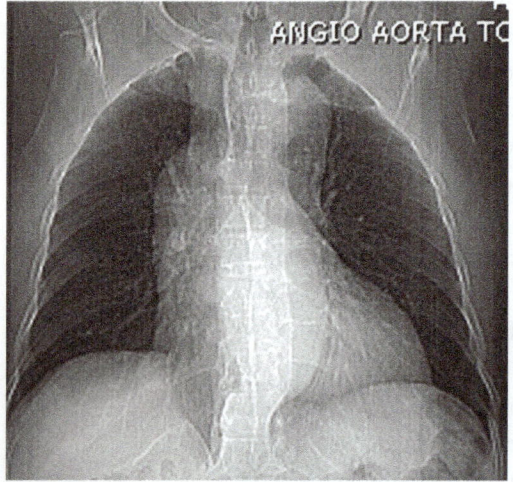

Fig. 7.10.1

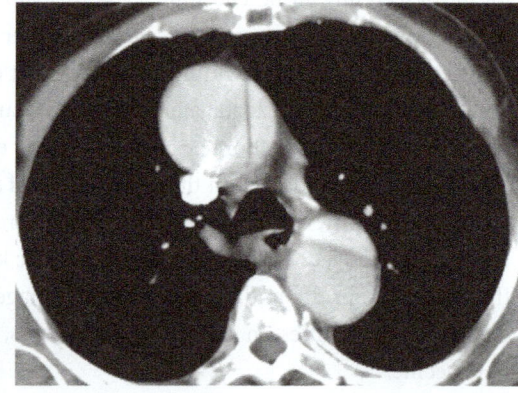

Fig. 7.10.2

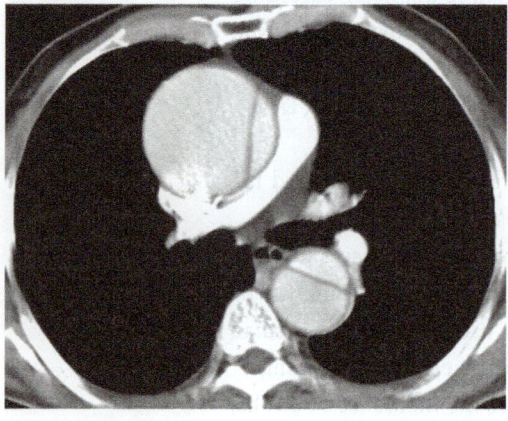

Fig. 7.10.3

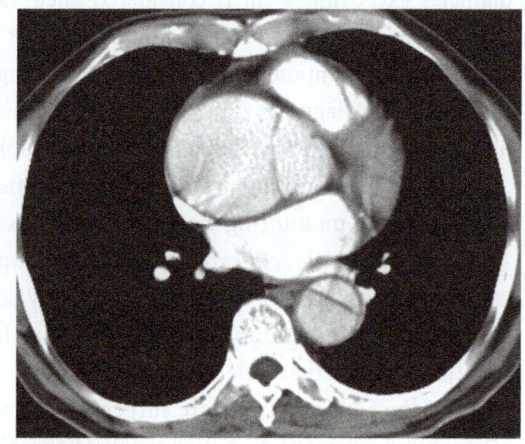

Fig. 7.10.4

A 68-year-old man with hypertension is referred for chest pain.

Comments Thoracic aortic dissection may be described as acute or chronic, depending on its clinical manifestation. Dissection is considered acute if the symptoms last less than 2 weeks and chronic if they last longer. Seventy-five percent of deaths from the condition occur within 2 weeks after the initial manifestation of symptoms. The dissection is classified according to the extent of involvement of the thoracic aorta. The original system for classification of aortic dissection, the DeBakey system, has been superseded by the Stanford system, which includes two types based on whether surgery is required. Dissection affecting the ascending aorta or the aortic arch is classified as Stanford type A (DeBakey types I and II) and accounts for 75 % of cases of aortic dissection.

At radiography, mediastinal widening is the most common plain radiographic finding in aortic dissection; it is noted in 80 % of patients. Other radiographic findings include the following: double aortic knob sign (present in 40 % of patients), diffuse enlargement of the aorta with poor definition or irregularity of the aortic contour, inward displacement of aortic wall calcification by more than 10 mm, tracheal displacement to the right, pleural effusion (more common on the left side; suggests leakage), pericardial effusion, cardiac enlargement, displacement of a nasogastric tube, and left apical opacity.

Transesophageal echocardiography (TOE) is highly accurate in detecting class 1 aortic dissection. All information necessary for decision making is provided by this technique. Sensitivity and specificity are more than 90 %. Duplex sonography can be used to detect involvement of abdominal arteries as well as carotid arteries. But the imaging quality in these areas rarely reaches the quality necessary for decision making. Importantly, the negative predictive accuracy of TOE is nearly 100 %.

CT is widely available and commonly used in patients with aortic dissection. The drawback of CT is the inability to diagnose aortic regurgitation and to localize entry tears precisely. The advantage of this technique is that the total extent of the aortic dissection and side branch involvement can be visualized as well as pericardial and pleura effusion. The sensitivity is not as high as for TOE, but the specificity is similar.

MRI seems to be the most sensitive method for diagnosing aortic dissection, and has the same specificity as TOE and CT. Until now only a few centers used the technique in acute dissections, owing to the difficulties in handling emergency cases, but in stable patients, particularly chronic dissection during follow-up, MRI seems to be the method of choice. Nearly all diagnostic requirements can be fulfilled; tears are detected and side branch involvement even of coronary arteries can be described.

For a long time, angiography was the gold standard for imaging patients with aortic dissection. It has now been replaced by the newer imaging methods, as they are noninvasive and avoid the use of radiographic contrast agents. The sensitivity and specificity of angiography is lower than that for the newer imaging techniques. In particular, there are problems in detecting class 2 and 4 dissection with angiography, but it has been helpful in detecting discrete or subtle class 3 dissection and traumatic class 5 dissection.

Imaging Findings

CRX film shows widened mediastinum due to increased size of the aortic arch (Fig. 7.10.1). CT scan (arterial phase) shows aortic dissection in the ascending aorta, aortic arch, and descending aorta (Figs. 7.10.2, 7.10.3, and 7.10.4).

Further Reading

Agarwal PP et al (2009) Multidetector CT of thoracic aortic aneurysms. Radiographics 29:537–552

Cohen A (2008) Risk of vascular events atherosclerosis of the thoracic aorta: further characterization for higher. J Am Coll Cardiol 52:862–864

Dotter CT et al (1950) Aortic length: angiocardiographic measurements. Circulation 2:915–920

Eva Castañer E et al (2003) CT in nontraumatic acute thoracic aortic disease: typical and atypical features and complications. Radiographics 23:S93–S110

Felson B (1982) Principios de Radiología torácica. Un texto programado 2ªEd, Lawrence Goodman, Mcgraw-Hill, Interamericana, pp 1–242

Fraser RS, Paré JAM, Fraser RG, Paré PD (1994) Sinopsis of diseases of the chest, 2nd edn. W.B. Saunders Company, Philadelphia

Gotway MB, Dawn SK (2003) Thoracic aorta imaging with multislice CT. Radiol Clin North Am 41(3):521–543

Hartnell GG (2001) Imaging of aortic aneurysms and dissection: CT and MRI. J Thorac Imaging 16(1):35–46

Hoffman RB, Rigler LG (1965) Evaluation of left ventricular enlargement in the lateral projection of the chest. Radiology 85:93

Hussein A et al (2009) Value of aortic arch analysis during routine transthoracic echocardiography in adults. Eur J Echocardiogr 10:625–629

Jefferies JL, Towbin JA (2010) Dilated cardiomyopathy. Lancet 375(9716):752–762

Joshi FR (2012) Non-invasive imaging of atherosclerosis. Eur Heart J Cardiovasc Imaging 13(3):205–218

Juan TM, Joseph FT (2000) Radiology: diagnosis, imaging, intervention. Lippincott William and Wilkins, Philadelphia

Kronzon I, Tunick PA (2006) Aortic atherosclerotic disease and stroke. Circulation 114:63–75

Lankipalli RS, Pellecchia M, Burke JF (2002) Magnetic resonance angiography in the evaluation of aortic pseudoaneurysm. Heart 87(2):157

Methodius-Ngwodo WC, Burkett AB, Kochupura PV, Wellons ED, Fuhrman G, Rosenthal D (2008) The role of CT angiography in the diagnosis of blunt traumatic thoracic aortic disruption and unsuspected carotid artery injury. Am Surg 74(7):580–585; discussion 585–586

Miller WT (2001) Thoracic aortic aneurysms: plain film findings. Semin Roentgenol 36(4):288–294

Mochida M (2006) Visceral fat obesity contributes to the tortuosity of the thoracic aorta on chest radiograph in poststroke Japanese patients. Angiology 57(1): 85–91

Moran E, Schwartz A, Ungar H (1963) A correlative study between the radiologic and pathologic diagnoses of atherosclerosis of the aorta. Am Heart J 65(2): 190–194

Nguyen BT (2001) Computed tomography diagnosis of thoracic aortic aneurysms. Semin Roentgenol 36(4): 309–324

Pereles FS, McCarthy RM, Baskaran V et al (2002) Thoracic aortic dissection and aneurysm: evaluation with nonenhanced true FISP MR angiography in less than 4 minutes. Radiology 223(1):270–274

Shah AK et al (2007) Aortic elongation induced aortic stenosis (AEAS). Ann Thorac Surg 84:1010–1012

Steiner RM (2001) Radiology of the heart and great vessels. Braunwald: heart disease: a textbook of cardiovascular medicine, 6th edn. W. B. Saunders Company, Philadelphia

Tunick PA et al (2000) Diagnostic imaging of thoracic aortic atherosclerosis. AJR Am J Roentgenol 174: 1119–1125

Yu T et al (2007) Revisión de la angio-TC de aorta. Radiol Clin North Am 45:461–484

John C. Pedrozo Pupo and Alvaro Coral Martinez

Contents

J.C. Pedrozo Pupo (ed.), *Learning Chest Imaging*, Learning Imaging,
DOI 10.1007/978-3-642-34147-2_8, © Springer-Verlag Berlin Heidelberg 2013

Case 1: Multiple Rib Fracture

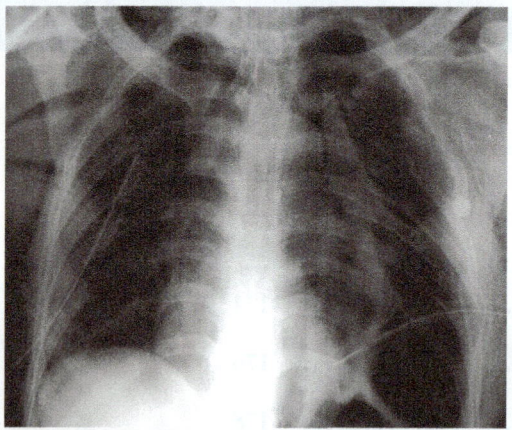

Fig. 8.1.1

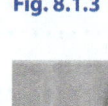

Fig. 8.1.3

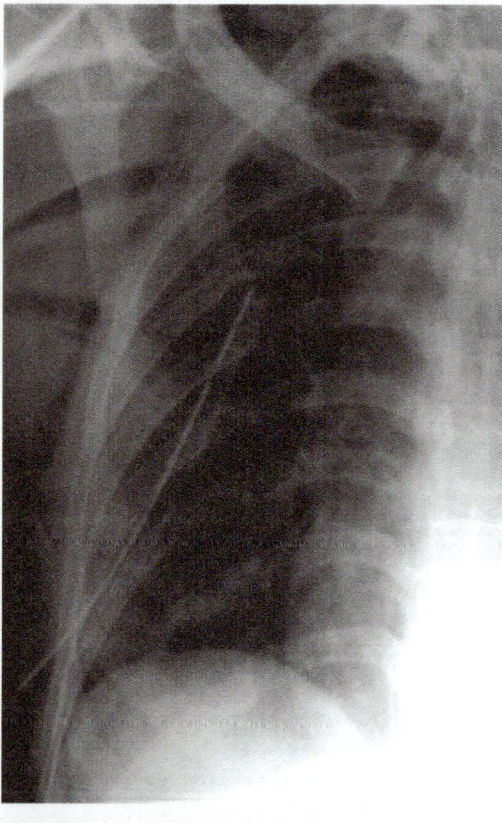

Fig. 8.1.2

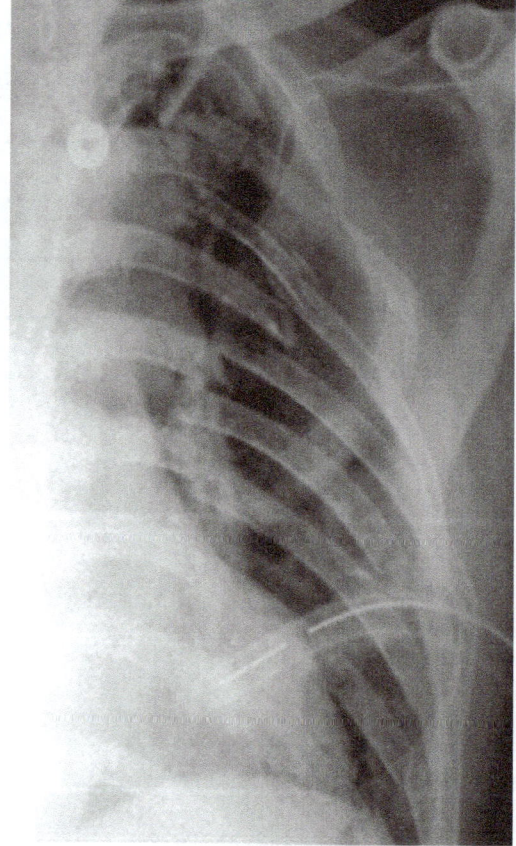

Fig. 8.1.4

A 45-year-old man seeks consultation for emergency car accident. He had chest trauma.

Rib fracture is the most common thoracic injury and is thought to be present in 10 % of all traumatic injuries and in almost 40 % of patients who sustain severe nonpenetrating trauma. Rib fractures typically affect the fifth through ninth ribs. This may be due to the fact that the shoulder girdle affords relative protection to the upper ribs and the lower ribs are relatively mobile and may deflect before fracturing.

The presence and number of rib fractures do carry prognostic significance, and detection of rib fractures may be indicated under certain circumstances. Rib fractures are associated with pulmonary dysfunction (atelectasis, shunting, impairment of clearance of secretions, pneumonia, and adult respiratory distress syndrome).

Fractures of the first through third ribs are considered to be high-energy trauma because these ribs are well protected by the scapulae, clavicles, and musculature. These fractures may be associated with brachial plexus injury or subclavian vascular injuries. Fractures of the lower three ribs may be associated with liver, spleen, and kidney injuries and, less frequently, with lung injuries. In elderly persons, rib fractures can be a significant source of pain and splinting.

Chest radiography is routinely used to assist in the diagnosis of rib fractures, even though it has limited sensitivity. Rib radiography can provide superior visualization of the ribs and rib fractures.

CT is the most sensitive technique for imaging rib fractures, since it can help determine the site and number of fractures and, more important, provide information regarding any associated injuries.

CRX film shows bilateral subcutaneous emphysema, multiple fractures in posterior rib, and collapsed lung associated with left pneumothorax (Figs. 8.1.1 and 8.1.2). CRX film shows appropriate bilateral lung expansion, persistence of left posterior multiple fractures, and bilateral chest tube (Figs. 8.1.3 and 8.1.4).

Case 2: Askin's Tumor

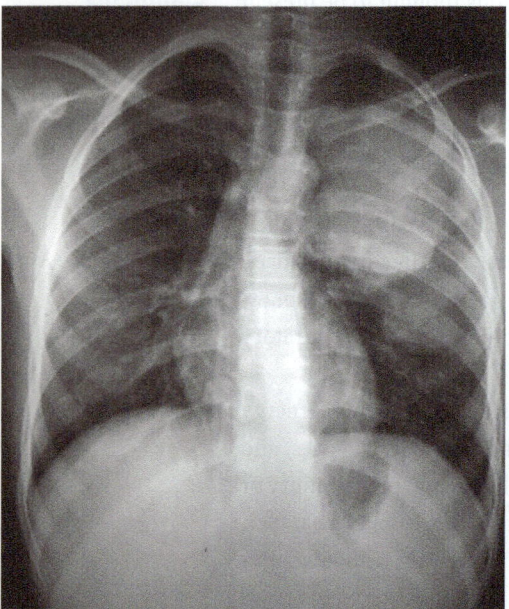

Fig. 8.2.1

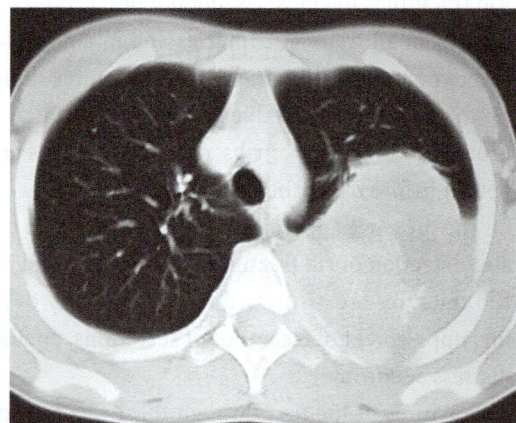

Fig. 8.2.2

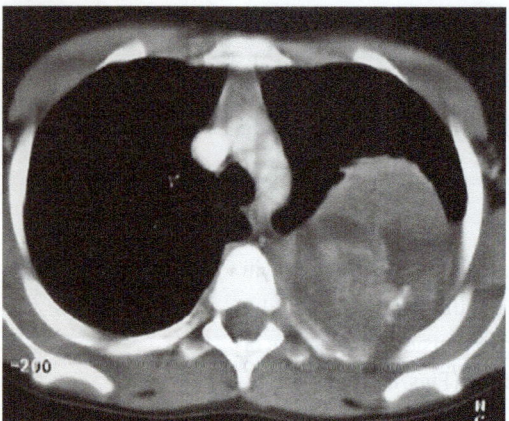

Fig. 8.2.3

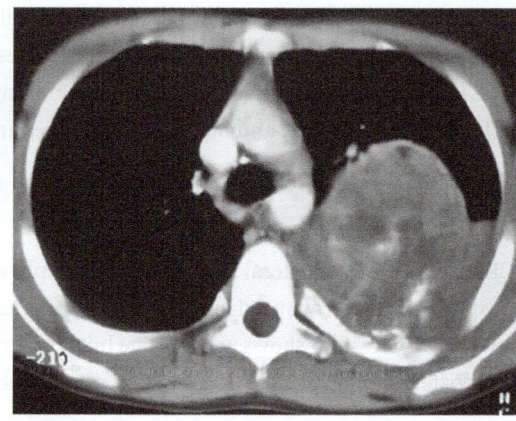

Fig. 8.2.4

A 14-year-old male has a 3-month history of chest pain and weight loss.

Askin's tumor, also known as PNET/extraskeletal Ewing sarcoma, is a malignant small round cell which originates from the soft tissues of the chest wall. It was first described by Askin et al., in 1979, in a study of 20 children and adolescents. About 80 % of cases have been found in patients under 20 years of age.

The chest radiograph shows a usually large extrapulmonary heterogeneous mass, which can completely opacify hemithorax. Are common spill or thickening associated pleural. The destruction of costal arches is observed in 25–63 % of cases. The expansion of the tumor may collapse or invade the lung.

At CT, Askin's tumor appears as a mass of heterogeneous soft tissue density that tends to shift and compress adjacent structures such as vessels, trachea, and bronchi, rather than wrap. Large tumors (greater than 5 cm in diameter) contain some cystic or necrotic areas and areas of hemorrhage that reflect the aggressive nature of tumor. The masses are large, often extending to intrathoracic compartments, cord, and retroperitoneal compartment. Rarely exhibit calcifications, unlike chondrosarcoma and osteosarcoma, showing a calcified matrix. This helps the spread of these tumors. The ribs may be intact, present erosion and periosteal reaction, or be displaced in a permeative pattern.

At MRI, the tumors have average intensity or high relative to muscle on T1 information, have a heterogeneous high signal intensity on T2 information, and present variable enhancement with gadolinium.

There are few reports of ultrasound findings in Askin's tumor, describing the appearance of a hypoechoic lesion containing some areas anechoic cystic.

The differential diagnosis of extraskeletal Ewing sarcoma approach includes malignancies such as Ewing sarcoma, neuroblastoma, rhabdomyosarcoma, lymphoma, chondrosarcoma, osteosarcoma, hemangiopericytoma, Langerhans cell histiocytosis, and benign tumors, such as lipoblastoma, fibroma, lymphangioma, and mesenchymal hamartoma.

CRX film shows pulmonary voluminous mass located in upper left lung (Fig. 8.2.1). CT scan (lung window) shows soft tissue mass of heterogeneous density dependent on posterior rib cage (Fig. 8.2.2). CT scan (arterial phase) shows soft tissue mass with heterogeneous density which undertakes the posterior rib (Figs. 8.2.3 and 8.2.4).

Case 3: Pectus Excavatum

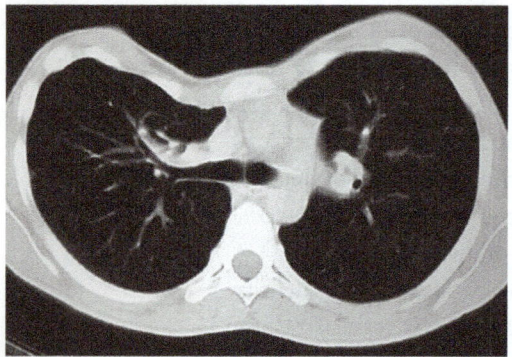

Fig. 8.3.1

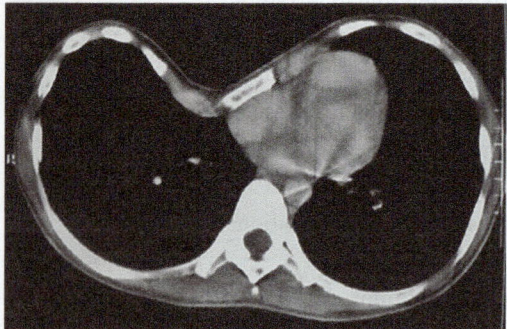

Fig. 8.3.2

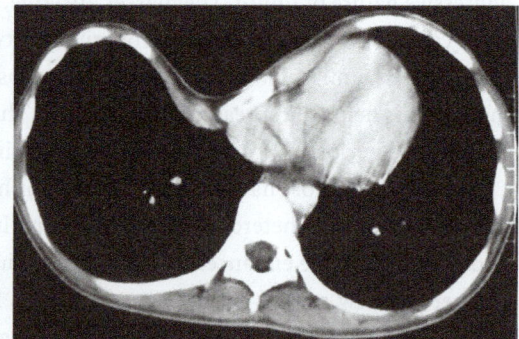

Fig. 8.3.3

Fig. 8.3.4

A 17-year-old male seeks consultation for chest deformity.

Pectus excavatum, also known as funnel chest, is the most common congenital deformity of the sternum. The anomaly is present in between 1 in 400 and 1 in 1,000 live births and is thought to result from rapid and misdirected growth of the lower costal cartilages. The sternum is displaced posteriorly, and as a consequence, the ribs protrude anteriorly. The aberrant position of these skeletal structures results in a reduction of prevertebral space, leftward displacement and axial rotation of the heart, and reduction of the space occupied by the left lung.

Males have an increased risk of this deformity, whereas females have an increased risk of associated scoliosis.

Posteroanterior radiography also depicts parasternal soft tissues of the anterior chest wall as an area of increased density in the inferomedial portion of the right hemithorax.

CT scans are very helpful, because they clearly show the degree of cardiac compression and displacement, the degree of pulmonary compression and atelectasis, asymmetry of the chest, sternal torsion, compensatory development of a barrel chest deformity in long-standing deformities, and ossification of the cartilages in patients with previous repairs.

The severity of the deformity is best quantified with CT. The quantitative measurement of the deformity is measured using cross-sectional imaging. In particular, the commonly used Haller index is the ratio between the lateral distance of the chest wall (inner margins) and the narrowest anteroposterior distance between the vertebrae and sternum (both measured at the same axial level). If this ratio is above 3.25, it is considered severe.

Determination of a severe pectus excavatum and the need for repair include two or more of the following criteria:

- A Haller CT index greater than 3.25
- Pulmonary function studies that indicate restrictive or obstructive airway disease
- A cardiology evaluation where the compression is causing murmurs, mitral valve prolapse, cardiac displacement, or conduction abnormalities on the echocardiogram or EKG tracings
- Documentation of progression of the deformity with associated physical symptoms other than isolated concerns of body image
- A failed Ravitch procedure
- A failed minimally invasive procedure

When using these criteria, approximately 50 % of patients are found to have a deformity severe enough to warrant surgery.

CT scan (lung and mediastinal window) shows posterior displacement of the sternum and costal arches (Figs. 8.3.1, 8.3.2, 8.3.3, and 8.3.4).

Case 4: Pectus Carinatum

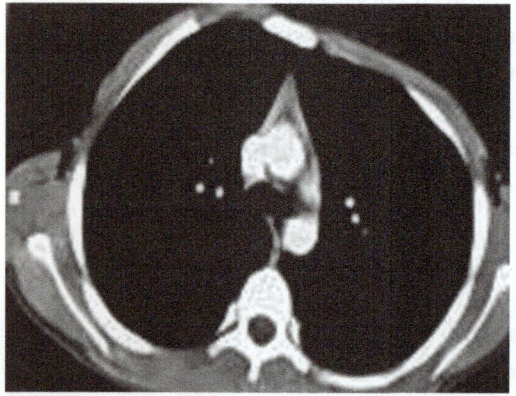

Fig. 8.4.1

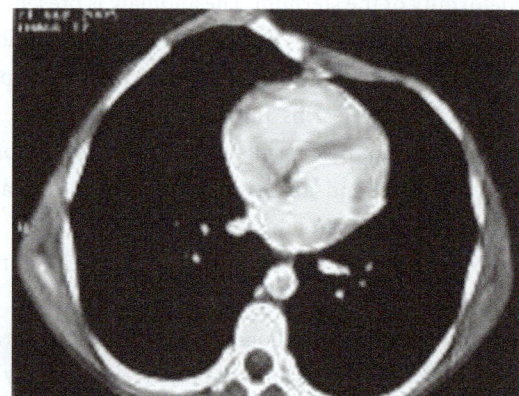

Fig. 8.4.2

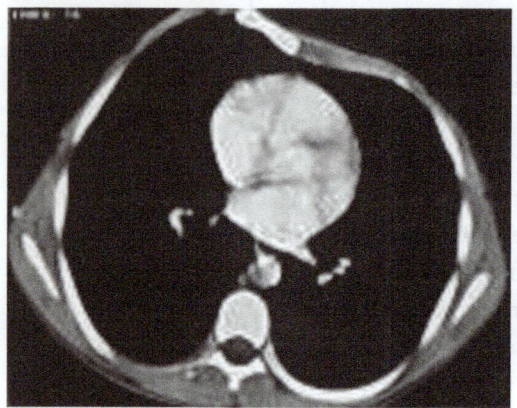

Fig. 8.4.3

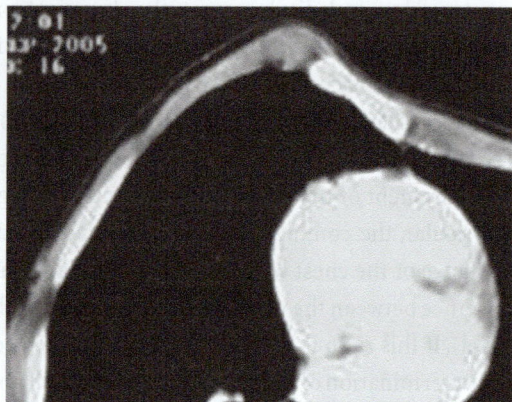

Fig. 8.4.4

A 16-year-old male consults for anterior chest deformity.

In pectus carinatum, the sternum is displaced anteriorly. This anomaly is less common than pectus excavatum. It occurs in approximately 1 per 1,500 live births, more commonly in males than in females (male-to-female ratio, 4:1). More than 30 % of cases of pectus carinatum are associated with scoliosis, and a small percentage is associated with congenital heart disease. Familial occurrence is reported in approximately 25 % of cases.

Clinical manifestations are frequent and include shortness of breath and exercise intolerance. Two different types of pectus carinatum deformity, with different surgical implications, have been identified. The less common variant is a chondromanubrial deformity (Currarino-Silverman syndrome) that produces manubrial and upper sternal protrusion, and the more common is a chondrogladiolar deformity that results in protrusion of the middle and lower sternum.

Chest radiographs show an increased anteroposterior diameter of the chest with anterior protrusion of the sternum. CT or MR imaging measurements may be used to calculate the pectus index. A pectus index value of 1.42–1.98 is indicative of pectus carinatum.

CT scan (mediastinal window) shows chest deformity by anterior displacement of the costal arches (Figs. 8.4.1, 8.4.2, 8.4.3, and 8.4.4).

Case 5: Recurrent Desmoid Tumor

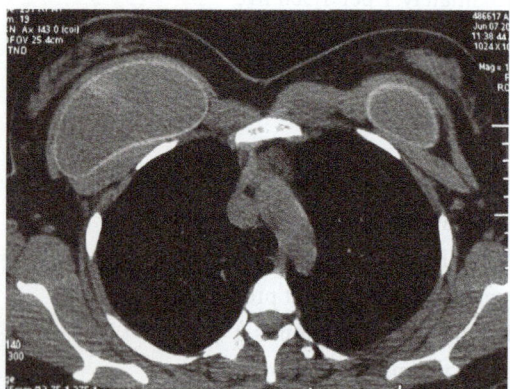

Fig. 8.5.1

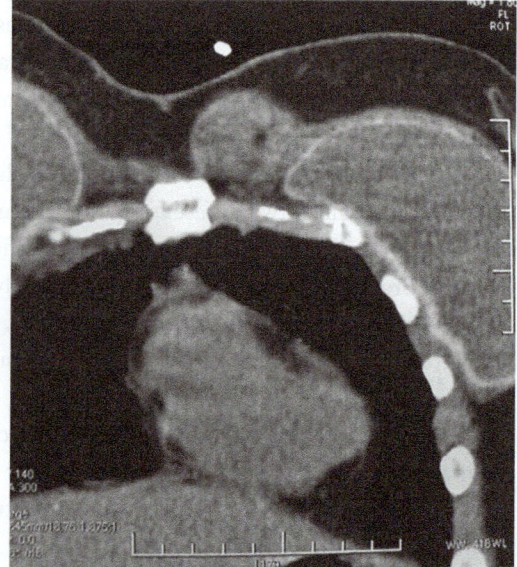

Fig. 8.5.2

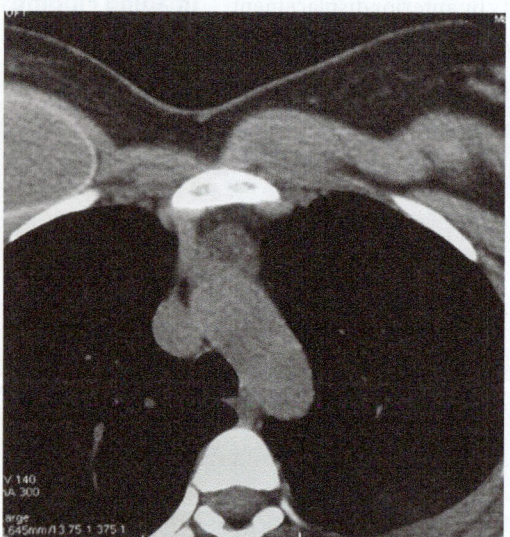

Fig. 8.5.3

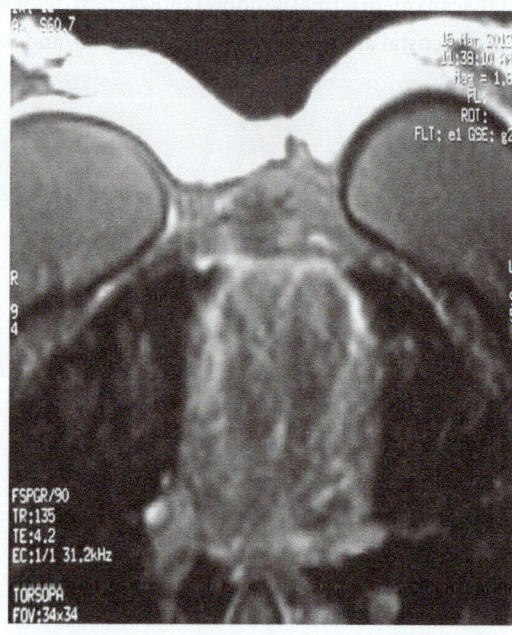

Fig. 8.5.4

A 34-year-old woman has a history of surgical resection of desmoid tumor in the chest wall.

Tumors of the chest wall are uncommon. They can be benign or malignant and can be divided based on skeletal versus soft tissue origin. Common soft tissue neoplasms and nonneoplastic chest wall masses include peripheral nerve tumors, lipomas, liposarcomas, hemangiomas, elastofibromas, lymphoma, metastases from distant tumors, infectious lesions, desmoid tumors, and malignant fibrous histiocytoma.

Desmoid tumors are cytologically bland fibrous neoplasms originating from the musculoaponeurotic structures throughout the body. Desmoid tumors, also known as aggressive fibromatosis, are rare connective tumors that account for only 0.03 % of all the neoplasms. These tumors are also locally aggressive and produce large exuberant masses characterized by local invasion and frequent recurrences, but they rarely metastasize. Desmoid tumors are usually noninflammatory asymptomatic masses that become symptomatic when they compress surrounding structures, especially nerves. These tumors arise from connective tissue of fascia, aponeurosis, or muscle striae; they do not show any significant mitotic activity or cytological features of malignancy.

At CT, findings of chest wall desmoid tumors have shown that these lesions have variable appearance and depend on the tumor composition, including the collagen content and amount of solid or necrotic tissue present. Lesions with higher solid tissue components have greater attenuation and enhancement, and most lesions are confined by the surrounding fascia. CT usually reveals the size and location of the tumor precisely, but MRI is probably more sensitive in detecting soft tissue infiltration and evidence of local recurrence.

On MRI, these lesions have a similar signal to muscle on T1-weighted images, with very high signal on T2-weighted images. Central areas of low signal are also seen on T2-weighted images, which is thought to be a result of the high collagen content. In our patient, the MRI study demonstrated such an imaging appearance on T1- and T2-weighted images, with mild heterogeneity seen on the postcontrast images.

CT scan (mediastinal window) shows solid lesion in the anterior chest (Figs. 8.5.1, 8.5.2, and 8.5.3). MRI (T1-weighted image) shows lesion with similar signal to muscle in the anterior chest (Fig. 8.3.4).

Case 6: Subclavian Artery Aneurysm

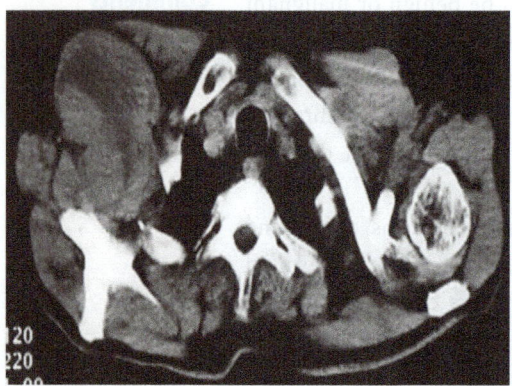

Fig. 8.6.1

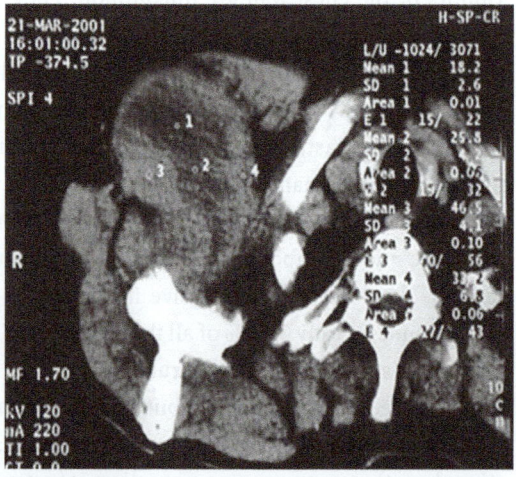

Fig. 8.6.2

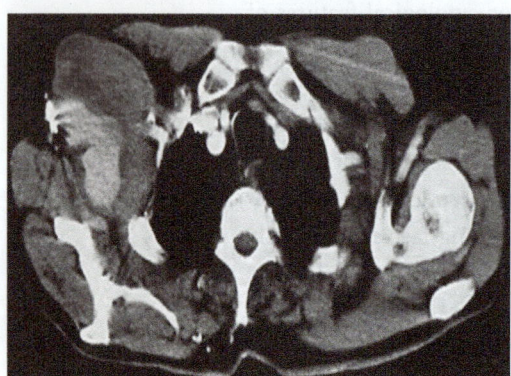

Fig. 8.6.3

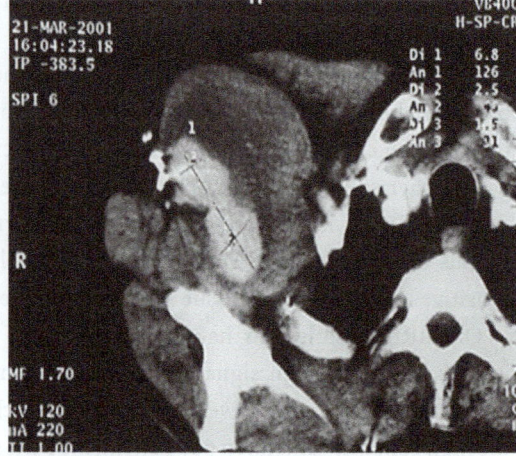

Fig. 8.6.4

A 65-year-old man complained of pain and mass in the chest and has a history of hypertension.

Aneurysms of the subclavian artery are uncommon, accounting for less than 1 % of all peripheral aneurysms. Isolated aneurysm in nonaberrant subclavian arteries is even rarer. The most common cause of subclavian artery aneurysm is atherosclerosis, posttraumatic; less common causes are mycotic aneurysm, cystic medial necrosis, and Marfan's syndrome. Various congenital syndromes may be associated, including Turner's syndrome, but are less frequent. Right sided aneurysm is more common, the male-to-female ratio is 2:1, and the mean age is years.

Approximately 50 % of the patients seen with a subclavian artery aneurysm are asymptomatic. For those experiencing symptoms, the most common include dyspnea, chest pain, hoarseness, dysphagia, and numbness in the fingers. Similarly, the chest pain and hoarseness result from compression on the neighboring trachea.

Compression of an adjacent nerve is the reason for symptoms of numbness of the extremities.

Typical sonographic appearance of a subclavian artery aneurysm is similar to aneurysms seen in the great vessels. A subclavian artery aneurysm is seen as a dilated pulsatile hypoechoic mass in the neck. Thrombus may be seen along the periphery of the aneurysm. Old thrombus is hyperechoic in comparison to the lumen of the vessel. With use of color Doppler imaging, turbulent flow and eddy currents may be visualized as well.

Arteriography is an accurate way to confirm the diagnosis. The MRI and CT scans may add useful information. A chest x-ray can be useful to find out about a first cervical rib (thoracic outlet syndrome) or other bony abnormality.

Patients diagnosed with a subclavian artery aneurysm are at risk of developing life-threatening complications. Subclavian artery aneurysm can lead to emolization, thrombosis, fatal rupture, or transient ischemic attack. In addition, patients with a subclavian artery aneurysm due to atherosclerosis have a 30 % likelihood of having an associated aneurysm in either a peripheral or major artery.

CT scan (mediastinal window) shows liquid density lesion with double contour inside (Figs. 8.6.1 and 8.6.2). CT scan (arterial phase) shows aneurysmal dilatation of the right subclavian artery (Figs. 8.6.3 and 8.6.4).

Case 7: Costal Chondroma

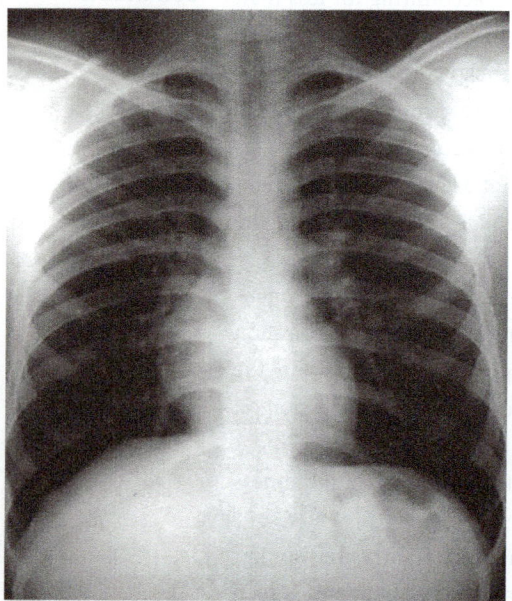

Fig. 8.7.1

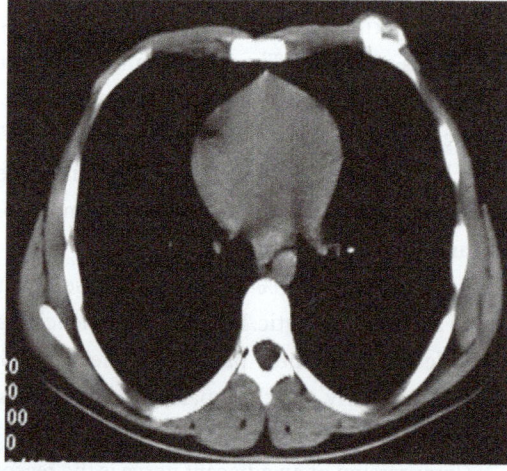

Fig. 8.7.2

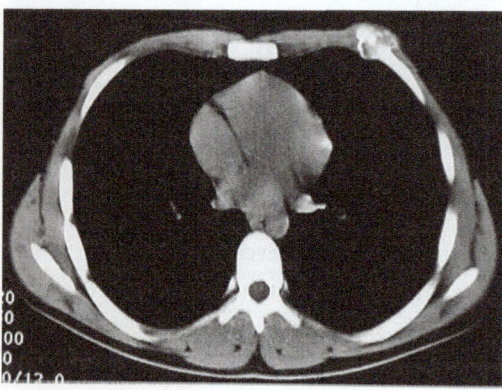

Fig. 8.7.3

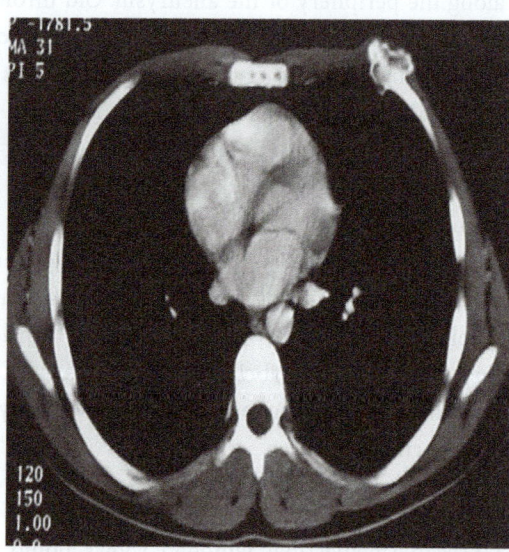

Fig. 8.7.4

A 36-year-old man has swelling and pain referred to left costal.

True primary neoplasms of the ribs are rare. Chondroid lesions are the most common primary tumors and nearly always arise at or near the anterior end of the rib. Therefore, lesions at the costochondral junction, especially if calcified, are suggestive of a chondroid origin. Osteochondroma (exostosis), although not a true neoplasm, is often classified as a tumor and is the most common of these lesions.

In cases of multiple familial exostoses, nearly half of patients have a rib lesion. The typical appearance is a deformity or expansion of the rib with calcification of the cartilaginous cap. CT allows more definitive evaluation of the mass. Spontaneous hemothorax associated with rib exostoses has been reported.

Plain radiography is the first examination that is required and can be characteristic of the lesion. An osteochondroma appears as a stalk or a flat protuberance emerging from the surface of the bone. A usual finding is that of calcified flakes or linear interruptions inside the cartilaginous component of the osteochondroma.

CT can depict the bony lesion in detail, as well as show the presence of calcifications. It has the ability of distinguishing an osteochondroma from an osteosarcoma. The criterion that is used is the thickness of the cartilaginous cap of the tumor, given that an osteosarcoma has a thicker one. CT is currently thought to be unreliable on this subject, as underestimation of the thickness is usual. The disadvantage of CT is that it cannot estimate the metabolic activity, a serious indication of malignancy of any tumor.

MRI is the most precise imaging method for symptomatic cases of bone masses as it can depict the exact morphology of a tumor, arterial and venous compromise, and nervous lesions. MRI is first of all used in order to verify the continuity of the palpable mass with the cortex of the affected bone and to differentiate an osteochondroma from other surface bone lesions. The cartilaginous cap, because it is rich in water, presents a high signal on T2-weighted MRI and a low one on T1-weighted MRI. It is usual to detect above it a low signal zone of the perichondrium. T2-weighted MRI is preferable because it provides better differentiation of signal intensities.

Rarely costal exostosis may cause some complications such as hemothorax; diaphragmatic and pericardial wounds are also reported. In case of symptomatic exostosis, a surgical removal is recommended to avoid severe complications.

CRX film shows nodular lesion that has calcium density in the left anterior fifth rib (Fig. 8.7.1). CT scan (mediastinal window) shows nodular lesion of the rib with the presence of calcium inside (Figs. 8.7.2, 8.7.3, and 8.7.4).

Case 8: Neurofibroma

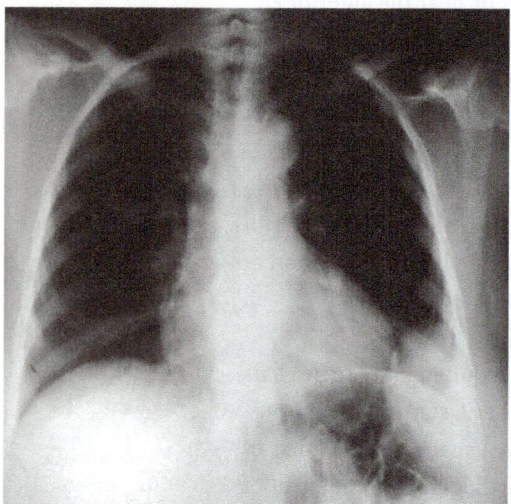

Fig. 8.8.1

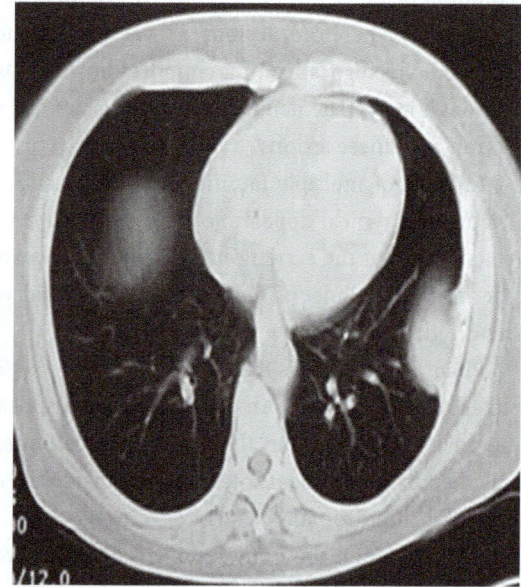

Fig. 8.8.2

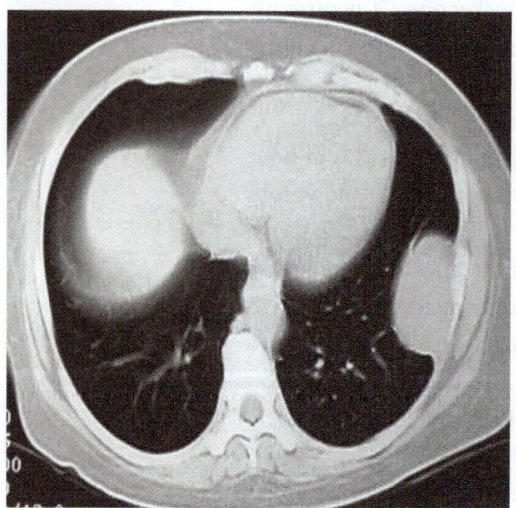

Fig. 8.8.3

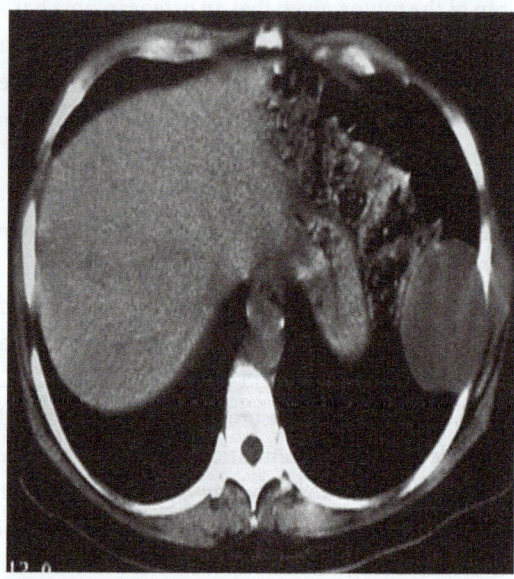

Fig. 8.8.4

A 44-year-old man is referred for 1 month of evolution left costalgia.

Comments

Neurogenic tumors may originate from the intercostal nerves of the thoracic cage or from the paraspinal ganglion of the sympathetic chain. Tumors that arise from nerve roots include neurilemmoma (benign schwannoma, neurinoma), neurofibroma, neurofibrosarcoma, and neuroma. Tumors that affect the sympathetic ganglion include neuroblastoma, ganglioneuroma, and ganglioneuroblastoma.

Neurofibromas most commonly develop in patients between 20 and 30 years of age and may demonstrate a localized, diffuse, or plexiform pattern. The localized type is by far the most common, representing approximately 90 % of lesions, with the vast majority being solitary and not associated with neurofibromatosis type I.

The extent of chest wall involvement is easily evaluated with MR imaging because neurofibromas and other neurogenic tumors have high signal intensity on T2-weighted images. A characteristic imaging feature of neurofibroma on T2-weighted MR images is the target sign, a central focus of low signal intensity within the bright tumor.

MR imaging has been proposed for the differential diagnosis of PNSTs. The classic target sign seen in T2-weighted imaging consists of relatively low signal intensity at the center of a lesion together with high signal intensity at the periphery. Typically, the central lower-signal-intensity region enhances on gadolinium-enhanced MR images, whereas the peripheral high-signal-intensity region does not. The target sign has been reported to be present in T2-weighted imaging in 50–70 % of neurofibromas and 0–54 % of schwannomas.

Imaging Findings

CRX film shows mass compromises the left rib cage (Fig. 8.8.1). CT scan (lung and mediastinal window) shows that the soft tissue mass in left rib cage elevates bone matrix (Figs. 8.8.2, 8.8.3, and 8.8.4).

Case 9: Clear Cell Sarcoma

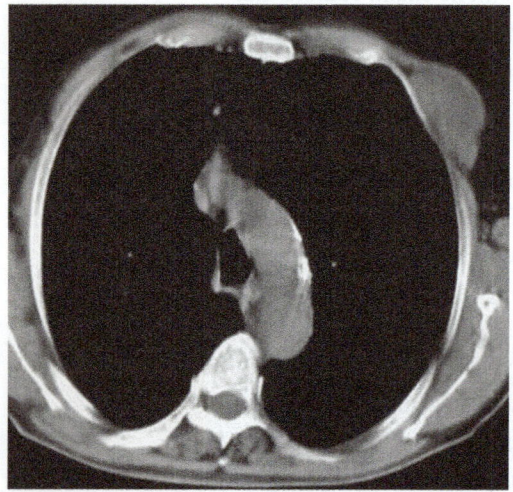

Fig. 8.9.1

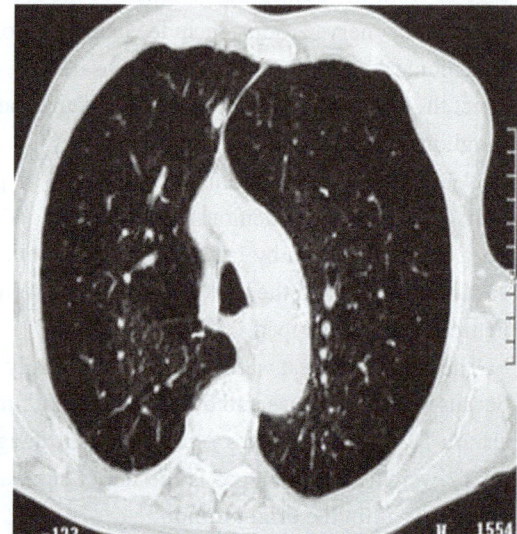

Fig. 8.9.2

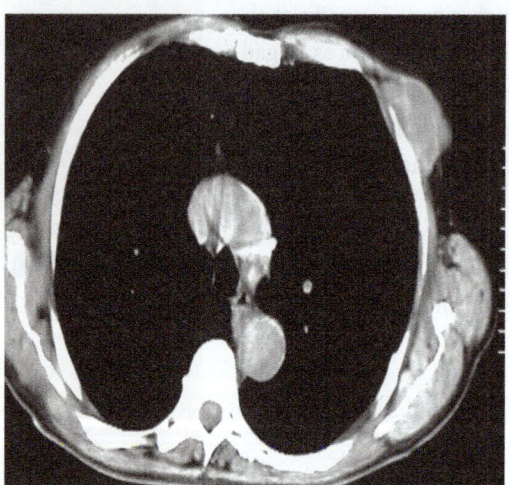

Fig. 8.9.3

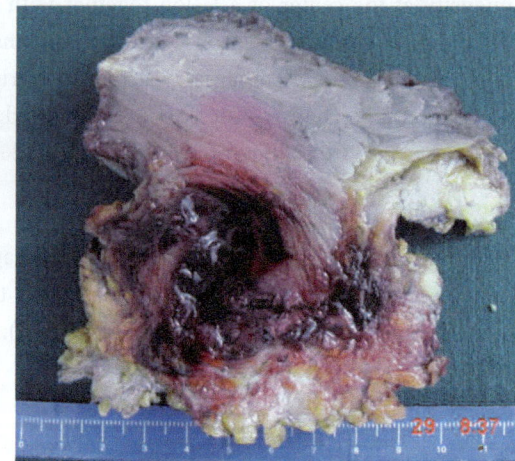

Fig. 8.9.4

A 67-year-old man is referred for left costalgia with Tru-Cut percutaneous needle biopsy that supports clear cell sarcoma.

Clear cell sarcoma (CCS) is a rare and highly malignant neoplasia which is difficult to diagnose and shows melanocytic differentiation. It is a tumor with a propensity for lymph node, lung, and bone metastasis. CCS mainly occurs in young adults between the ages of 20 and 40 years. The male-to-female ratio is almost equal. Its prevalence ranges between 0.5 and 1 % of all malignancies of the musculoskeletal system.

Conventional radiographs of CCS are usually normal but may reveal a deep-seated radiopaque soft tissue mass. Calcification in the tumor and local bone invasion are uncommon.

MR imaging is required to detect and characterize CCS. Due to the paramagnetic effect of the melanin pigment in CCS, most of the tumors show a hyperintense signal to muscle on T1- and hypointense signal on T2-weighted images. The signal on T1 images is more specific for tumors displaying melanocytic differentiation, whereas the signal on T2 images is rather variable. The high signal intensity on T1 images can help to differentiate CCS from other strongly enhancing soft tissue tumors.

CT scan (lung and mediastinal window) shows soft tissue mass and the density of the liquid inside (Figs. 8.9.1, 8.9.2, and 8.9.3). Anatomical specimen shows costal mass and presence of bleeding inside (Fig. 8.9.4).

Case 10: Poland Syndrome

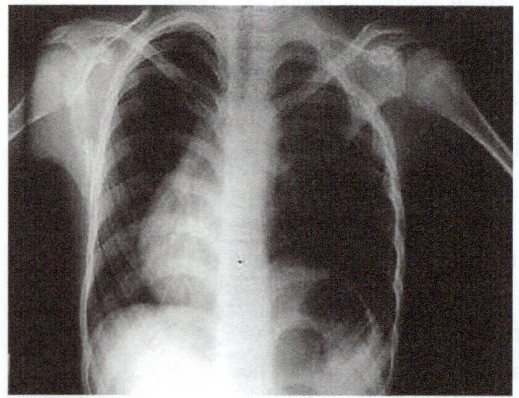

Fig. 8.10.1

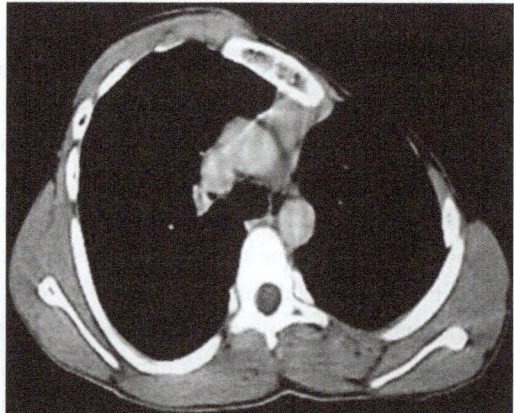

Fig. 8.10.2

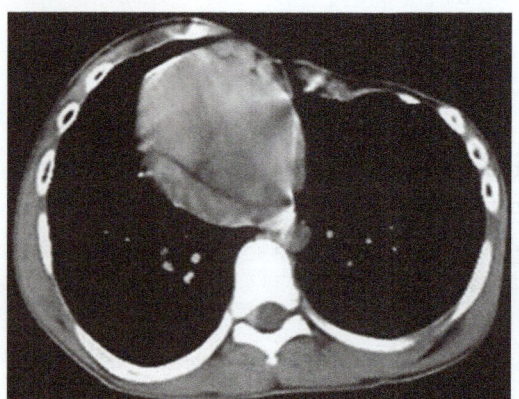

Fig. 8.10.3

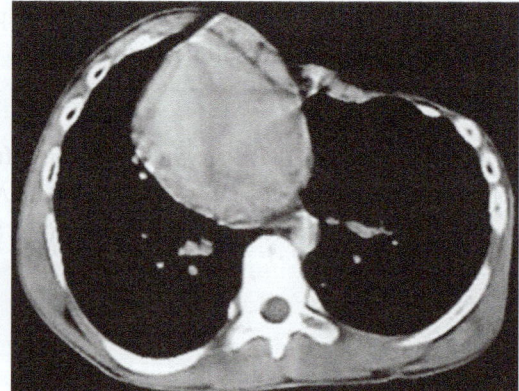

Fig. 8.10.4

A 17-year-old man seeks consultation for asymmetry in the left chest.

Comments

Poland's syndrome is a rare congenital anomaly characterized by hypoplasia of the breast and nipple, scarcity of subcutaneous tissue, absence of the costosternal portion of the pectoralis major muscle, lack of the pectoralis minor muscle, aplasia or deformity of the costal cartilages or ribs II to IV or III to V, alopecia of the axillary and mammary region, and unilateral brachysyndactyly.

The reported incidence of Poland's syndrome ranges from 1 in 7,000 to 1 in 100,000. Males are affected more frequently by a 2:1 to 3:1 ratio. Poland's syndrome has also been diagnosed in 1 of 19,000 mammograms. The right side of the body was found to be involved in 60–75 % of patients.

The role of radiology is to confirm diagnosis and aid in surgical management. Radiographic examination of the chest reveals hyperlucency of the affected side, mimicking a radical mastectomy. A dense ascending line as a result of the absence of the pectoralis major muscles replaces the normal downward curve of the axillary fold.

At CT, ipsilateral partial or complete absence of chest wall musculature is seen. Ipsilateral mammary tissue may appear hypoplastic (compared with the contralateral breast) or completely absent. Both chest radiography and CT depict absent or hypoplastic ipsilateral ribs and scoliosis when present.

CRX film shows hyperlucency left thoracic (Fig. 8.10.1). CT scan (mediastinal window) shows absence of pectoralis major muscle and breast tissue in the left chest (Figs. 8.10.2, 8.10.3, and 8.10.4).

Imaging Findings

Further Reading

Multiple Rib Fracture

Alkadhi H, Wildermuth S, Marincek B, Boehm T (2004) Accuracy and time efficiency for the detection of thoracic cage fractures: volume rendering compared with transverse computed tomography images. J Comput Assist Tomogr 28(3):378–385

Bansidhar BJ, Lagares-Garcia JA, Miller SL (2002) Clinical rib fractures: are follow-up chest X-rays a waste of resources? Am Surg 68(5):449–453

Kaewlai R, Avery LL, Asrani AV, Novelline RA (2008) Multidetector CT of blunt thoracic trauma. Radiographics 28:1555–1570

Lee RB, Bass SM, Morris JA Jr, MacKenzie EJ (1990) Three or more rib fractures as an indicator for transfer to a Level I trauma center: a population-based study. J Trauma 30(6):689–694

Askin's Tumor/Ewing Sarcoma/pPNET

Askin F, Rosai J, Sibley R et al (1979) Malignant small cell tumor of the thoracopulmonary region in childhood. A distinctive clinicopathologic entity of uncertain histogenesis. Cancer 43:2438–2451

Dick E, McHuhg K, Kimber C et al (2001) Imaging of non-central nervous system primitive neuroectodermal tumours: diagnostic features and correlation with outcome. Clin Radiol 56:206–215

Gladish G, Sabloff B, Munden R et al (2002) Primary thoracic sarcomas. Radiographics 22:621–637

Hari S, Jain P, Thulkar S et al (2008) Pictorial review. Imaging features of peripheral primitive neuroectodermal tumours. Br J Radiol 81:975–983

Iribarren MA, Carnerero V, Domínguez A et al (2011) Tumor neuroectodérmico primitivo (tumor de Askin) en la pared torácica. An Pediatr (Barc) 75:343–344

Khong P, Chan G, Shek T et al (2002) Imaging of peripheral PNET: common and uncommon locations. Clin Radiol 57:272–277

Krassas A, Mallios D, Kalkandi P et al (2010) Primitive neuroectodermal tumor of the thoracic wall in a 48-year-old man. Asian Cardiovasc Thorac Ann 18:285–287

Laskar S, Nair C, Mallik S et al (2011) Prognostic factors and outcome in Askin-Rosai tumor: a review of 104 patients. Int J Radiat Oncol Biol Phys 79:202–207

Suárez M, Osorio M (2008) Tumor de Askin: Presentación de un caso y revisión de la literatura. Ann Radiol México 1:55–60

Winer-Muram H, Kauffman W, Gronemeyer S et al (1993) Primitive neuroectodermal tumors of the chest wall (Askin tumors): CT and MR findings. AJR Am J Roentgenol 161:265–268

Pectus Excavatum

Goretsky MJ, Kelly RE, Croitoru D, Nuss D (2004) Chest wall anomalies: pectus excavatum and pectus carinatum. Adolesc Med 15:455–471

Haller JA Jr, Kramer SS, Lietman SA et al (1987) Use of CT scans in selection of patients for pectus excavatum surgery: a preliminary report. J Pediatr Surg 22:904–906

Restrepo CS, Martinez S, Lemos DF, Washington L, McAdams HP, Vargas D, Lemos JA, Carrillo JA, Diethelm L (2009) Imaging appearances of the sternum and sternoclavicular joints. Radiographics 29:839–859

Pectus Carinatum

Fonkalsrud EW, Beanes S (2001) Surgical management of pectus carinatum: 30 years' experience. World J Surg 25:898–903

Haller JA Jr, Kramer SS, Lietman SA (1987) Use of CT scans in selection of patients for pectus excavatum surgery: a preliminary report. J Pediatr Surg 22:904–906

Jeung MY, Gangi A, Gasser B et al (1999) Imaging of chest wall disorders. Radiographics 19:617–637

Shamberger RC (1998) Congenital chest wall deformities. In: O'Neill J, Rowe MI, Grosfeld JL et al (eds) Pediatric surgery, 5th edn. Mosby, St. Louis, pp 787–817

Shamberger RC, Welch KJ, Castaneda AR, Keane JF, Fyler DC (1988) Anterior chest wall deformities and congenital heart disease. J Thorac Cardiovasc Surg 96:427–432

Williams AM, Crabbe DC (2003) Pectus deformities of the anterior chest wall. Paediatr Respir Rev 4:237–242

Recurrent Desmoid Tumor

Klein DL, Gamsu G, Gant TD (1977) Intrathoracic desmoid tumor of the chest wall. AJR Am J Roentgenol 129:524–525

Munden RF, Kemp BL (1999) Desmoid tumor of the chest wall. AJR Am J Roentgenol 172:1149

O'Sullivan P, O'Dwyer H, Flint J, Munk P, Muller N (2007) Soft tissue tumours and mass-like lesions of the chest wall: a pictorial review of CT and MR findings. Br J Radiol 80:574–580

Souza FF et al (2010) PET/CT appearance of desmoid tumour of the chest wall. Br J Radiol 83:e39–e42

Tateishi U, Gladish G, Kusumoto M, Hasegawa T, Tsuchiya R, Moriyama N et al (2003) Chest wall tumors: radiologic findings and pathologic correlation: part 1. Benign tumors. Radiographics 23:1477–1490

Subclavian Artery Aneurysm

Dicle O et al (1999) Subclavian artery aneurysm with oesophagoarterial fistula. Br J Radiol 72:1208–1210

Dougherty MJ, Calligaro KD et al (1995) Atherosclerosis aneurysm of the intrathoracic subclavian artery: a case report and review of the literature. J Vasc Surg 21:521–529

Riley JT (2009) Right subclavian artery aneurysm: an incidental finding. J Diagn Med Sonog 25:255–258

Costal Chondroma

Guttentag AR, Salwen JK (1999) The spectrum of normal variants and diseases that involve the ribs. Radiographics 19:1125–1142

Kenney PJ, GlIula LA, Murphy WA (1981) The use of computed tomography to distinguish osteochondroma and chondrosarcoma. Radiology 139:129–137

Murphey MD, Choi JJ, Kransdorf MJ (2000) Imaging of osteochondroma: variants and complications with radiologic-pathologic correlation. Radiographics 20:1407–1434

Neurofibroma

Jeung MY (1999) Imaging of chest wall disorders. Radiographics 19:617–637

Kuhlman JE, Bouchardy L, Fishman EF, Zerhouni EA, Janet E (1994) Imaging evaluation of chest wall disorders. Radiographics 14:571–595

Nam SJ, Kim S et al (2011) Imaging of primary chest wall tumors with radiologic-pathologic correlation. Radiographics 31:749–770

Clear Cell Sarcoma in the Chest Wall

Kim DH et al (2009) Clear cell sarcoma of the upper thoracic back muscle. J Korean Neurosurg Soc 45: 112–114

Poland Syndrome

Dillman JR, Sanchez R, Ladino-Torres MF, Yarram SG, Strouse PJ, Lucaya J (2011) Expanding upon the unilateral hyperlucent hemithorax in children. Radiographics 31:723–741

Fokin AA, Robicsek F (2002) Poland's syndrome revisited. Ann Thorac Surg 74:2218–2225

Jeung MY (1999) Imaging of chest wall disorders. Radiographics 19:617–637

Jorge Carrillo Bayona, Liliana Arias Álvarez, and Paulina Ojeda León

Contents

J.C. Pedrozo Pupo (ed.), *Learning Chest Imaging*, Learning Imaging,
DOI 10.1007/978-3-642-34147-2_9, © Springer-Verlag Berlin Heidelberg 2013

Case 1: Pulmonary Alveolar Proteinosis

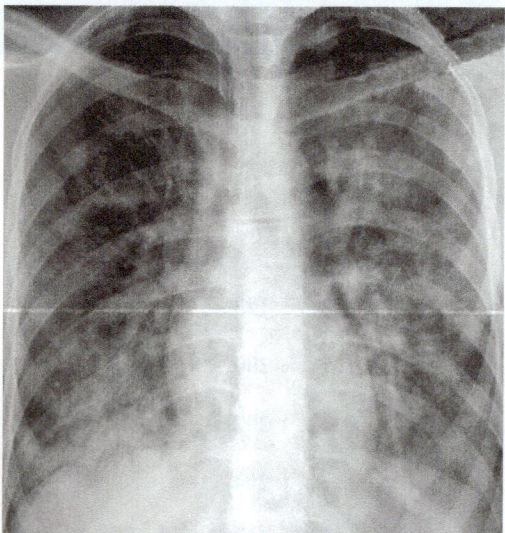

Fig. 9.1.1

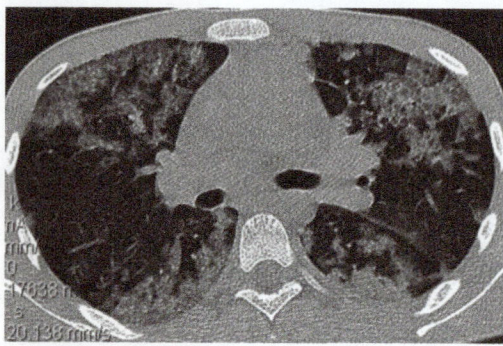

Fig. 9.1.2

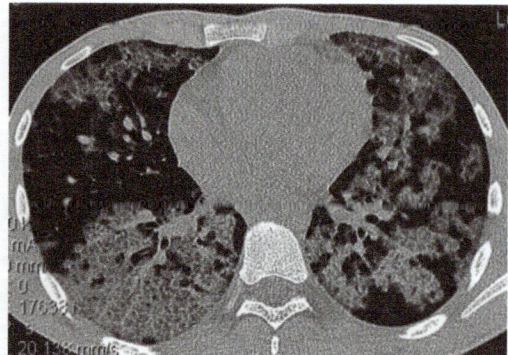

Fig. 9.1.3

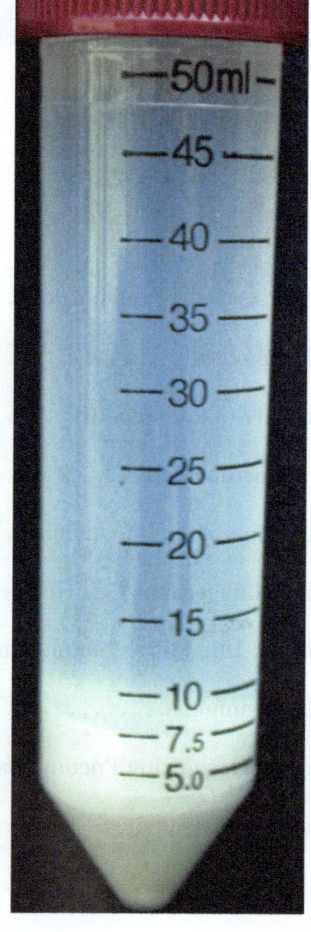

Fig. 9.1.4

A 19-year-old patient with an 8-month history of dyspnea and productive cough with mucoid sputum. The diagnosis of pulmonary alveolar proteinosis was confirmed by bronchoalveolar lavage (BAL).

Pulmonary alveolar proteinosis (PAP) is an uncommon disease, characterized by alveolar accumulation of lipoproteinaceous material. PAP is classified in two main types: congenital and acquired. Congenital PAP (2 % of the cases) appears in the neonatal period as a clinical picture of acute respiratory distress. Acquired PAP is divided into idiopathic or autoimmune (90 % of the cases) and secondary, associated to exposure conditions (inhalation of silica, cotton, aluminum), infections (*P. asteroids*, cytomegalovirus), and immune disorders (human immunodeficiency virus infection, posttransplant immunosuppression).

PAP prevalence is 6.2 cases per million people, the disease is more prevalent in the male gender (3:1), and 39 years is the mean age at diagnosis.

The idiopathic or autoimmune type seems to be associated to the presence of antibodies against the granulocyte-macrophage colony-stimulating factor (GM-CSF), which alters the pulmonary surfactant metabolism.

Clinical features are nonspecific and the approximate average time between the onset of symptoms and the diagnosis is 7 months.

Radiological manifestations are diverse. The radiographic appearance most frequently described in the series consists of symmetrical central and basal consolidations. However, predominantly central reticular opacities, mixed opacities with reticulation and consolidation, and asymmetrical patchy parenchymal opacities may be found. In high-resolution computed tomography (HRCT), the most frequent finding is a "crazy paving" pattern (combination of ground-glass and linear opacities). Areas of "crazy paving" are typically bilateral, extensive, and follow a geographic pattern. Nevertheless, in some cases, the distribution can be asymmetrical, predominantly central, peripheral, or patchy. Other HRCT findings in patients with PAP include ground-glass opacities, consolidation, and airway irregularity.

CRX film shows multilobar consolidation (Fig. 9.1.1). HRCT shows crazy paving pattern with lower lobes predominance (Figs. 9.1.2 and 9.1.3). Gross photo of bronchoalveolar fluid shows the characteristic milky aspect (Fig. 9.1.4).

Case 2: Silicone Embolism

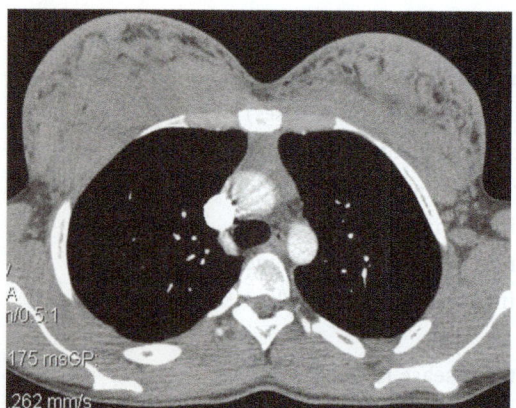

Fig. 9.2.1

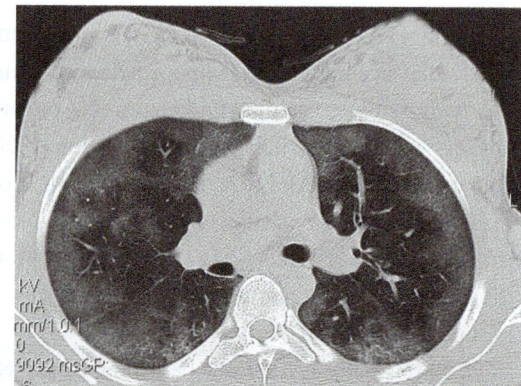

Fig. 9.2.2

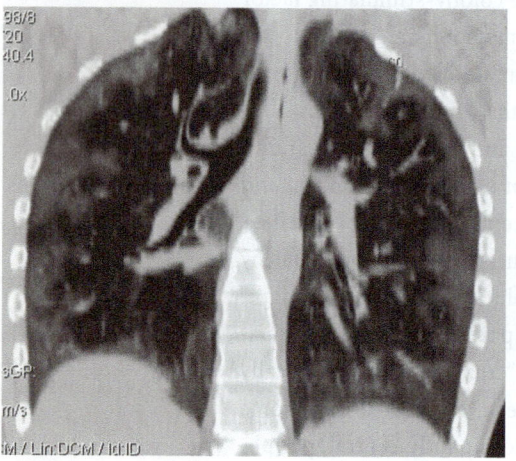

Fig. 9.2.3

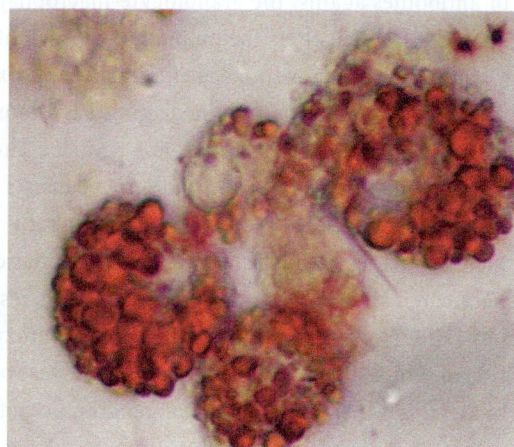

Fig. 9.2.4

A 24-year-old patient with a 24-h history of progressive dyspnea and dry cough, which started after an injection of liquid silicone in the pectoral region. The diagnosis of silicone pulmonary embolism was confirmed by the history, alterations in imaging studies, and the findings of a bronchoalveolar lavage (BAL).

Comments

Liquid silicone is a highly stable polymer, with minimum tissue reaction, widely used in the cosmetic industry. Subcutaneous injection of liquid silicone can be associated to pulmonary embolism. The preferred sites for subcutaneous injection of liquid silicone are the breasts and gluteus. Silicone pulmonary embolism (SPE) after a subcutaneous injection has been associated to the volume injected and to the local massages following the procedure.

The mechanism of pulmonary injury in these patients is similar to that described in fatty embolism with alveolar hemorrhage and fat globules in lung microcirculation and macrophages.

Sixty percent of the patients with SPE develop acute respiratory distress syndrome (ARDS), and 20 % die due to respiratory insufficiency.

All patients with SPE have abnormal chest x-rays with bilateral and peripheral ground-glass opacities, as the characteristic feature.

The most frequent HRCT abnormality in these patients is the presence of bilateral subpleural ground-glass opacities. Other findings in HRCT include thickening of interlobular septum and subpleural reticulation.

Imaging Findings

CT scan shows breast enlargement in male patient with increased density and nodular appearance of subcutaneous fat. Left axillary lymphadenopathy (Fig. 9.2.1). HRCT shows subpleural ground-glass opacity (Figs. 9.2.2 and 9.2.3). Bronchoalveolar lavage shows fat droplets and silicone within macrophages (Sudan stain, 40×; Fig. 9.2.4).

Case 3: Hypersensitivity Pneumonitis

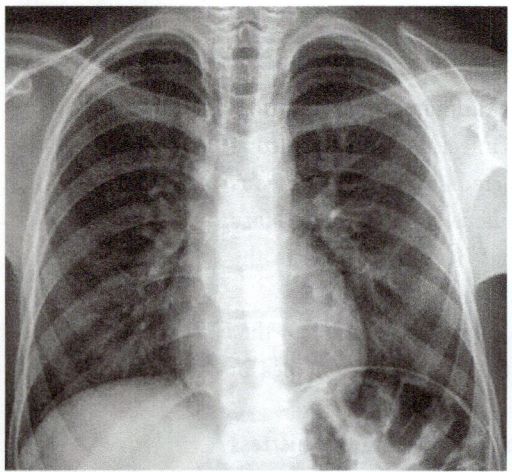

Fig. 9.3.1

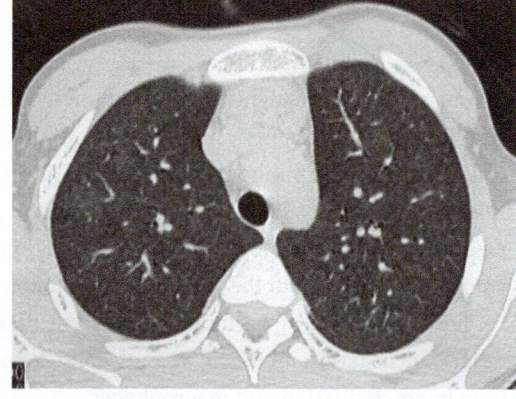

Fig. 9.3.2

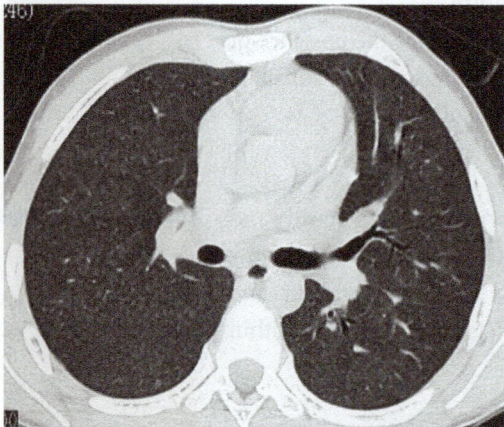

Fig. 9.3.3

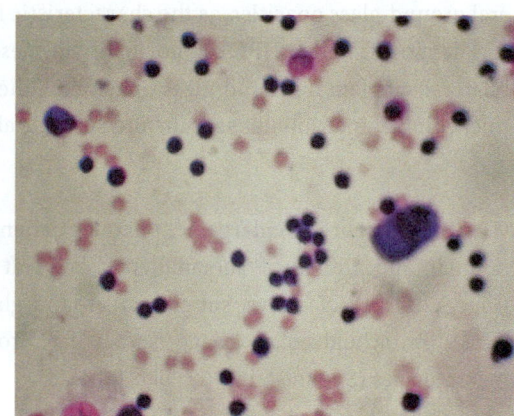

Fig. 9.3.4

A 16-year-old patient with repeated episodes of cough and dyspnea, which subsided spontaneously. There was a history of occasional contact with pigeons. The diagnosis of hypersensitivity pneumonitis was confirmed by the clinical findings, diagnostic images, and BAL findings.

Comments

Hypersensitivity pneumonitis (HN) is a pulmonary disease with symptoms of cough and dyspnea, produced by the inhalation of an allergen by a previously sensitized individual. Most antigens related with HN originate in bacteria (*Saccharopolyspora rectivirgula*), mold (*Penicillium* species), yeast, or poultry (pigeon proteins). Chemical agents such as isocyanates, zinc, tinctures, and dyes can act as haptens to induce NH.

In a study carried out in three European countries, HN represented between 4 and 15 % of pulmonary interstitial diseases.

HN has traditionally been classified in acute, subacute, and chronic. However, recent trials by the HN study group have had difficulties classifying patients in these groups and particularly in cases previously described as subacute.

In the acute phase, radiological abnormalities are similar to those described in pulmonary edema, with multilobar areas of consolidation. In the subacute phase, the main HRCT manifestations are: centrilobular nodule (ill defined), areas of ground-glass opacity (variable distribution and extension), and cystic lesions in 13 % of the cases. In the chronic phase, changes associated to pulmonary fibrosis are found, usually respecting lung bases, with reticular opacities, traction bronchiectasis, and limited areas of honeycombing.

Imaging Findings

CRX film shows diffuse micronodular opacities (Fig. 9.3.1). CT scan shows multiple ground-glass nodules with centrilobular distribution (Figs. 9.3.2 and 9.3.3). Bronchoalveolar lavage with lymphocyte proliferation (Diff-Quick stain, 10×; Fig. 9.3.4).

Case 4: *P. jiroveci* Pneumonia

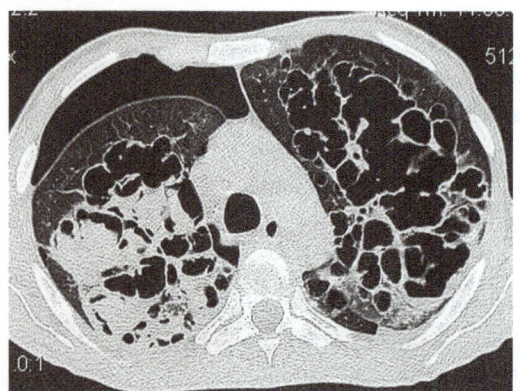

Fig. 9.4.1

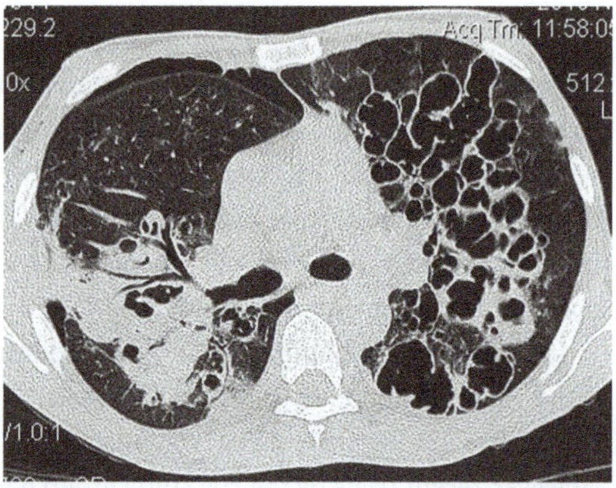

Fig. 9.4.2

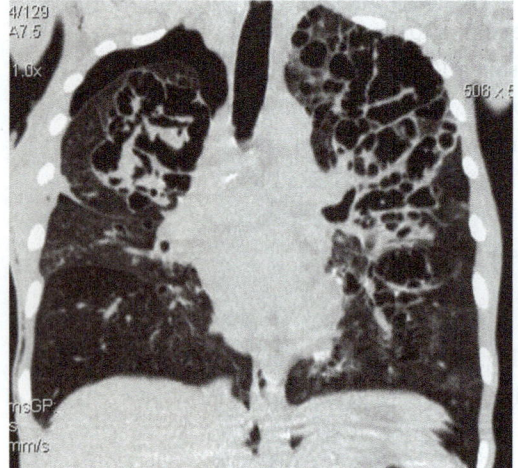

Fig. 9.4.3

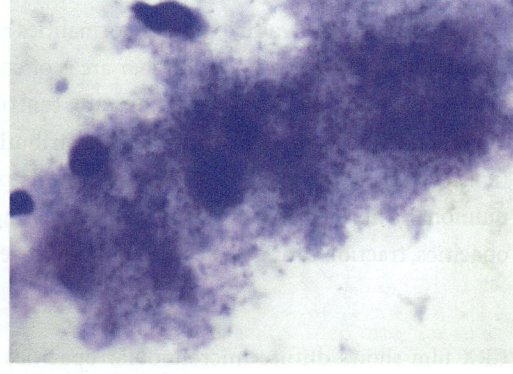

Fig. 9.4.4

A 23-year-old patient with acute chest pain (4 h before consulting the emergency room) and a 1-month history of dry cough and progressive dyspnea. The diagnosis or *P. jiroveci* pneumonia was confirmed by bronchoalveolar lavage.

Comments

P. jiroveci pneumonia (PJP) has been described in immunocompromised patients and particularly in patients with human immunodeficiency virus (HIV) infection. The current incidence of PCP in HIV (+) patients has decreased due to the use of high impact antiretroviral therapy and prophylaxis with trimethoprim/sulfamethoxazole. Nevertheless, PJP incidence remains high in HIV (+) patients in underdeveloped countries.

The clinical picture of PJP in HIV (+) patients is subacute and characterized by dry cough and progressive dyspnea (2–4 weeks).

Radiologic manifestations of *P. jiroveci* pneumonia include: predominantly central reticular opacities, ground-glass opacities, and mixed opacities. In HRCT, the predominant manifestation is the presence of ground-glass opacities with diverse distributions: central, in a "mosaic" pattern, or diffuse. As the infection progresses, areas of consolidation and reticular opacities may appear. The presence of cystic lesions in PJP is variable according to the series (10–20 % of patients). Cysts appear mainly in apical segments; have variable sizes, irregular margins, and thin or thick walls; and are associated with spontaneous pneumothorax.

Imaging Findings

HRCT shows thin-walled cystic appearance lesions without communication with airway. Peribronchial consolidation adjacent cystic lesions. Right pneumothorax. Upper lobes predominance of cystic appearance lesions (Figs. 9.4.1, 9.4.2, and 9.4.3). Bronchoalveolar fluid shows numerous trophozoites of pneumocystis (Diff-Quick stain, 40×; Fig. 9.4.4).

Case 5: Chronic Eosinophilic Pneumonia

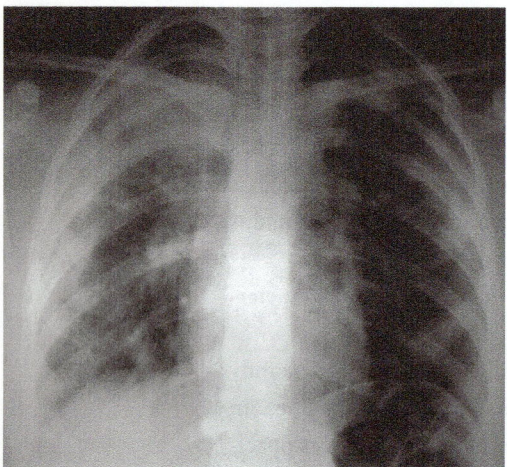

Fig. 9.5.1

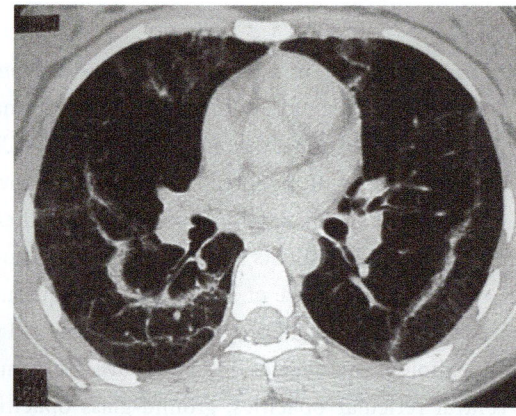

Fig. 9.5.3

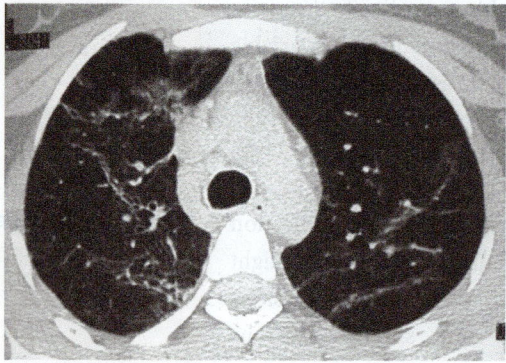

Fig. 9.5.2

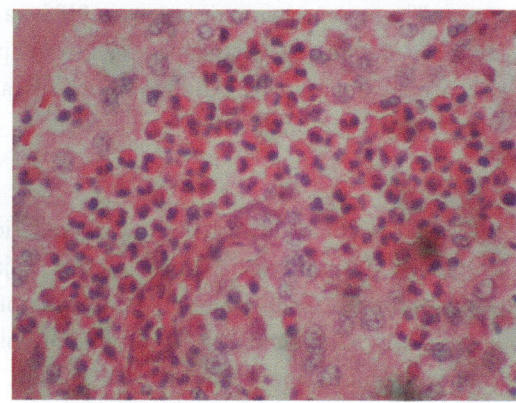

Fig. 9.5.4

A 32-year-old patient with a 6-month history of episodic productive cough with mucoid sputum and dyspnea. Eosinophilia was found in BAL and the diagnosis of chronic eosinophilic pneumonia was confirmed by open lung biopsy.

Comments

Chronic eosinophilic pneumonia (CEP) is an uncommon idiopathic disorder characterized by subacute or chronic respiratory and systemic symptoms, blood and/or alveolar eosinophilia, and peripheral opacities in the chest x-ray.

CEN is considered to represent between 0 and 2.5 % of pulmonary interstitial disease cases. This disorder is more frequent in women (2:1) and between one-third and half of the patients with CEP have a history of asthma.

Most CEP patients are symptomatic and the most frequent manifestations are: progressive dyspnea, cough, and general symptoms (asthenia, weight loss, and night sweats).

Eosinophilia is found in BAL (12–95 % of cellular count, with an average of 59 %). Lung biopsy shows evidence of predominantly eosinophilic alveolar and interstitial inflammatory infiltration.

The classic radiographic finding is the "inverse pulmonary edema" (peripheral, mainly apical, nonsegmental consolidation). However, this finding is seen in less than 50 % of the patients. HRCT manifestations are variable and related to disease evolution. Predominantly peripheral areas of ground-glass opacities and/or consolidation are more common in early stages. With disease progression, septal lines, reticular opacities, nodules, and subpleural parenchymal bands may be found.

Imaging Findings

CRX film shows multilobar and peripheral consolidation (Fig. 9.5.1; HRCT). Pulmonary architecture distortion. Parenchymal bands with traction bronchiectasis, ground-glass and subpleural consolidation (Figs. 9.5.2 and 9.5.3). Lung biopsy shows numerous eosinophils filling an alveolar space (HE, 40×; Fig. 9.5.4).

Case 6: Pulmonary Langerhans Cell Histiocytosis

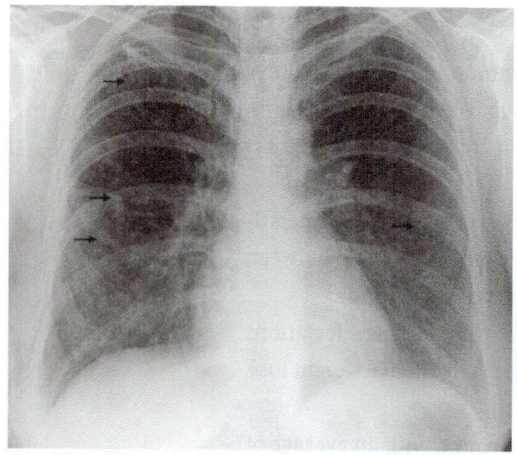

Fig. 9.6.1

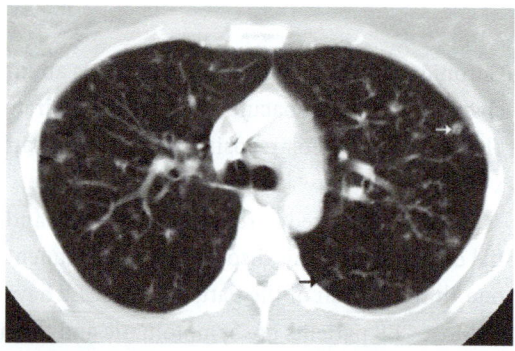

Fig. 9.6.2

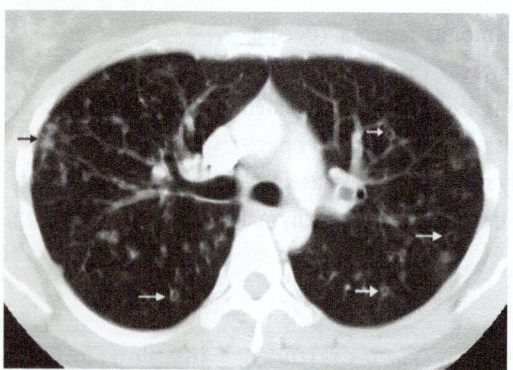

Fig. 9.6.3

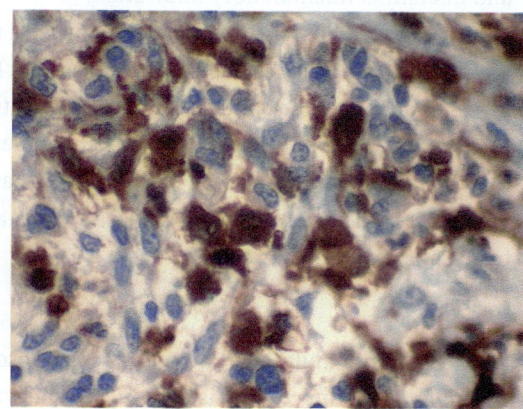

Fig. 9.6.4

A 40-year-old patient with progressive dyspnea starting 6 months before and a history of smoking. The diagnosis of Langerhans cell histiocytosis was made by an open lung biopsy.

Comments

Pulmonary Langerhans cell histiocytosis (PLCH) is an isolated form of Langerhans cell histiocytosis (LCH) that mainly affects smokers. Disease pathogenesis remains uncertain. LCH represents a clonal proliferation of cells similar to that typical of neoplastic diseases. In the particular case of the pulmonary type, pathogenesis may be different, as it has been demonstrated that most nodules do not follow clonal proliferation. It has been suggested that this disorder corresponds to an exaggerated immune response to an antigen, in which Langerhans cells can serve as accessory cells in T lymphocyte activation.

From the histological viewpoint, histiocytosis is a temporary heterogeneous disorder characterized by peribronchiolar proliferation of Langerhans cells, which form nodules. Nodular lesions frequently cavitate forming thick- or thin-walled cysts according to the evolutional stage. These cysts represent the lumen of the dilated airway. In the most severe cases, the presence of fibrosis can reach the alveolar wall, forming scars and distorting pulmonary architecture.

It is a clinically rare disease (5 % of interstitial diseases). Patients are sometimes asymptomatic. However, the most frequent symptoms are cough and dyspnea. Other clinical manifestations can be hemoptysis, fever, weight loss, and night sweats. Pneumothorax, sometimes recurrent, can occur in one out of every four patients.

Radiological manifestations depend on the evolution of the disease.

Chest x-rays can be interpreted as normal in early stages of disease. In advanced cases, the most frequent semiological findings are reticular opacities corresponding to the visualization of the walls of contiguous cystic lesions and predominantly apical small nodules.

In HRCT, the most frequent manifestation of early disease is the presence of small, irregular, peribronchiolar nodules, with different degrees of cavitation in an otherwise healthy lung. With disease progression, cystic lesions increase in number and size and their walls become thinner. The presence of cystic lesions larger than 1 cm, with irregular margins, and distortion of pulmonary architecture suggests an advanced stage of the disease. Related findings include ground-glass opacities and changes due to emphysema associated to the habit of smoking.

Imaging Findings

CRX film shows ill-defined nodular opacities (arrows). Peribronchial thickening (Fig. 9.6.1).

CT scan shows ground-glass small nodules (black arrows) and soft tissue nodules (arrowheads), with varying degree of cavitation (white arrows) and random distribution (Figs. 9.6.2 and 9.6.3). Lung biopsy shows the typical nuclear and cytoplasmic staining of Langerhans cells (S-100 stain, 40×; Fig. 9.6.4).

Case 7: Lymphocytic Interstitial Pneumonia

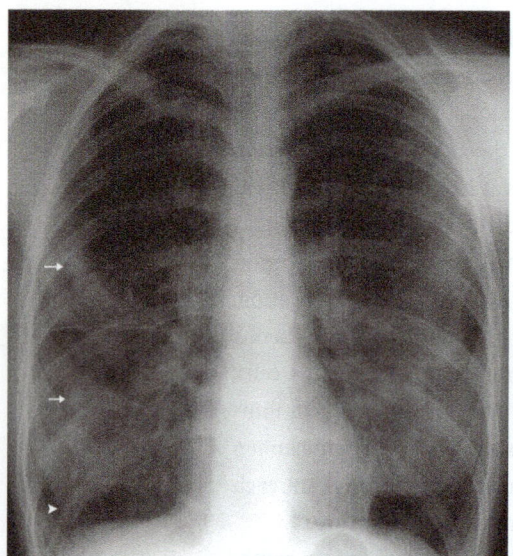

Fig. 9.7.1

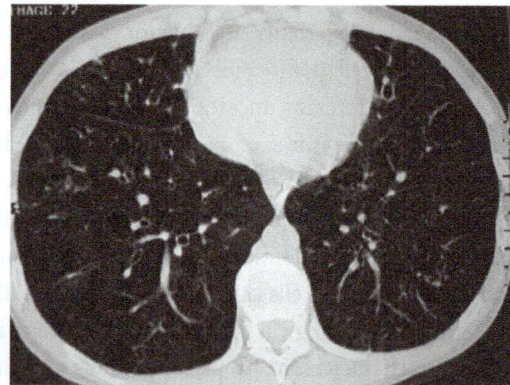

Fig. 9.7.2

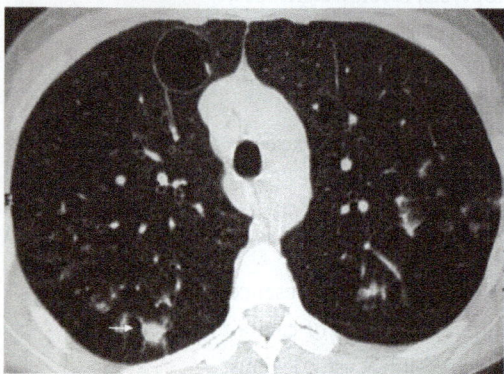

Fig. 9.7.3

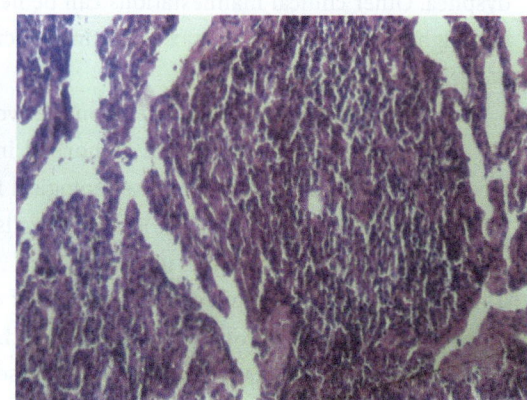

Fig. 9.7.4

A 43-year-old patient with a 1-year clinical picture consisting of cough and dyspnea and a 3-month history of weight loss and fever. After an open lung biopsy, the diagnosis of lymphocytic interstitial pneumonia was made.

Comments

Lymphocytic interstitial pneumonia (LIP) is considered a nonneoplastic inflammatory reaction of bronchial associated lymphoid tissue (BALT). This pattern of pulmonary response can be associated to systemic diseases (Sjögren syndrome, systemic lupus erythematosus), dysproteinemias, human immunodeficiency virus infection, and adverse reaction to drugs (diphenylhydantoin). In its idiopathic presentation, it is included in the group of idiopathic interstitial pneumonias, due to the presence of fibrosis during the course of the disease in some patients.

LIP may appear in pediatric population associated to HIV infection. Most adults with LIP are women between the 5th and 7th decades of life. Clinical manifestations are nonspecific and include cough and dyspnea of gradual onset. Less frequently, weight loss, chest pain, fever, and arthralgia are described.

Histologically, LIP is characterized by a lymphocitary infiltrate extensively compromising alveolar septa. Hyperplasia of type II pneumocytes and granuloma formation are described. Immunohistochemistry using CD20 shows that B cells are predominantly located in germ centers.

Radiological findings described in LIP are nonspecific, with predominantly basal reticular or reticulonodular opacities as the main manifestations. Areas of consolidation and ill-defined nodules may also be found. The most frequent alterations found in HRCT are ground-glass opacities, centrilobular nodules, thickening of peribronchovascular interstitium, interlobular septum thickening, areas of consolidation, and cysts. Pathogenesis of cysts is related to partial obstruction of bronchioles and air trapping due to peribronchial lymphocytic infiltration and occasionally due to focal amyloid deposits.

Imaging Findings

Chest x-ray film shows ill-defined nodules (arrow) and ground-glass patchy areas. Thin-walled cystic appearance lesion in right lower lobe (arrowhead) (Fig. 9.7.1). HRCT shows soft tissue nodules and diffuse ground-glass and thin-walled cystic lesions of variable size (Figs. 9.7.2 and 9.7.3). This photomicrograph shows the typical densely cellular appearance of widened alveolar septa (HE stain, 10×; Fig. 9.7.4).

Case 8: Varicella Pneumonia

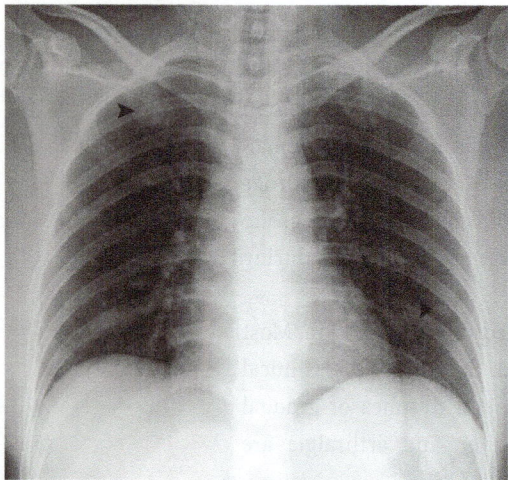

Fig. 9.8.1

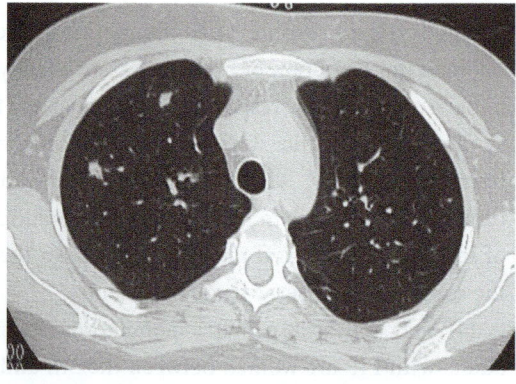

Fig. 9.8.2

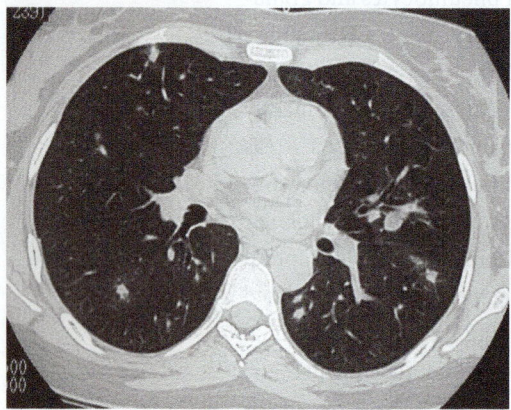

Fig. 9.8.3

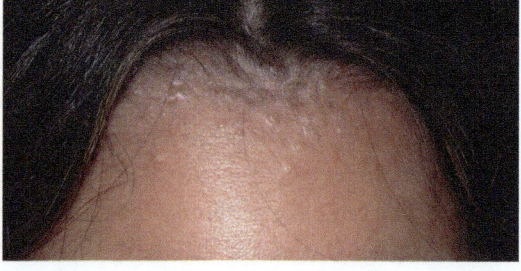

Fig. 9.8.4

A 16-year-old patient with acute lymphocytic leukemia under treatment and a 6-day history of fever, dry cough, and cutaneous vesicular lesions. Considering the clinical picture and imaging study findings, the diagnosis of varicella pneumonia was made.

Pneumonia due to Varicella-Zoster virus is the most severe complication of a systemic infection, with a mortality rate ranging between 9 and 50 %.

Disease course in children is self-limited and benign. However, in adults, it tends to be a significant cause of complications. More than 90 % of cases of viral pneumonia due to Varicella-Zoster occur in immunocompromised adult patients and pregnant women.

There is no gender predilection. Conditions causing immunosuppression as leukemia, lymphoma, and corticosteroid therapy are considered risk factors. Pregnancy, advanced age, chronic obstructive pulmonary disease, and severe cutaneous eruption are other predisposing conditions.

Symptoms of pneumonia develop a few days after cutaneous vesicles appear and include cough, dyspnea, hemoptysis, tachypnea, pleuritic pain, and fever.

Histologically, they are nodules formed by areas of hyalinized collagen or necrotic tissue with a fibrous capsule that can resolve and calcify in various ways or form areas of mononuclear inflammatory interstitial infiltration with an intra-alveolar proteinaceous exudate and hyaline membrane formation (diffuse alveolar damage).

Radiological findings include ill-defined nodules, randomly distributed, ranging between 5 and 10 mm in diameter. Nodules can disappear or calcify late after cutaneous lesions have disappeared. Nodular lesions of soft tissue density, ranging between 1 and 10 mm in diameter, which may have a perilesional ground-glass halo, are described in HRCT. Nodular lesions can coalesce and combine with patchy ground-glass opacities.

Chest x-ray film shows nodular opacities, ill defined (arrowhead) (Fig. 9.8.1). Random soft tissue small nodules with ground-glass halo (Figs. 9.8.2 and 9.8.3). Vesicular lesions in the patient's forehead (Fig. 9.8.4).

Case 9: Cryptogenic Organizing Pneumonia

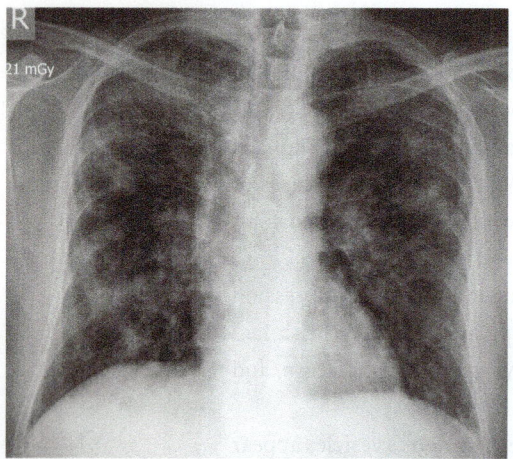

Fig. 9.9.1

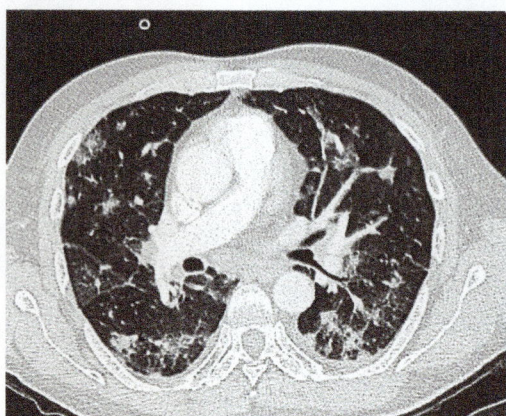

Fig. 9.9.2

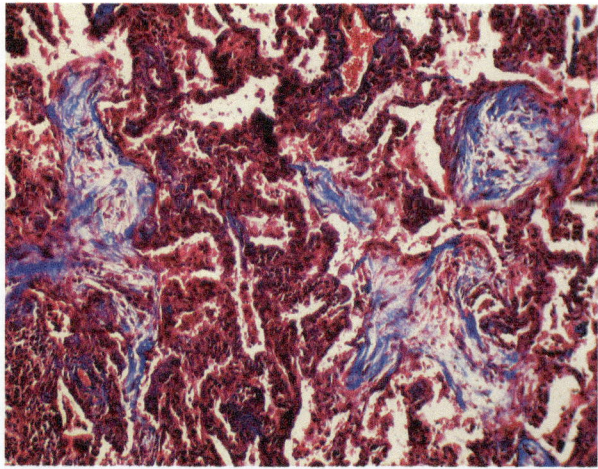

Fig. 9.9.3

Fig. 9.9.4

A 39-year-old patient with a 3-month clinical picture consisting of fever, adynamia, weight loss, and cough. Open lung biopsy was interpreted as a pattern of organizing pneumonia. In the absence of an etiological factor or associated condition, the diagnosis of cryptogenic organizing pneumonia was made.

Comments

Organizing pneumonia (OP) is a nonspecific histopathological pattern of pulmonary response to injuries of diverse nature, characterized by the presence of granulation tissue buds in the distal airways. This process occurs mainly in alveoli, but may extend to alveolar duct lumen and bronchioles. OP can be classified in three categories: idiopathic (cryptogenic organizing pneumonia), of known cause (infection, radiation), or of unknown cause associated to a specific clinical context (collagen vascular disease, posttransplant).

The histological hallmark of organizing pneumonia is a distinct, usually patchy type of fibrosis that predominantly involves bronchiolar lumen and peribronchiolar airspaces. The fibrosis is composed of elongated fibroblasts and myofibroblasts arranged in parallel and embedded in a myxoid or pale staining matrix.

The typical or classical presentation of OP described in chest x-rays consists of bilateral patchy airspace consolidations, most prominent in the peripheral lower lung zones, with a tendency to progress and change location over time. CT reflects the findings of the chest x-ray demonstrating that the areas of consolidation are predominantly peribronchovascular and/or subpleural. Bronchial dilation in consolidated areas is described in 55 % of patients. Other findings in HRCT of patients with OP pattern are: nodule(s) – mass(es), ground-glass opacities, parenchymal bands, nodules with halo and reverse halo signs, and reticular opacities.

Imaging Findings

Chest x-ray film shows consolidation and ground-glass patchy (Fig. 9.9.1). CT scan (lung window) shows multilobar consolidation and ground-glass halo sign (Figs. 9.9.2 and 9.9.3). Lung biopsy shows fibroblast plugs within alveolar spaces (trichrome stain, 10×; Fig. 9.9.4).

Case 10: Lymphangioleiomyomatosis

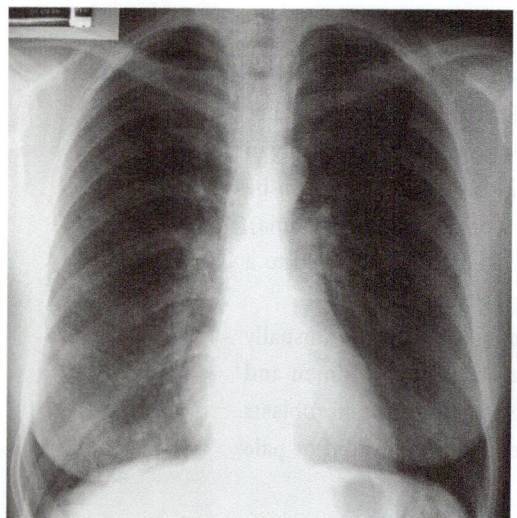

Fig. 9.10.1

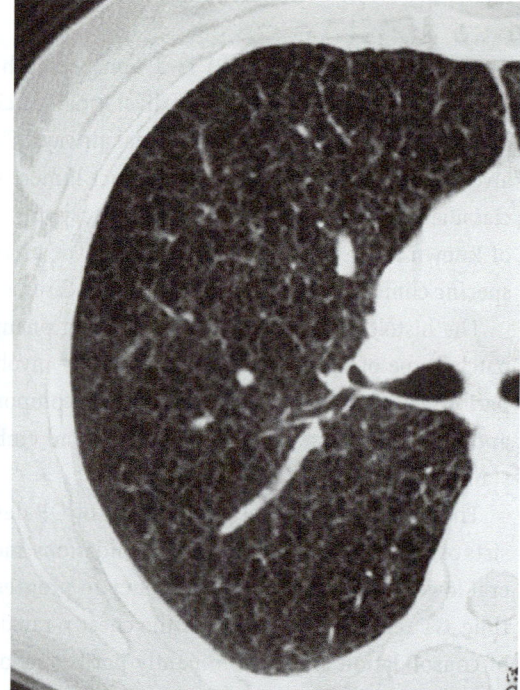

Fig. 9.10.2

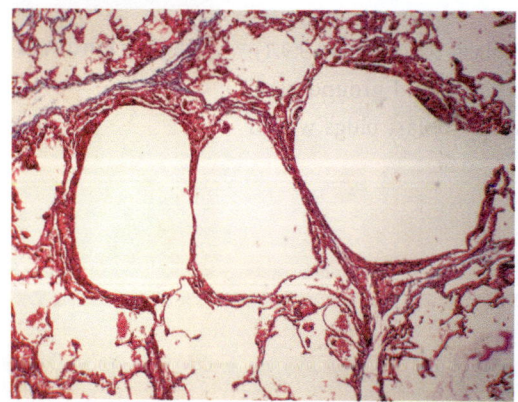

Fig. 9.10.3

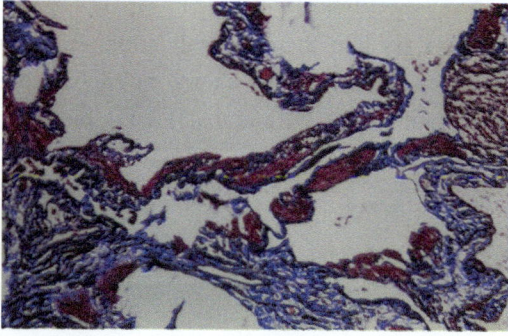

Fig. 9.10.4

A 28-year-old female patient with progressive dyspnea and a history of spontaneous pneumothorax. Open lung biopsy showed lymphangioleiomyomatosis.

Comments

Lymphangioleiomyomatosis (LLM) is a rare, progressive, multisystemic disorder characterized by the proliferation of pulmonary parenchyma bronchiolar, venular, and lymphatic smooth muscle. The pathogenesis is not clearly established but it probably has its bases in TSC2 gene mutations of the tuberous sclerosis complex located in chromosome 16.

Although classified as a different entity, LLM shares its physiopathology with tuberous sclerosis, and LLM patients may have extrapulmonary manifestations such as angiomyolipomas (15–30 % of patients). These similarities lead some researchers to consider LLM as a frustrated form of tuberous sclerosis or that both entities correspond to the same disease with a different degree of expression.

LLM affects almost exclusively women of childbearing age and can occur as a complication associated to tuberous sclerosis in women (men with tuberous sclerosis usually do not develop cystic changes of LLM in the lung).

Histologically, abnormal proliferation of immature smooth muscle cells within the airway, lymph vessels, and blood vessels causes mechanic obstruction with secondary cyst formation, pneumothorax, lymphatic flow obstruction, lymph node enlargement, chylothorax, and pulmonary arterial and venous hypertension that can lead to hemorrhage and hemothorax. A biochemical explanation for cyst formation in this disease is metalloprotease production by LAM cells, which destroy pulmonary collagen and elastin. LAM cells can be identified by immunohistochemistry techniques that demonstrate the presence of antigens to smooth muscle actin- and melanoma-associated HMB-45.

In chest x-rays, the most frequent manifestations are an increase in pulmonary volume and reticular opacities in relation to cyst overlapping.

HRCT shows multiple thin-walled cysts, of similar size and regular margins, uniformly distributed in lungs. Lung parenchyma in between cystic lesions is normal. These findings can simulate changes due to emphysema; the diagnostic key relies on the identification of cyst walls and the population group.

Imaging Findings

Chest x-ray film shows fine reticular opacities (Fig. 9.10.1). CT scan (lung window) shows diffuse and uniform small thin-walled cystic lesions (Fig. 9.10.2). Lung biopsy shows the characteristic smooth muscle in the cyst wall (HE and trichrome stain, 10×; Figs. 9.10.3 and 9.10.4).

Further Reading

Pulmonary Alveolar Proteinosis

Borie RC et al (2011) Pulmonary alveolar proteinosis. Eur Respir Rev 20(120):98–107

Godwin JD, Muller NL, Takasugi JE (1988) Pulmonary alveolar proteinosis: CT findings. Radiology 169:609–613

Holbert JM et al (2001) CT features of pulmonary alveolar proteinosis. AJR Am J Roentgenol 176:1287–1294

Johkoh T, Itoh H, Muller NL et al (1999) Crazy-paving appearance at thin-section CT: spectrum of disease and pathologic findings. Radiology 211:155–160

Lee CH (2007) The crazy-paving sign. Radiology 243:905–906

Muller NL, Fraser RS, Lee KS, Johkoh T (2003) Diseases of the lung: radiologic and pathologic correlations. Lippincott Williams & Wilkins, Philadelphia, pp 219–222

Murrayama S, Murakami J, Yabuuchi H, Soeda H, Masuda K (1999) Crazy-paving appearance on high resolution CT in various diseases. J Comput Assist Tomogr 23:749–752

Trapnell BC, Whitsett JA, Nakata K (2003) Pulmonary alveolar proteinosis. N Engl J Med 349:2527–2539

Silicone Embolism

Bartsich S, Wu JK (2010) Silicon emboli syndrome: a sequela of clandestine liquid silicone injections. A case report and review of the literature. J Plast Reconstr Aesthet Surg 63:1–3

Han D, Lee KS, Franquet T, Müller NL, Kim TS, Kim H et al (2003) Thrombotic and nonthrombotic pulmonary arterial embolism: spectrum of imaging findings. Radiographics 23:1521–1539

Jorens PG, Van Marck E, Snoeckx A, Parizel PM (2009) Nonthrombotic pulmonary embolism. Eur Respir J 34:452–474

Martínez JC, Manrique C, Sáenz O, Ojeda P, Nicolás Rocha N et al (2009) Silicone pulmonary embolism. Report of a case and review of the literature. Rev Colomb Neumol 21(2):84–88

Price EA, Schueler H, Perper JA (2006) Massive systemic silicone embolism: a case report and review of literature. Am J Forensic Med Pathol 27:97–102

Restrepo CS, Artunduaga M, Carrillo JA, Rivera AL, Ojeda P, Martinez-Jimenez S et al (2009) Silicone pulmonary embolism: report of 10 cases and review of the literature. J Comput Assist Tomogr 33:233–237

Schmid A, Tzur A, Leshko L, Kriege BP (2005) Silicone embolism syndrome. Chest 127:2276–2281

Hypersensitivity Pneumonitis

Glazer CS, Rose CS, Lynch DA (2002) Clinical and radiologic manifestations of hypersensitivity pneumonitis. J Thorac Imaging 17:261–272

Hanak V, Golbin JM, Hartman TE et al (2008) High-resolution CT findings of parenchymal fibrosis correlate with prognosis in hypersensitivity pneumonitis. Chest 134:133–138

Hansell DM, Wells AU, Padley SP et al (1996) Hypersensitivity pneumonitis: correlation of individual CT patterns with functional abnormalities. Radiology 199:123–128

Hirschmann JV, Pipavath SN, Godwin JD (2009) Hypersensitivity pneumonitis: a historical, clinical, and radiologic review. Radiographics 29:1921–1938

Lynch DA, Rose CS, Way D et al (1992) Hypersensitivity pneumonitis: sensitivity of high-resolution CT in a population-based study. Am J Roentgenol 159: 469–472

Lynch DA, Newell JD, Logan PM et al (1995) Can CT distinguish hypersensitivity pneumonitis from idiopathic pulmonary fibrosis? Am J Roentgenol 165: 807–811

Ranks TJ, Galvin JR, Frazier AA (2004) The impact and use of high-resolution computed tomography in diffuse lung disease. Curr Diagn Pathol 10:279–290

Silva CI, Churg A, Müller NL (2007) Hypersensitivity pneumonitis: spectrum of high-resolution CT and pathologic findings. AJR Am J Roentgenol 188: 334–344

Silva CI, Muller NL, Lynch DA et al (2008) Chronic hypersensitivity pneumonitis: differentiation from idiopathic pulmonary fibrosis and nonspecific interstitial pneumonia by using thin-section CT. Radiology 246:288–297

P. jiroveci Pneumonia

Boiselle PM, Crans CA, Kaplan MA (1999) The changing face of Pneumocystis carinii pneumonia in AIDS patients. AJR Am J Roentgenol 172(5):1301–1309

Hartman TE, Primack SL, Müller NL et al (1994) Diagnosis of thoracic complications in AIDS: accuracy of CT. AJR Am J Roentgenol 162(3):547–553

Hidalgo A, Falcó V, Mauleón S et al (2003) Accuracy of high-resolution CT in distinguishing between Pneumocystis carinii pneumonia and non-Pneumocystis carinii pneumonia in AIDS patients. Eur Radiol 13(5):1179–1184

Kanne JP, Yandow DR, Meyer CA (2012) Pneumocystis jiroveci pneumonia: high-resolution CT findings in patients with and without HIV infection. AJR Am J Roentgenol 198:W555–W561

Opravil M, Marincek B, Fuchs WA et al (1994) Shortcomings of chest radiography in detecting Pneumocystis carinii pneumonia. J Acquir Immune Defic Syndr 7(1):39–45

Shah RM, Kaji AV, Ostrum BJ et al (1997) Interpretation of chest radiographs in AIDS patients: usefulness of CD4 lymphocyte counts. Radiographics 17(1):47–58

Chronic Eosinophilic Pneumonia

Ebara H, Ikezoe J, Johkoh T, Kohno N, Takeuchi N, Kozuka T et al (1994) Chronic eosinophilic pneumonia: evolution of chest radiograms and CT features. J Comput Assist Tomogr 18(5):737–744

Gaenster EA, Carrington B (1977) Peripheral opacities in chronic eosinophilic pneumonia: the photographic negative of pulmonary edema. AJR Am J Roengenol 128:1–13

Jeong YJ et al (2007) Eosinophilic lung diseases: a clinical, radiologic, and pathologic overview. radiographics 27:617–639

Johkoh T, Müller NL, Akira M et al (2000) Eosinophilic lung diseases: diagnostic accuracy of thin-section CT in 111 patients. Radiology 216(3):773–780

Mayo JR, Muller NL, Sisler J, Lillington G (1989) Chronic eosinophilic pneumonia: CT findings in six cases. AJR Am J Roentgenol 153:727–730

Pulmonary Langerhans Cell Histiocytosis

Abbott GF, Rosado-de-Christenson ML et al (2004) Pulmonary Langerhans cell histiocytosis. Radiographics 24:821–841

Brauner MW, Grenier P, Tijani K et al (1997) Pulmonary Langerhans cell histiocytosis: evolution of lesions on CT scans. Radiology 204(2):497–502

Ko S-M et al (2008) Atypical radiological manifestations of pulmonary Langerhans cell histiocytosis in a 12-year-old girl. Br J Radiol 81:e238–e241

Leatherwood DL, Heitkamp DE, Emerson RE (2007) Pulmonary Langerhans cell histiocytosis. Radiographics 27:265–268

Moore AD, Godwin JD, Müller NL et al (1989) Pulmonary histiocytosis X: comparison of radiographic and CT findings. Radiology 172(1):249–254

Schmidt S, Eich G, Geoffray A et al (2008) Extraosseous Langerhans cell histiocytosis in children. Radiographics 28(3):707–726

Suri H et al (2012) Pulmonary Langerhans cell histiocytosis. Orphanet J Rare Dis 7:16

Tazi A (2006) Adult pulmonary Langerhans' cell histiocytosis. Eur Respir J 27:1272–1285

Tazi A, Soler P, Hance AJ (2000) Adult pulmonary Langerhans' cell histiocytosis. Thorax 55:405–416

Lymphocytic Interstitial Pneumonia

Honda O, Johkoh T, Ichikado K et al (1999) Differential diagnosis of lymphocytic interstitial pneumonia and malignant lymphoma on high-resolution CT. AJR Am J Roentgenol 173(1):71–74

Johkoh T, Muller NL et al (1999) Lymphocytic interstitial pneumonia: thin-section CT findings in 22 patients. Radiology 212:567–572

Kim TS, Lee KS, Chung MP et al (1998) Nonspecific interstitial pneumonia with fibrosis: high-resolution CT and pathologic findings. AJR Am J Roentgenol 171(6):1645–1650

Swigris JJ, Berry GJ, Raffin TA, Kuschner WG (2002) Lymphoid interstitial pneumonia: a narrative review. Chest 122(6):2150–2164

Varicella Pneumonia

Aquino SL, Dunagan DP, Chiles C, Haponik EF (1998) Herpes simplex virus I pneumoniae patterns on CT scans and conventional chest radiographs. J Comput Assist Tomogr 22:795–800

Franquet T (2011) Imaging of pulmonary viral pneumonia. Radiology 260:18–39

Kim EA et al (2002) Viral pneumonias in adults: radiologic and pathologic findings. Radiographics 22:S137–S149

Maher TM et al (2007) CT findings of varicella pneumonia after lung transplantation. AJR Am J Roentgenol 188:W557–W559

Umans U, Golding RP, Duraku S, Manoliu RA (2001) Herpes simplex virus I pneumonia: conventional chest radiograph pattern. Eur Radiol 11:990–994

Cryptogenic Organizing Pneumonia

Cordier JF (2000) Organising pneumonia. Thorax 55:318–328

Greenberg-Wolff I et al (2005) Cryptogenic organizing pneumonia: variety of radiologic findings. Isr Med Assoc J 7:568–570

King TE Jr, Mortenson RL (1992) Cryptogenic organizing pneumonitis. The North American Experience. Chest 102:8S–13S

Lee KS, Kullnig P, Hartman TE, Muller NL (1994) Cryptogenic organizing pneumonia: CT findings in 43 patients. Am J Roentgenol 162:543–546

Thurlbeck WM, Miller RR, Muller NL, Rosenow ECI (1991) Diffuse diseases of the lung: a team approach. BC Deckler, Philadelphia

Ujita M et al (2004) Organizing pneumonia: perilobular pattern at thin-section CT. Radiology 232:757–761

Lymphangioleiomyomatosis

Abbott GF, Rosado-de-Christenson ML, Frazier AA, Franks TJ, Pugatch RD, Galvin JR (2005) Lymphangioleiomyomatosis: radiologic-pathologic correlation. Radiographics 25:803–828

Avila NA, Dwyer AJ, Moss J (2011) Imaging features of lymphangioleiomyomatosis: diagnostic pitfalls. AJR Am J Roentgenol 196:982–986

Johnson SR, Cordier JF et al (2010) European Respiratory Society guidelines for the diagnosis and management of lymphangioleiomyomatosis. Eur Respir J 35:14–26

Lim KE et al (2004) Pulmonary lymphangioleiomyomatosis high-resolution CT findings in 11 patients and compared with the literature. J Clin Imaging 28:1–5

Medical Device and Monitoring of the Chest

John C. Pedrozo Pupo, Ana María Pizarro,
Alvaro Coral Martinez, and Joel Zabaleta Arroyo

Contents

J.C. Pedrozo Pupo (ed.), *Learning Chest Imaging*, Learning Imaging,
DOI 10.1007/978-3-642-34147-2_10, © Springer-Verlag Berlin Heidelberg 2013

Case 1: Chest Tube

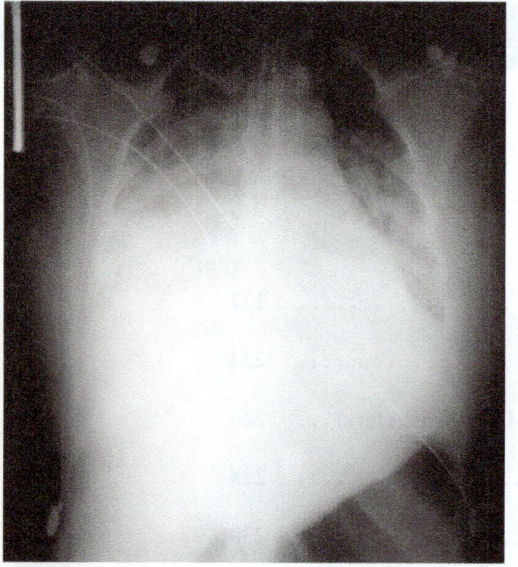

Fig. 10.1.1

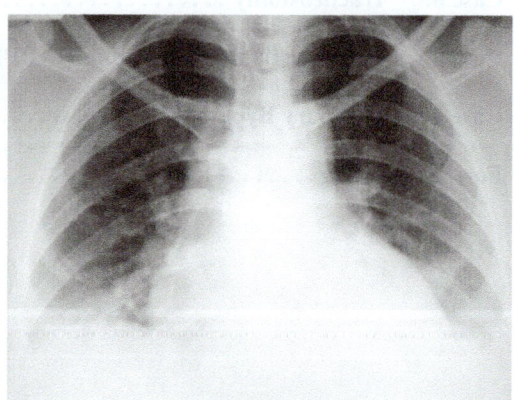

Fig. 10.1.2

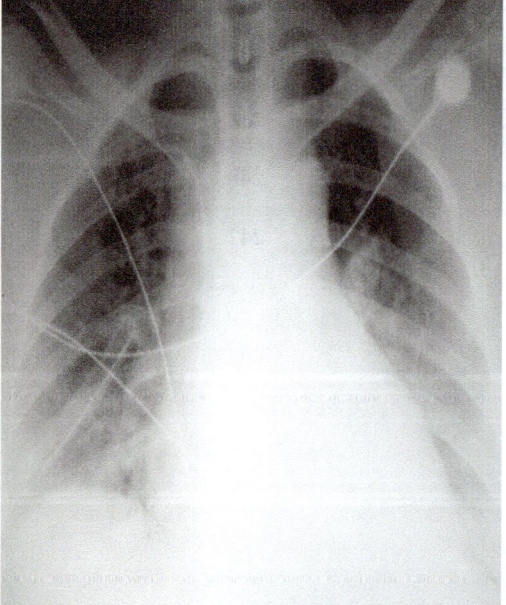

Fig. 10.1.3

Fig. 10.1.4

 A 24-year-old woman with approximately 1 h of evolution characterized by generalized tonic-clonic seizures for about 5 min and later accompanied by severe headache and nausea. She reports that postpartum blood pressure remained high. Background: 6 days back severe post-caesarean preeclampsia.

Comments

Tube thoracostomy is the most commonly performed surgical procedure in thoracic surgery. As a life-saving procedure, general surgeons, intensivists, emergency physicians, and respiratory physicians may at one time or the other be required to perform tube thoracostomy.

After placing the chest tube, the first thing to confirm is their location within the pleural cavity, as in some cases can be located at the subcutaneous cellular tissue, intra-abdominal, or within the lung parenchyma. The ideal location of closed thoracostomy tube should be anterior to the drainage of the posterior pneumothorax and hydrothorax drainage whatever the etiology. A chest tube very introduced in the pleural cavity can cause injury on mediastinal structures. Chest radiograph is also used to evaluate the presence of subcutaneous emphysema and, in this case, track length.

The practice of post-tube thoracostomy chest radiography is supported based on the 29 % incidence of misplacement of such tubes into a fissure.

Complications of tube thoracostomy can be classified as either technical or infective. Technical causes include tube malposition, blocked drain, chest drain dislodgement, reexpansion pulmonary edema, subcutaneous emphysema, nerve injuries, cardiac and vascular injuries, esophageal injuries, residual/post-extubation pneumothorax, fistulae, tumor recurrence at insertion site, herniation through the site, chylothorax, and cardiac dysrhythmias. Infective complications include empyema and surgical site infection including cellulitis and necrotizing fasciitis.

Tube malposition is the commonest complication of tube thoracostomy. It is more common when tubes are inserted under suboptimal conditions and in urgent tube thoracostomy. Trocar technique of chest tube insertion has been shown to increase the risk of tube malposition compared with the blunt dissection techniques. Complication rates of tube thoracostomy have been found to be higher in the critically ill patients with about 21 % of tubes placed intrafissurally and 9 % intraparenchymally. Tube malposition has been defined by CT confirmation in four locations: intraparenchymal, fissural, extrathoracic, and angulation of the drain in the pleural space. Tube malposition will be classified as intraparenchymal tube placement, fissural tube placement, chest wall tube placement, mediastinal tube placement, and abdominal tube placement.

Malposition may sometimes be along the major fissures or less. Other complications that can occur are the reexpansion pulmonary edema unilaterally by rapid drainage of fluid from the pleural cavity. This clearly established that the frontal projection only is insufficient to assess cases of malposition of chest tube, being very useful and necessary lateral projection.

Imaging Findings

CRX film shows pulmonary edema associated with right pleural effusion (Fig. 10.1.1). CRX film shows chest tube in proper position (Figs. 10.1.2 and 10.1.3). CRX film shows the absence of chest tube and resolution of pulmonary edema (Fig. 10.1.4).

Case 2: Mechanical Ventilation

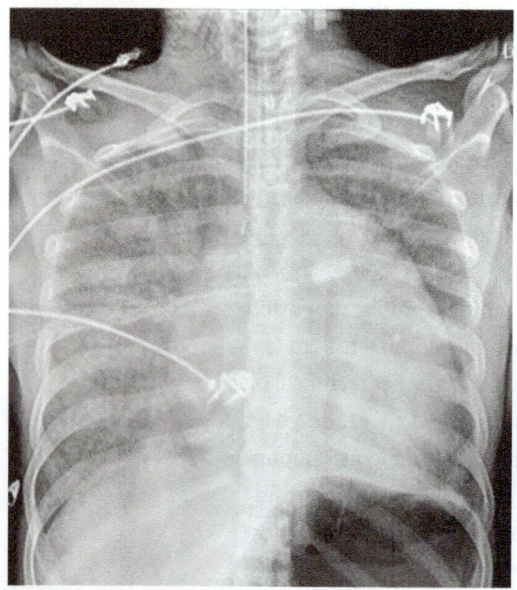

Fig. 10.2.1

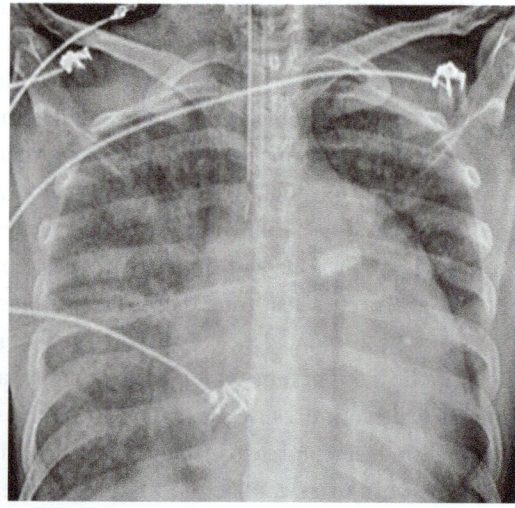

Fig. 10.2.2

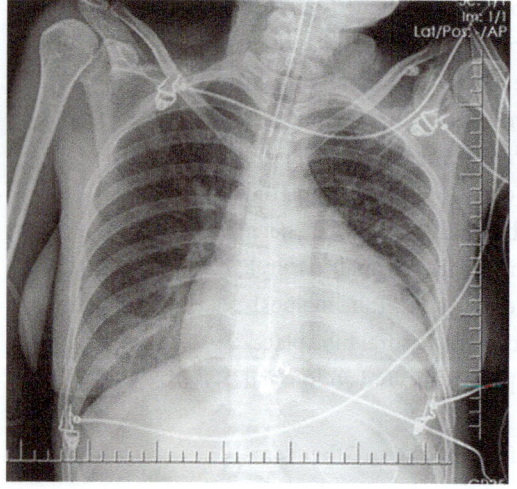

Fig. 10.2.3

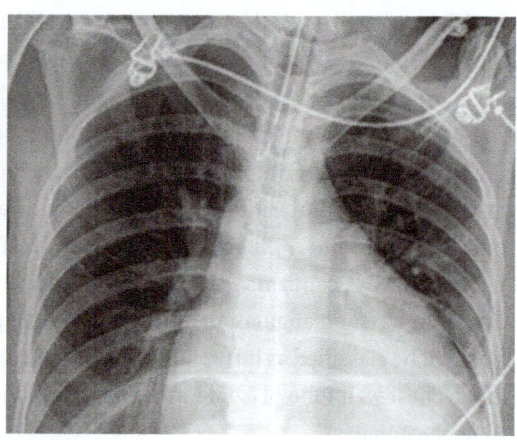

Fig. 10.2.4

A 57-year-old woman with pulmonary edema.

Comments

It is common for a patient in the intensive care unit (ICU) to undergo chest radiography on a daily basis, especially those who are mechanically ventilated. Daily routine chest radiographs are obtained in an attempt to find a relevant abnormality that would otherwise not be detected. It is clear that the American College of Radiology's Appropriateness Criteria recommend daily chest radiography for patients with acute cardiopulmonary problems and for patients on mechanical ventilation, but lately in a meta-analysis, it demonstrates that the elimination of daily routine chest radiography did not adversely affect hard outcomes, such as hospital or ICU mortality, hospital or ICU length of stay, and ventilator days.

Positive pressure ventilation, especially with positive end-expiratory pressure (PEEP), has an effect known as alveolar overdistension, which can be viewed as a radiographically apparent increase in lung volumes. This makes infiltrators hide or suffer the cosmetic effect (they are infiltrators who improve with the use of ventilatory support). The effect of PEEP produces cosmetic changes such as increase in the appearance of lung volumes and improved alveolar infiltrates, and it negates the cardiac silhouette sign unless the pulmonary vessels are displayed. Among the most important complication is barotrauma, which is associated with using high PEEP.

Barotrauma has an impact on the patient ventilated at 4–15 % with a very high rate of 60 % in patients with underlying lung disease, especially in ARDS (acute respiratory distress syndrome). The development of barotrauma in patients in intensive care is associated with high mortality rate of 60 %. Barotrauma is very likely to occur when there is an excess in the peak inspiratory pressure of 40 cm H_2O and the use and duration of PEEP.

Pulmonary interstitial emphysema occurs when there is alveolar rupture, air dissects along the perivascular connective tissue to the hilum resulting in pneumomediastinum and pulmonary interstitial emphysema. The mediastinal pleura is thin and can be changed as a result of overdistension leading to pneumothorax. Subpleural cysts are also formed by progressive air dissection from interlobular septum to adjacent subpleural connective tissue. Air cysts are very common in the medial, inferior, and anterior lung. The rupture of subpleural cysts can weigh to the formation of pneumothorax.

Imaging Findings

CRX film shows cardiomegaly and pulmonary congestion associated with cardiogenic pulmonary edema (Figs. 10.2.1 and 10.2.2). CRX film after the application of PEEP clearance of the lung fields is shown (Figs. 10.2.3 and 10.2.4).

Case 3: Pulmonary Artery Catheters (Swan-Ganz Catheters)

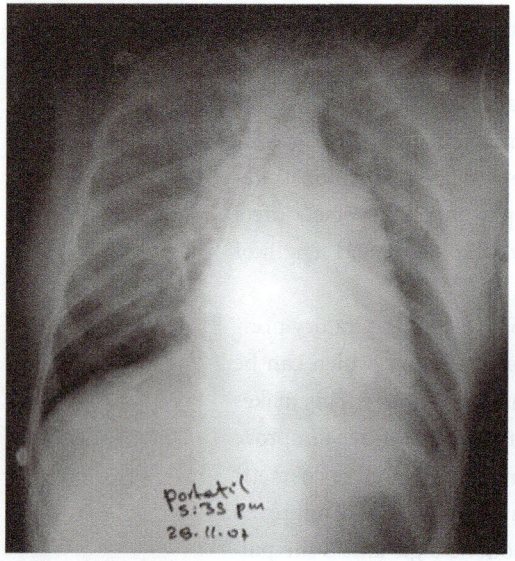

Fig. 10.3.1

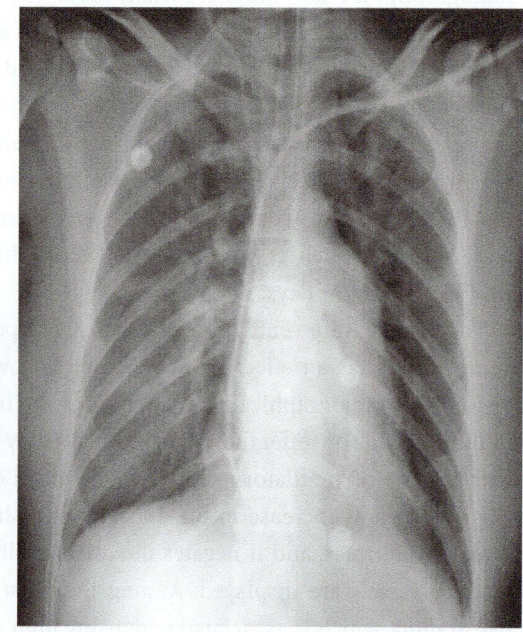

Fig. 10.3.3

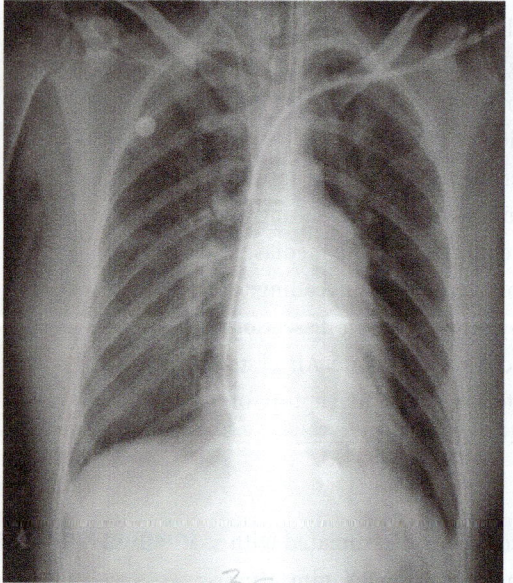

Fig. 10.3.2

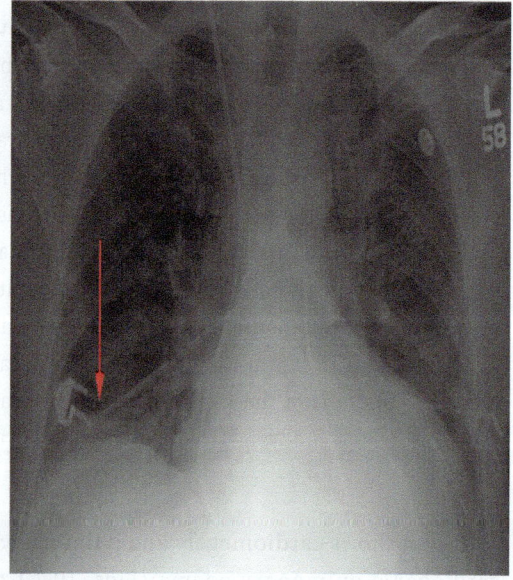

Fig. 10.3.4

A 49-year-old woman with cardiogenic pulmonary edema and a history of mitral stenosis

Comments

The flow-directed balloon-tipped pulmonary artery catheter (PAC) (also known as the Swan-Ganz or right heart catheter) has been in clinical use for more than 30 years. Initially developed for the management of acute myocardial infarction (AMI), it gained widespread use in the management of a variety of critical illnesses and surgical procedures.

The Swan-Ganz catheter is used to measure pressure in the pulmonary capillary wedge. This catheter allows the intensivist to accurately measure the patient's blood volume and differentiate between pulmonary edema and cardiogenic, cardiogenic.

The location of the catheter in the chest radiograph should ideally be located proximal to the interlobar artery, hopefully in the posterior branches of the lower lobe, 3 cm from the midline on the west zone III. If placed very distal, it increases the possibility of pulmonary infarction or rupture. For 25 years, it was widely used in intensive care until 1996, when its routine use was questioned in the study by Connors et al. We show that its use increased mortality and hospitalization costs. As invasive element is not innocuous, its complications among those presented are: bad position (25 %), pneumothorax (0.5–6 %), pulmonary infarction, cardiac arrhythmias, rupture of the pulmonary artery (10 %), pulmonary artery pseudoaneurysm (late complication seen at 2 weeks), endocarditis, and sepsis.

Imaging Findings

CRX film shows postcapillary pulmonary hypertension and increased left atrial size (Fig. 10.3.1). CRX film shows pulmonary artery catheters (Swan-Ganz catheters) located in the right pulmonary artery (Figs. 10.3.2 and 10.3.3). CRX film shows different patients showing abnormal localization of Swan-Ganz (arrow) (Fig. 10.3.4).

Case 4: Pacemaker

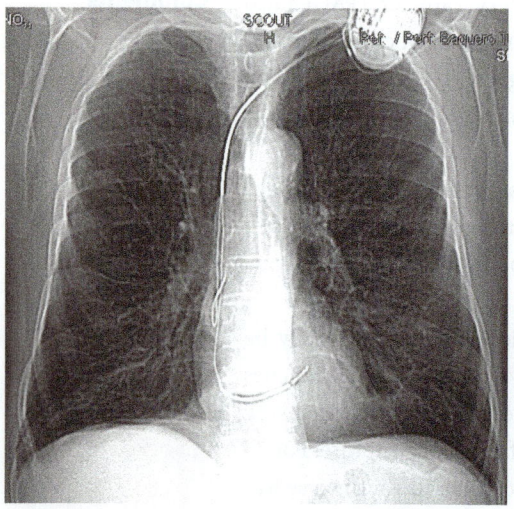

Fig. 10.4.1

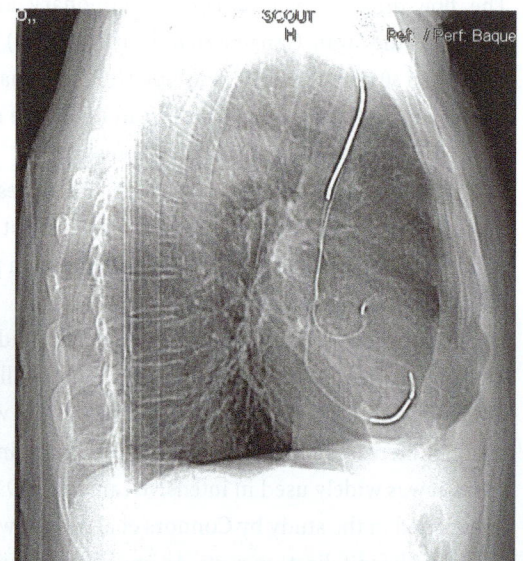

Fig. 10.4.2

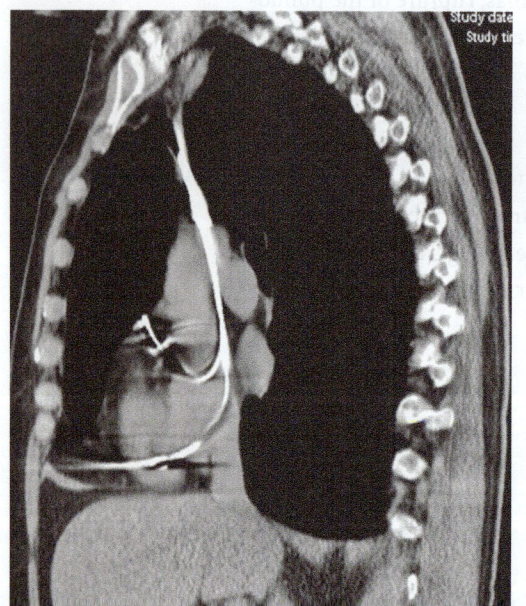

Fig. 10.4.3

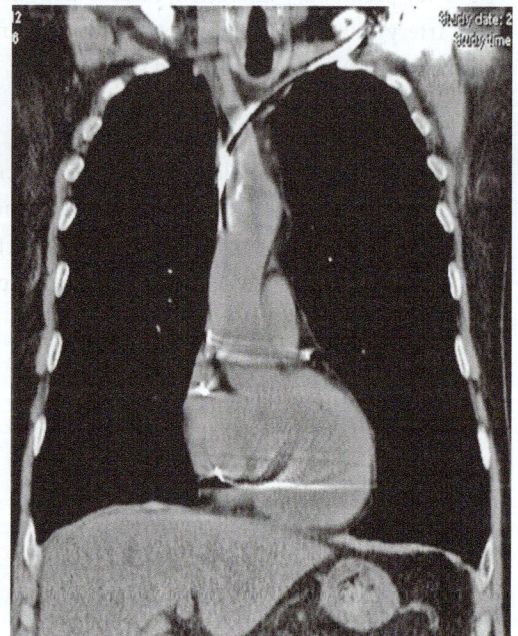

Fig. 10.4.4

A 68-year-old man with pacemaker, congestive heart failure, and COPD phenotype emphysema, with a history of 9 years of evolution cough, dyspnea, and weight loss. He is a smoker of 35 pack years.

Intensive care patients with bradyarrhythmias or atrioventricular block require placement of cardiac pacemakers. This should be introduced through the cephalic vein or subclavian and the tip must be located at right ventricular apex. The frontal and lateral projections are required to evaluate the placement of the pacemaker. In the frontal projection, the tip of the pacemaker must be located at the apex without any angle, and on the lateral tip, it must be located within the ventricular trabecula to 3–4 mm of the epicardial fat. Among the complications are rupture of the electrode with distal embolism and fracture of the electrode which cannot be visualized on plain radiographs of the chest, and fluoroscopic studies are required for its location. If the pacemaker is a DDD, there must be an electrode in the right atrium and the other in the right ventricle.

Comments

CRX film shows bicameral pacemaker's normal location (Figs. 10.4.1 and 10.4.2). CT scan (mediastinal window) shows bicameral pacemaker located in the heart chambers (Figs. 10.4.3 and 10.4.4).

Imaging Findings

Case 5: Nasogastric and Duodenal Probe

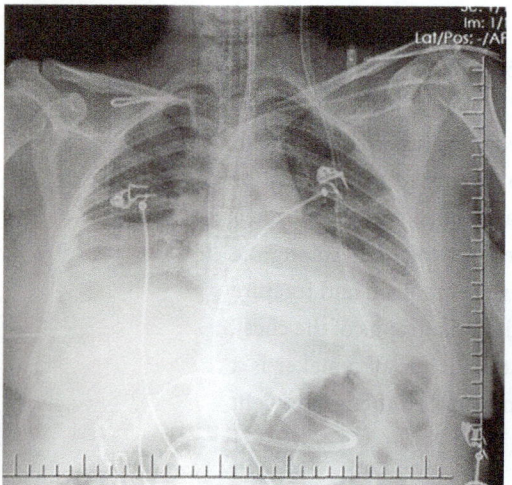

Fig. 10.5.1

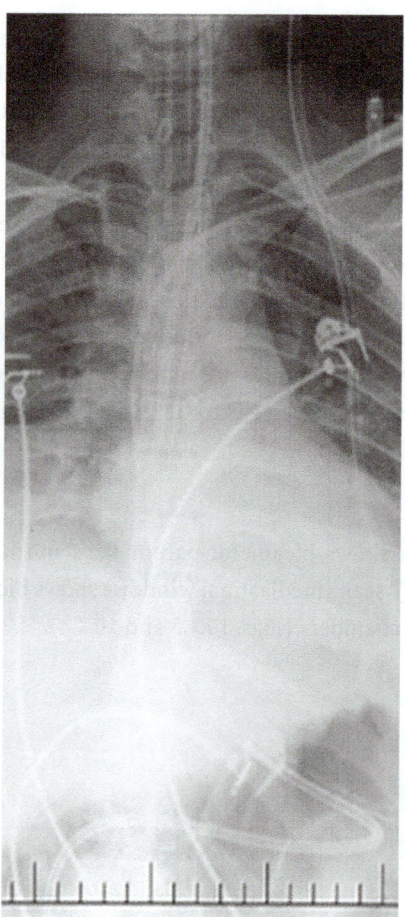

Fig. 10.5.2

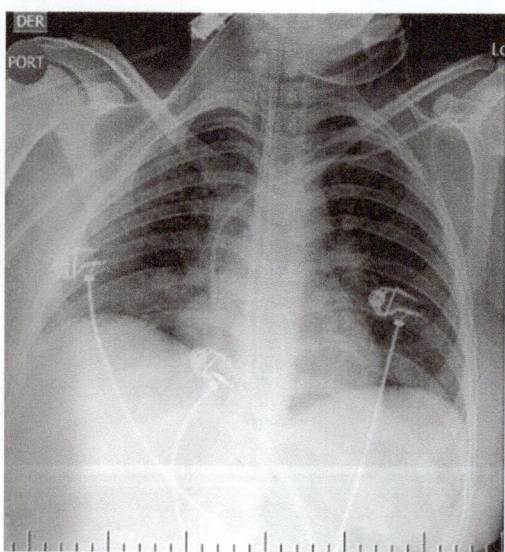

Fig. 10.5.3

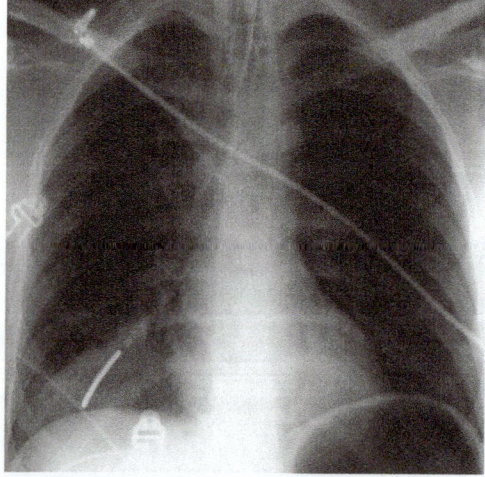

Fig. 10.5.4

A 52-year-old woman with renal sepsis

Comments

The collected opinions of ICU physicians on the appropriateness of a systematic CRX after placement of a nasogastric tube for enteral nutrition were highly variable. However, ensuring correct enteral feeding tube (EFT) position is of paramount importance for patients in the ICU.

Accidental placement of EFT in the tracheobronchial tract can lead to potentially lethal complications, and tracheal intubation does not always prevent this misplacement. When used alone, epigastric auscultation after air injection through the EFT is not a reliable test for confirming the adequate placement of EFT. Some studies have suggested testing the pH of an aspirate obtained from the EFT to ensure proper placement, but this test can be inconclusive in patients with small-bore EFT or those on acid-suppression therapies. Therefore, most guidelines recommend confirmation of EFT placement with a CRX before starting enteral nutrition. Nevertheless, two interesting alternatives to CRX might be considered: ultrasonography and capnography combined with epigastric auscultation.

Bedside ultrasonography, a noninvasive procedure is increasingly used in ICU by non-radiologist physicians who can obtain reliable results after a short training in various organ explorations. Within 5 min, a 2- to 5-MHz probe-based ultrasonography was shown to allow the display of a small-bore EFT in the digestive tract with a sensitivity of 97 % and to assess whether it is properly placed in the stomach. If the EFT is not immediately visible by ultrasound, injection of 5 ml of normal saline mixed with 5 ml of air into the tube increases the sensitivity. This radiation-free procedure is more rapid than conventional radiography and can be taught to ICU physicians during a short training period. Radiography might be only reserved for the rare cases of ultrasonography failures due to gas interposition, for example.

Capnography often is used to assess expiratory CO_2. However, it is possible to connect the capnography device to the EFT via the tip of an endotracheal tube and to assess the correct placement of the EFT by the absence of CO_2 detection.

Finally, to check that the EFT is not coiled in the esophagus after its complete insertion, nurses perform epigastric auscultation. Radiography is required only when epigastric auscultation is inconclusive (10.1 % of cases).

A 0.2 % incidence of complications associated with placement of these probes, including pneumothorax, hydropneumothorax, lung abscess, pneumonia, and empyema secondary to food or medication infusion intrapleurally or intrabronchially has been reported.

Imaging Findings

CRX film shows nasogastric probe in proper position (Figs. 10.5.1, 10.5.2 and 10.5.3). CRX film shows another patient's duodenal probe, located intrabronchially (right lower lobe) (Fig. 10.5.4).

Case 6: Central Venous Catheter

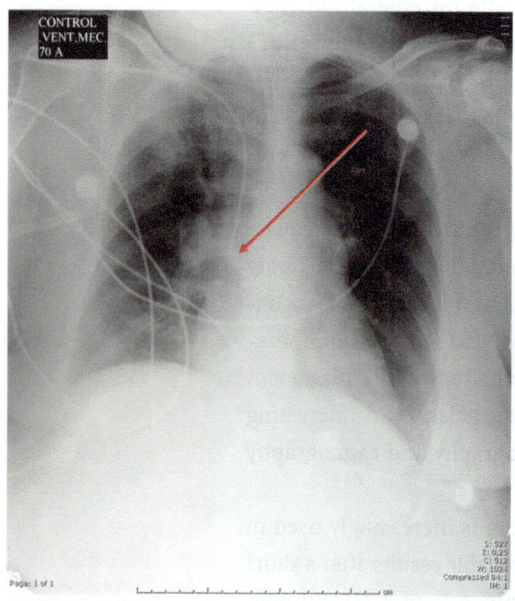

Fig. 10.6.1

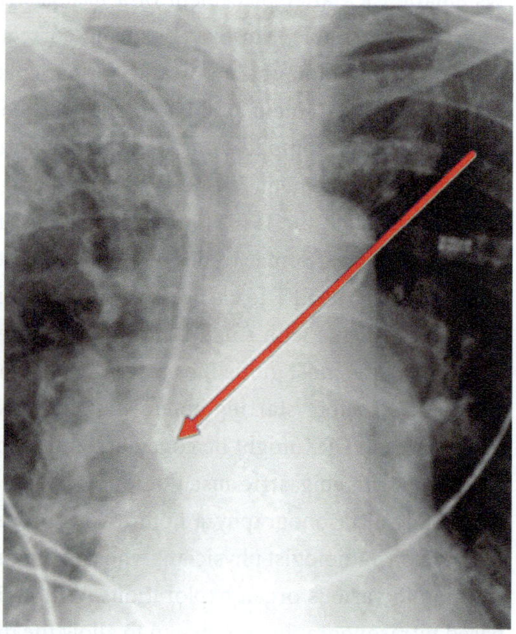

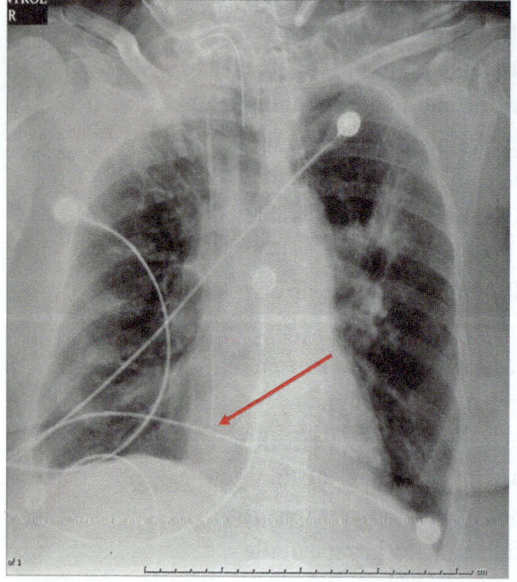

Fig. 10.6.3

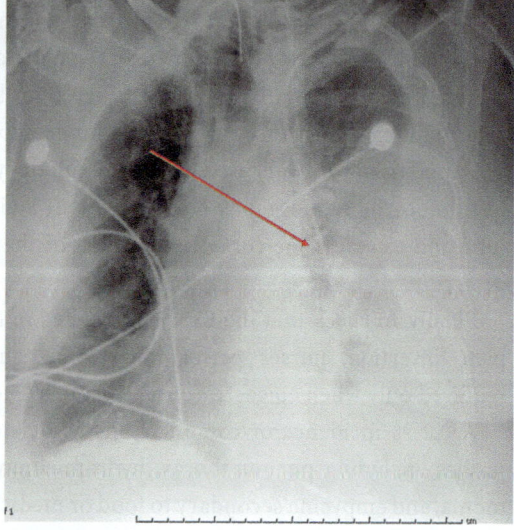

Fig. 10.6.2

Fig. 10.6.4

A 70-year-old woman with Guillain-Barre syndrome and pneumonia was admitted to the hospital with purulent productive cough, dyspnea, right pleuritic chest pain, fever, fatigue, weakness, and malaise, with a history of hypertension.

Comments

The French ICU physicians who participated in the Delphi study agreed on the appropriateness of performing a CRX after central venous catheter (CVC) insertion in the superior vena cava system. The access roads are used more commonly, the subclavian vein, the internal jugular veins, and the right and left femoral veins, respectively. Each time you insert a central catheter, it is mandatory to evaluate routine chest radiograph to establish the location of the catheter and detect complications associated with such placement.

The chest radiograph of the patient showed the central catheter placed properly. Compared with aberrant catheter positions, one has a central catheter at the level of the inferior vena cava and the other catheter is moving in the ascending jugular.

After catheterization of the subclavian or internal jugular vein, CVC tip misplacement occurs in 5–6 % and pneumothorax occurs in 1.5–3.1 % and 0.1–0.2 %, respectively. Clinical evaluation of the patient to predict the absence of complications after CVC insertions via the subclavian vein or internal jugular vein was very accurate in Gray and colleagues' study. However, Gladwin and colleagues showed that the clinical impression of the operator (based on the number of needle passes; difficulty establishing access; operator experience; poor anatomical landmarks; number of previous catheter placements; resistance to wire or catheter advancement; resistance to aspiration of blood or flushing of the catheter ports; sensations in the ear, chest, or arm; and development of signs or symptoms suggestive of pneumothorax) had a poor sensitivity (44 %) and specificity (55 %) for predicting a complication. Gladwin and colleagues concluded that postprocedural CRX remains necessary because clinical factors alone cannot reliably identify tip misplacement.

Nevertheless, as mentioned, numerous pneumothoraces can be missed by bedside CRX, whereas ultrasonography showed excellent sensitivity and specificity for diagnosing pneumothorax within a few minutes. Postprocedural ultrasonography and CRXs were compared after insertion of 85 central venous catheters (70 subclavian and 15 internal jugular). Ultrasonic examination feasibility was 99.6 %. Ten misplacements and one pneumothorax occurred. This pneumothorax and all misplacements except one were diagnosed by ultrasound. Taking into consideration signs of misplacement and pneumothorax, ultrasonic examination did not give any false-positive results.

Imaging Findings

CRX film shows central venous catheter in proper position. Catheter tip is located in the cavo-atrial (Figs. 10.6.1 and 10.6.2). CRX film shows central venous catheter in the same patient in different aberrant positions (Figs. 10.6.3 and 10.6.4).

Case 7: Endotracheal Tube

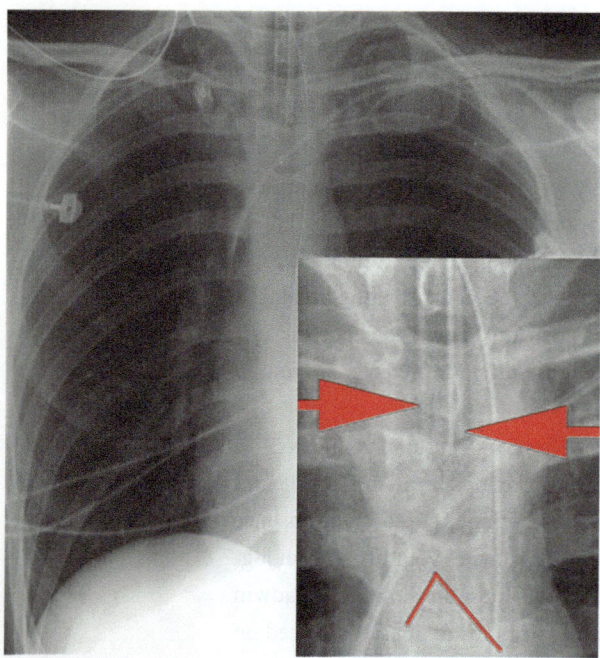

Fig. 10.7.1

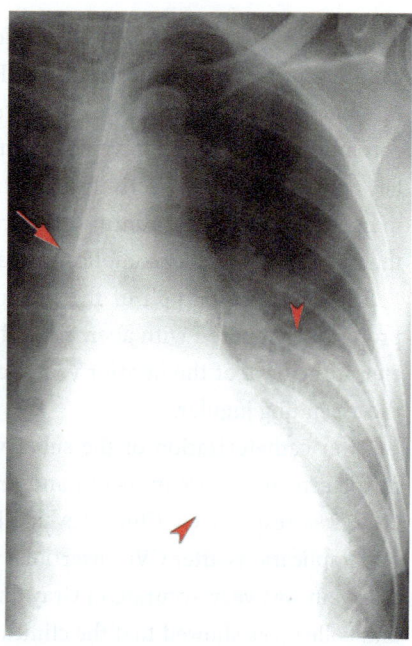

Fig. 10.7.3

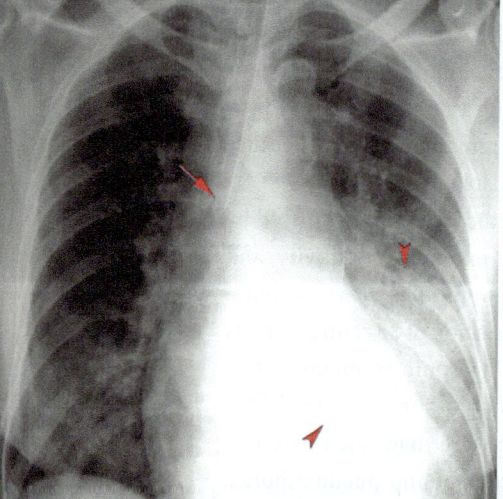

Fig. 10.7.2

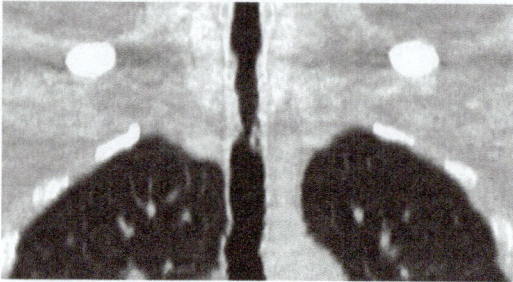

Fig. 10.7.4

After all endotracheal intubation of a patient, it is mandatory to make a radiograph as auscultation by itself cannot adequately assess lung expansion, breath sounds, or malposition (12 % of cases are diagnosed only with malposition radiography). Approximately 10 % of all intubations are selective. The daily control of the position is representative, and that even with good fixation of the tube, there is the possibility of displacement of this. The tip of the endotracheal tube should ideally be 4–6 cm above the carina with the neck in a neutral position. If the neck is flexed, the tube can migrate up to 2 cm inferiorly, while extension of the neck can cause migration of the tube up to 2 cm superiorly. If the endotracheal tube is advanced too far, it will typically extend into the right main bronchus. The balloon should be assessed to ensure that it is not overinflated. The balloon should not be greater than the diameter of the trachea. A ratio of the cuff to tracheal lumen >1.5 leads to an increased risk of tracheal damage.

Also the chest radiograph detects frequent complications associated with endotracheal intubation as 10 % malposition, pneumothorax, atelectasis, and sinusitis, and unusual complications include tracheal stenosis, ruptured trachea, vocal cord paralysis, cervical mediastinal emphysema, hematoma, and abscess formation.

CRX film shows endotracheal tube located in the middle third of the trachea (Fig. 10.7.1). CRX film shows atelectasis in the left lower lobe associated with selective intubation (right bronchus) (Figs. 10.7.2 and 10.7.3). CT scan (sagittal view) shows late complication associated with prolonged intubation tracheal stenosis (Fig. 10.7.4).

Comments

Imaging Findings

Case 8: Tracheostomy

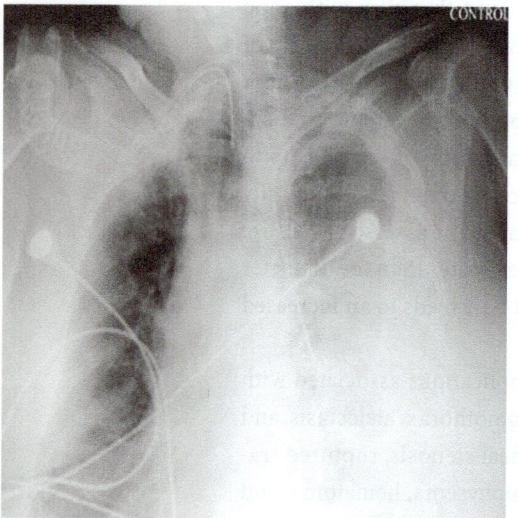

Fig. 10.8.1

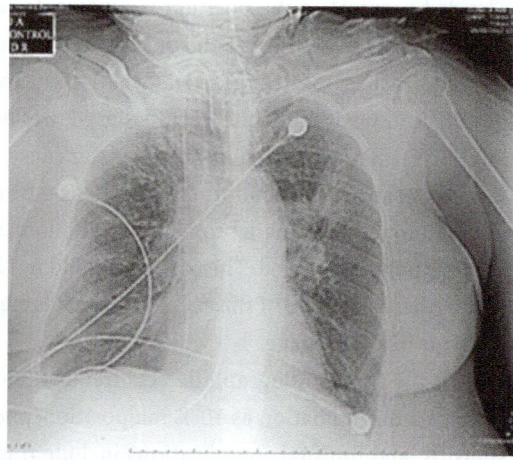

Fig. 10.8.2

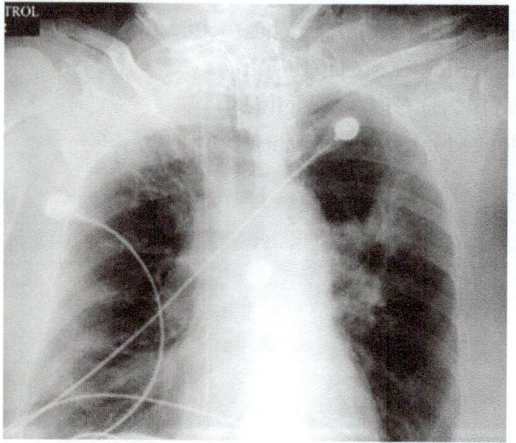

Fig. 10.8.3

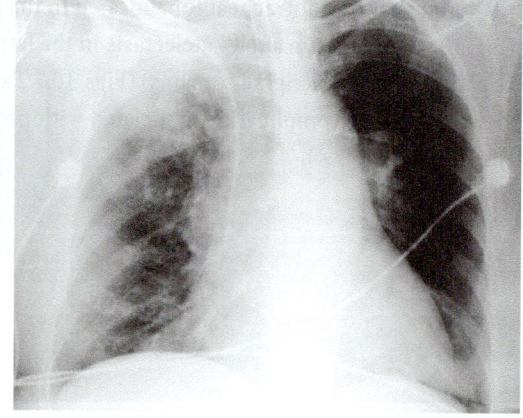

Fig. 10.8.4

A 70-year-old woman with Guillain-Barre syndrome.

Comments

In the case of tracheostomy in the critically ill patient, it is indicated when there is obstruction of the upper airway, ventilated patients with spinal cord injury, and polyneuropathies. The normal position of the chest plate should be in the middle of the 2/3 of the length of the trachea.

Indications for tracheotomy for critically ill patients include relief of upper airway obstruction after initial airway stabilization with translaryngeal intubation or an emergency cricothyroidotomy, assistance with removal of airway secretions, and provision of airway access for long-term mechanical ventilation.

Abnormalities revealed by routine chest radiography after tracheostomy did not appear to alter patient management frequently enough to warrant the costs.

Tracheostomy may be associated with numerous acute, perioperative complications, some of which continue to be relevant well after the placement of the tracheostomy.

The most frequent late complication is the development of granulation tissue, a complication that can be subclinical or may present as failure to wean from the ventilator or failure to decannulate, or may manifest as upper airway obstruction with respiratory failure after decannulation. Granulation tissue may cause airway occlusion or result in airway stenosis.

CRX film shows tracheostomy tube in proper position (Figs. 10.8.1, 10.8.2, 10.8.3 and 10.8.4).

Imaging Findings

Case 9: Intra-Aortic Balloon Pumps (IABP)

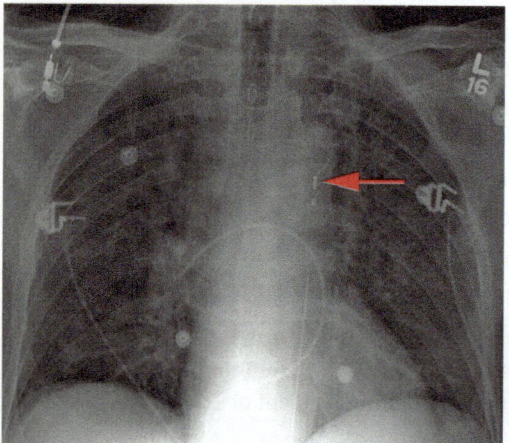

Fig. 10.9.1

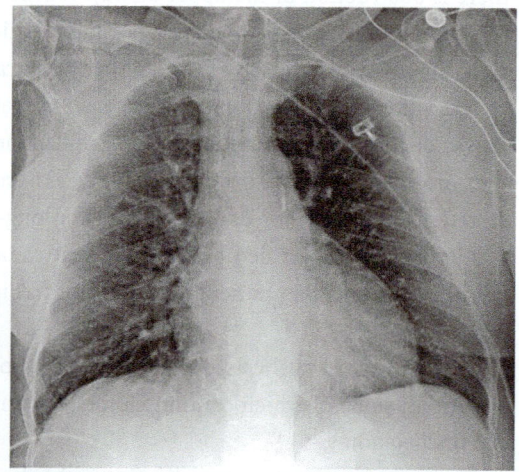

Fig. 10.9.3

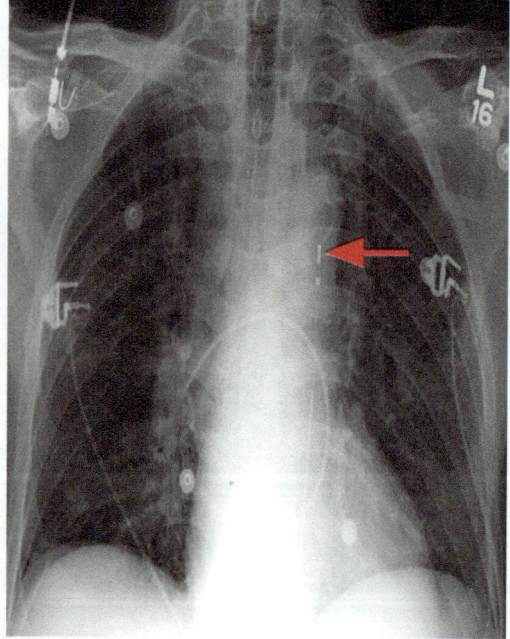

Fig. 10.9.2

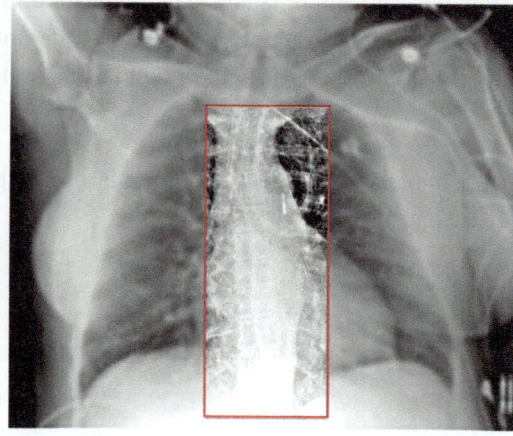

Fig. 10.9.4

Intra-aortic balloon counterpulsation is a method of temporary mechanical circulatory support that attempts to create more favorable balance of myocardial oxygen supply and demand by using the concepts of systolic unloading and diastolic augmentation. As a consequence, cardiac output, ejection fraction, and coronary perfusion are increased, with a concomitant decrease in left ventricular (LV) wall stress, systemic resistance to LV ejection, and pulmonary capillary wedge pressure. Intra-aortic balloon pumps (IABP) are used for the treatment of cardiogenic shock.

The American College of Cardiology/American Heart Association (ACC/AHA) guidelines for the management of ST elevation myocardial infarction (STEMI) and European Society of Cardiology (ESC) guidelines for the management of acute heart failure favor the use of IABP therapy in the setting of acute myocardial infarction where cardiogenic shock cannot be quickly reversed with pharmacologic therapy (class I indication). It is to be used as a temporary stabilizing measure prior to revascularization.

Other class I indications for IABP support include the following conditions: acute mitral regurgitation, ventricular septal defect (VSD), intractable ventricular arrhythmias, unstable angina refractory to medical therapy, and decompensated systolic heart failure.

The use of aortic balloon counterpulsation is to decrease preload and increase myocardial perfusion in patients who are in cardiogenic shock. It synchronizes with the aortic pressure or the patient's EKG and is inflated during diastole and deflated during systole. The path is usually the right and left common femoral artery percutaneously, and its ideal location should be at a distance of approximately 1–2 cm below the left subclavian artery, being displayed at the aortic arch and above the left main bronchus frontal projections of the thorax. Major complications include thromboembolism, neurological disorders by cerebral ischemia, systemic cholesterol embolization, infection, stroke, and aortic dissection. Repeated radiological control of the ball position is necessary because the mobilization of the patient also could affect the location.

CRX film shows intra-aortic balloon pumps (IABP) (Figs. 10.9.1, 10.9.2, 10.9.3 and 10.9.4).

Comments

Imaging Findings

Case 10: Coronary Bypass

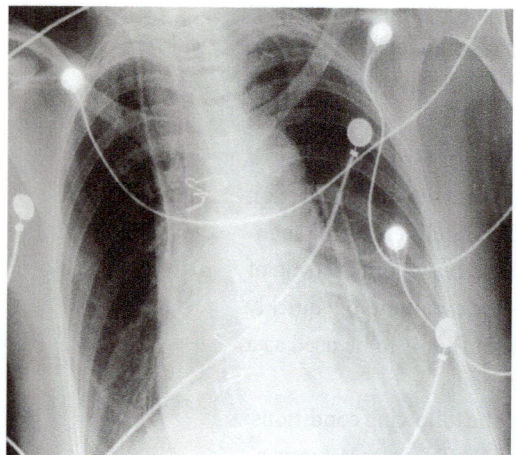

Fig. 10.10.1

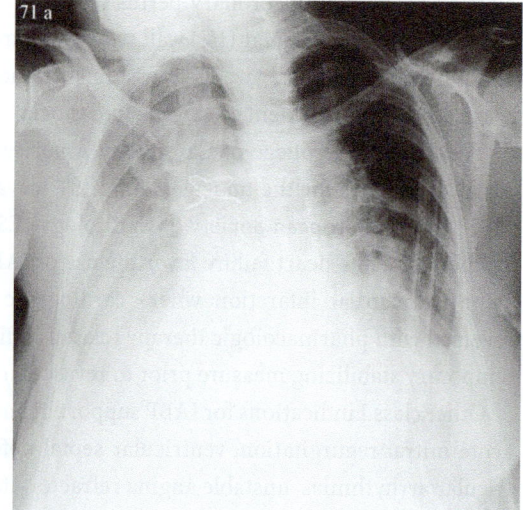

Fig. 10.10.2

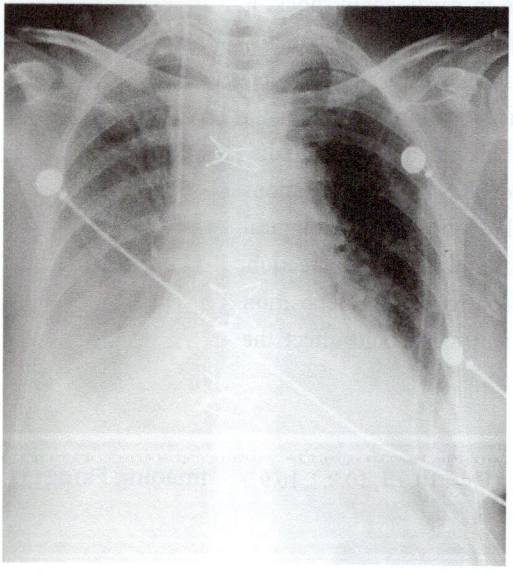

Fig. 10.10.3

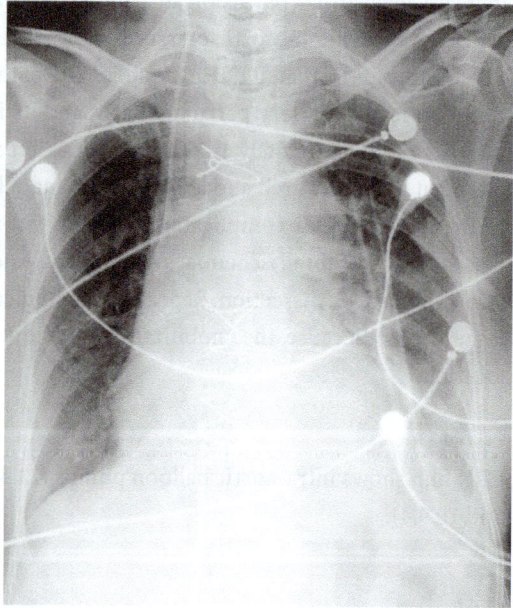

Fig. 10.10.4

A 71-year-old woman postoperative myocardial revascularization.

Comments

Omission of routine postoperative chest tube removal CRXs in postoperative cardiac patients is safe. The removal of chest tubes in these patients is not an indication for CRXs.

In the first days after placement of coronary bypass, keep in mind that over 75 % of patients experience some degree of atelectasis in LLL; 20 % are bilateral and resolve within a few days. The contour of the mediastinum may be slightly wider, and that any significant increase in the diameter may reflect mediastinal bleeding. Small pleural effusions are expected and that any increase in leakage compromises ventilation and oxygenation. Over 50 % of patients have pleural effusion after abdominal surgery.

Imaging Findings

CRX film shows cambios radiologicos asociados a edema pulmonar post revascularización miocardica (Figs. 10.10.1, 10.10.2, 10.10.3, and 10.10.4).

Further Reading

Bekemeyer WB et al (1985) Efficacy of chest radiography in a respiratory intensive care unit. A prospective study. Chest 88:691

Burns SM, Carpenter R, Truwit JD (2001) Report on the development of a procedure to prevent placement of feeding tubes into the lungs using end-tidal CO$_2$ measurements. Crit Care Med 29:936–939

Carrillo JA (2003) La radiografía de tórax en el paciente en ventilación mecánica. Capitulo No.14, Paginas 93–97. En Ventilación Mecánica – Aplicación en el paciente crítico. Editores Carmelo Dueñas Castell, Guillermo Ortiz Ruiz, Marco A. González © 2003 Editorial Distribuna Ltda. ISBN: 958-33-4600-4

Chalumeau-Lemoine L, Baudel JL, Das V, Arrive L, Noblinski B, Guidet B, Offenstadt G, Maury E (2009) Results of short-term training of naive physicians in focused general ultrasonography in an intensive-care unit. Intensive Care Med 35:1767–1771

Connors AF, Sporoff T, Dawson NV et al (1996) The effectiveness of right catheterization in the initial care of critically ill patients. JAMA 276:889–897

Epstein SK (2005) Late complications of tracheostomy. Respir Care 50(4):542–549

Fraser RS, Paré MJA, Fraser RG, Paré PD (1994) Sinopsis of diseases of the chest, 2nd edn. W.B. Saunders Company, Philadelphia

Galbois A, Ait-Oufella H, Baudel JL, Kofman T, Bottero J, Viennot S, Rabate C, Jabbouri S, Bouzeman A, Guidet B, Offenstadt G, Maury E (2010) Pleural ultrasound compared with chest radiographic detection of pneumothorax resolution after drainage. Chest 138:648–655

Galbois A, Vitry P, Ait-Oufella H, Baudel JL, Guidet B, Maury E, Offenstadt G (2011) Colorimetric capnography, a new procedure to ensure correct feeding tube placement in the intensive care unit: an evaluation of a local protocol. J Crit Care 26(4):411–414

Gladwin MT, Slonim A, Landucci DL, Gutierrez DC, Cunnion RE (1999) Cannulation of the internal jugular vein: is postprocedural chest radiography always necessary? Crit Care Med 27:1819–1823

Godman LR, Curtin JJ (1994) Imaging the mechanical ventilated patient. In: Tobin MJ (ed) Principles and practice of mechanical ventilation. McGraw-Hill, New York

Goodman L, Putman C (1992) Critical care imaging, 3rd edn. W.B. Saunders Company, Philadelphia

Gray P, Sullivan G, Ostryzniuk P, McEwen TA, Rigby M, Roberts DE (1992) Value of postprocedural chest radiographs in the adult intensive care unit. Crit Care Med 20:1513–1518

Heffner JF. (2003) Tracheotomy application and timing. Clin Chest Med 24(3):1–12

Hejblum G, Ioos V, Vibert JF, Boelle PY, Chalumeau-Lemoine L, Chouaid C, Valleron AJ, Guidet B (2008) A web-based Delphi study on the indications of chest radiographs for patients in ICUs. Chest 133:1107–1112

Herman P, Khan A (1998) Radiología en Cuidado Crítico. In Cuidados Intensivos Cardiopulmonares. Dantzker-Scharf. 3era. Edición McGraw-Hill Interamericana, México

Hind D, Calvert N, McWilliams R, Davidson A, Paisley S, Beverley C, Thomas S (2003) Ultrasonic locating devices for central venous cannulation: meta-analysis. BMJ 327:361

Hunter TB, Taljanovic MS et al (2004) Medical devices of the chest. Radiographics 24:1725–1746

Jolliet P, Pichard C, Biolo G, Chiolero R, Grimble G, Leverve X, Nitenberg G, Novak I, Planas M, Preiser JC, Roth E, Schols AM, Wernerman J (1998) Enteral nutrition in intensive care patients: a practical approach. Working Group on Nutrition and Metabolism, ESICM. European Society of Intensive Care Medicine. Intensive Care Med 24:848–859

Kefalides P (1998) Pulmonary artery catheters on trial. Ann Intern Med 128(2):161–162

Kesieme EB, Dongo A et al (2012) Tube thoracostomy: complications and its management. Pulm Med Article ID 256878:1–10

Krivopal M, Shlobin OA, Schwartzstein RM (2003) Utility of daily routine portable chest radiographs in mechanically ventilate patients in the medical ICU. Chest 123:1607–1614

Kunis K (2007) Confirmation of nasogastric tube placement. Am J Crit Care 16:19, author reply 19

Londoño N, Uriza A, Pedrozo Pupo J (2001) Radiología del Tórax en UCI. Rev Colomb Neumol 13:46–53

Maury E, Guglielminotti J, Alzieu M, Guidet B, Offenstadt G (2001) Ultrasonic examination: an alternative to chest radiography after central venous catheter insertion? Am J Respir Crit Care Med 164:403–405

McCormick JT, O'Mara MS et al (2002) The use of routine chest X-ray films after chest tube removal in postoperative cardiac patients. Ann Thorac Surg 74:2161–2164

McGee WT, Ackerman BL, Rouben LR, Prasad VM, Bandi V, Mallory DL (1993) Accurate placement of central venous catheters: a prospective, randomized, multicenter trial. Crit Care Med 21:1118–1123

Metheny NA (2006) Preventing respiratory complications of tube feedings: evidence-based practice. Am J Crit Care 15:360–369

Meyer P, Henry M, Maury E, Baudel JL, Guidet B, Offenstadt G (2009) Colorimetric capnography to ensure correct nasogastric tube position. J Crit Care 24:231–235

Oba Y, Zaza T (2010) Abandoning daily routine chest radiography in the intensive care unit: meta-analysis. Radiology 255(2):386–395. doi:10.1148/radiol.10090946

Sagristá JS, Boneta LA et al (2000) Guías de práctica clínica de la Sociedad Española de Cardiología en patología pericárdica. Rev Esp Cardiol 53:394–412

Stroud M, Duncan H, Nightingale J (2003) Guidelines for enteral feeding in adult hospital patients. Gut 52(Suppl 7):vii1–vii12

Tarnoff M, Moncure M, Jones F, Ross S, Goodman M (1998) The value of routine posttracheostomy chest radiography. Chest 113:1647–1649

Trotman-Dickenson B (2003a) Radiology in the intensive care unit (part I). J Intensive Care Med 18:198–210

Trotman-Dickenson B (2003b) Radiology in the intensive care unit (part II). J Intensive Care Med 18:239–252

Vigneau C, Baudel JL, Guidet B, Offenstadt G, Maury E (2005) Sonography as an alternative to radiography for nasogastric feeding tube location. Intensive Care Med 31:1570–1572

Batch number: 09636588

Printed by Printforce, the Netherlands